Dental Maintenance for Patients with Periodontal Diseases

Thomas G. Wilson, Jr, DDS
Private Practice of Periodontics, Dallas, Texas
Visiting Associate Professor in Graduate Periodontics,
Baylor University School of Dentistry
Clinical Associate Professor, University of Texas at San Antonio Dental School
Affiliate Assistant Professor, University of Washington

Quintessence Publishing Co, Inc   1989
Chicago, London, Berlin, São Paulo, Tokyo, and Hong Kong

Dedication

I love my family immensely, but I could never understand why authors
dedicated books to their families.
Now I do.

> To: Penny
> Trey
> John
> My Mother
> And in memory of my Father

Library of Congress Cataloging-in-Publication Data

Dental maintenance for patients with periodontal diseases / [edited
   by] Thomas G. Wilson, Jr.
      p.   cm.
   Includes bibliographical references.
   ISBN 0-86715-209-5
   1. Periodontal disease—Treatment.   2. Therapeutics, Dental.
I. Wilson, Thomas G.
   [DNLM: 1. Periodontal Diseases—therapy. WU 240 D413]
RK361.D46   1989
617.6′32—dc20
DNLM/DLC
for Library of Congress   89-10635
                                 CIP

© 1989 by Quintessence Publishing Co, Inc, Chicago, Illinois.
All rights reserved.

Books Editor: Laura G. Peppers
Production Manager: Kim Vander Steen
Production Editor: Kristen Trotter

Lithography: SCANTRANS Pte Ltd, Singapore
Composition: Midwest Technical Publications, St. Louis, MO
Printing: The Ovid Bell Press, Inc, Fulton, MO
Binding: Zonne Bookbinders, Inc, Chicago, IL
Printed in U. S. A.

Contents

Contributors

Fred E. Aurbach, DDS, FAGD, FACD, FICD
Private Practice of Dentistry, Dallas, Texas.

Justin E. Aurbach, BA, MS, DDS, CAGS
Private Practice of Endodontics, Dallas, Texas.

Janice Barone, RDH
Dental Hygiene, Dallas, Texas.

Reta Carlson, RDH
Dental Hygiene, Dallas, Texas.

Eugene W. Dahl, DDS
Associate Professor of Maxillofacial Prosthodontics (Graduate Division) and Associate Professor, Removable Prosthodontics, Baylor College of Dentistry; Private Practice of Prosthodontics and Maxillofacial Prosthetics, Dallas, Texas.

Pat Fallon, RDH, MS
Lecturer, Dental Hygiene Program, Texas Woman's University, Denton, Texas; Dental Hygiene, Dallas, Texas.

Mark E. Glover, DDS, MSD
Adjunct Professor, Texas Woman's University, Denton, Texas; Private Practice of Periodontics, Dallas, Texas.

Frank L. Higginbottom, DDS
Private Practice of Restorative Dentistry, Baylor University Medical Center, Dallas, Texas.

Charles Holt, DDS
Guest lecturer in The Department of Orthodontics, Baylor College of Dentistry; Private Practice limited to Temporomandibular Joint Dysfunction and Craniofacial Pain, Bedford, Texas.

Robert E. (Gene) Lamberth, DDS, MSD
Private Practice of Orthodontics, Dallas, Texas.

Leonard J. Ledet, Jr, BS, DDS, FAGD
Private Practice of Dentistry, Irving, Texas.

Steven A. Levy, DDS
Private Practice of Dentistry, Dallas, Texas.

Arvinder K. Malik, RDH
Dental Hygiene, Dallas, Texas.

Francis L. Miranda, DDS, MS
Associate Professor, Department of Pediatric Dentistry, Baylor College of Dentistry, Dallas, Texas; Private Practice of Orthodontics and Pediatric Dentistry, Dallas, Texas.

Michael J. Newman, DDS
Private Practice of Dentistry, Dallas, Texas.

Jan Schoen, RDH
Lecturer, Dental Hygiene Program, Texas Woman's University, Denton, Texas; Dental Hygiene, Lewisville, Texas.

Thomas G. Wilson, Jr, DDS
Private Practice of Periodontics, Dallas, Texas; Visiting Associate Professor in Graduate Periodontics, Baylor University School of Dentistry; Clinical Associate Professor, University of Texas at San Antonio Dental School; Affiliate Assistant Professor, University of Washington.

Preface

The demand for information about periodontics is increasing. This has come about because of recent scientific discoveries, emphasis in the mass media on the subject, and a flood of litigation against health care professionals for nondiagnosis and treatment of various periodontal lesions.

A great deal of knowledge is currently available about periodontal diseases and their treatment. Choosing pertinent data that were written with a minimum of bias and keeping up with the subject can be a full-time occupation. This has been complicated by the entry into the commercial marketplace of new and often untested products and services, each with claim and counterclaim, often poorly substantiated.

Our book attempts to sift through this material and present concepts and data that can be readily applied to daily practice. The work is written by a group of dental professionals who have worked together over a long period. We share mutual respect and the desire to provide proven, state-of-the-art care for our patients. Most of our contributors are in private practice and have struggled with maintenance care for years. We found that communications between our offices often included details of active therapy and its immediate results but rarely covered information on how best to maintain the healthy environment we had helped to create. To address this problem, each of us wrote on his or her area of expertise. We attempted to answer two basic questions: how best to maintain health, and how to monitor patients to determine when and whether their problems recur.

It is our hope that this work will be of assistance to those in private practice as well as to students of dentistry and dental hygiene, and that its use will provide information that will ultimately result in less stressful environments for our colleagues and better dental health for all our patients.

Acknowledgments

This book is the sum of many parts. The germ of the idea came from Pat Fallon, and it took many twists and turns to reach its final form. The work of my many contributors expanded greatly on the original notion and I want to thank each one for his or her contribution.

Along the way, I asked for and received much aid and assistance. Among those who reviewed sections of the book are Dr Jim Gartrell, Dr Ken Kornman, Dr Ed Zinman, Dr Louise Higgins, Dr Myron Nevins, and Dr Gene Savitt. All of the osseointegrated implants in chapter 11 were placed with Dr Hilton Israelson as my co-surgeon. Special thanks go to Dr Mark Glover for his continued attempts to keep me on the straight and narrow path, and of course, thanks to the people in my office who gave me time to write and a testing ground for my ideas and especially to Georgia Wright for her constant dedication and continued vigilance.

How to Use This Book

Dental Maintenance for Patients with Periodontal Diseases works on two levels. First, the "At a glance" sections are for quick reference. These should be used when a patient (or the practitioner) has a question in a specific area that demands a quick answer. These sections are the authors' conclusions based on a review of the pertinent literature and the writers' clinical experience. The whys and wherefores of these ideas are discussed in depth in the section preceding the summaries. These more detailed areas spell out the reasons for the conclusions and should be read when the reader has the opportunity.

A caveat: Making our information more relevant to the clinician in daily practice often required us to give specific parameters. These numbers should be tempered with experience. As an example, you would be more likely to perform periodontal surgery on a 26-year-old patient with a 6-mm pocket around a normal-length tooth than on the same defect in a 75-year-old patient with short roots.

The reader wishing to start with an overview is referred to chapter 6, which is an outline of a typical maintenance visit and contains references to other chapters with more information on subjects of interest.

In addition we recommend that the first three chapters be among the first covered by the reader because these set the background on which much of the book is based.

Chapter 1

Maintenance: An Overview

Thomas G. Wilson, Jr

Changes in the way we perceive periodontal diseases

"Brush your teeth twice a day and see your dentist twice a year" was the advice of one toothpaste commercial—a simple statement, but one with little or no scientific background. Unfortunately, until recently it set a standard of care for both the general public and the dental community. Recently we have begun to question this and other long-held beliefs about maintenance care. Because dental plaques have been found to grow virulent at different rates, brushing twice a day may not be necessary for some yet not frequent enough for others. In addition, other studies have shown that the most efficient method for removing plaque may be with devices other than the toothbrush,[1] and that waiting 6 months between cleanings may lead to increased bone loss for most periodontal patients.[2] These are a few examples of the many ways that our knowledge of periodontal maintenance is evolving. New findings such as these will be explored throughout this book, with the present chapter concentrating on an overview of maintenance for the periodontal patient.

Our goal in dentistry is to maintain the dentition in a state of optimal function and comfort throughout the patient's life. Many barriers arise to stop us short of this goal, the most important being the patient's level of compliance. From the dentist's perspective, when patients' lifespans increase, maintaining their dental health becomes more difficult. In the anthropologic sense, our teeth were not designed for the stresses of modern life or for our greater longevity. People in our society bombard their mouths with diets that promote dental caries, use local and systemic toxins that are detrimental to the periodontium, overuse their muscles of mastication, and then expect the dental professional to make the whole stomatognathic system work years longer than it was designed to. In addition, most patients would like this accomplished with minimal dental visits, minimal expense, and minimal expenditure of energy on their part. Unfortunately, there

is not yet a "magic bullet" that meets these requirements. This means that the patient must participate in maintaining dental health.

Successful maintenance, then, must involve educating the patient about his or her problem, helping him or her understand that permanent aftercare will usually be needed, and encouraging the acceptance of greater responsibility for personal health.

Increasingly our patients want to be healthier, and this simplifies our task. The whole "wellness" trend is having positive effects on dentistry. This movement is being aided by the manufacturers of commercially available dental products as they use the mass media to sell their wares. In addition, these manufacturers have placed more sophisticated information before the consumer. We have seen a movement on the consumer's part from toothbrushing as the answer to all dental ills, toward a recognition of "plaque" and "tartar" and their unwholesome effects on our mouths and our social lives. As a result, when patients are asked to use dental floss or come in more often for cleanings, these concepts are often no longer as foreign as they once were. Despite these positive trends, we are still dealing with an underinformed or often misinformed public, and much work remains before the average patient's dental knowledge reaches the level necessary to create motivation for behavioral change.

The professional environment, too, is changing rapidly, and the volume of new information that must be absorbed by the dental professional is swiftly expanding. This creates two problems. The first is the sheer volume of information, which makes it difficult to keep abreast of developments. The second is the question of whom to believe when new products or techniques are introduced. Most of us have a shelf full of materials that we used a few times and discarded. We have also been driven to the heights of ecstasy by a new product or procedure as demonstrated by an "expert" in the field, only to find that it may have worked well for him or her but not at all for us.

My solution to this problem has been to develop a

taste for the dental literature. When you begin to read this material, much of it seems bewildering; but if you persevere, patterns begin to emerge. You find that certain individuals really are knowledgeable and honest, and that practical benefit can be derived from their findings. For those wishing to explore this area, two refereed journals are recommended: *The Journal of Prosthetic Dentistry* and *Journal of Periodontology*. A relative newcomer that relates well to clinicians and is also refereed is *The International Journal of Periodontics & Restorative Dentistry*. The professional who subscribes to these journals and reads them soon will be able to judge new techniques and products on their merit and not from someone else's biased opinion. Although most authors strive for objectivity, one should avoid far-reaching conclusions from positive articles funded by the product's manufacturer or published in nonrefereed journals.

Periodontal maintenance

The more one reads and the longer one practices, the more important the subject of periodontal maintenance becomes. When our practices are young we are often more interested in new procedures, new instruments, and new materials that we hope will make our labors simple, our offices prosperous, and our patients disease-free. To be sure, our profession has made great strides toward achieving these goals, but almost without exception our best works in the area of periodontics are doomed without maintenance. Successful maintenance requires two well-informed, participating parties—the health professional and the patient. The professional's task is to establish a healthy state and then inform the patient what constitutes proper maintenance; the patient's job is to comply. This sounds so very simple, but how incredibly difficult it is to translate to reality! To comply often means behavioral change, and this is difficult for all of us, professional and patient alike; it requires information, the desire to change, and a helping atmosphere—an environment that does not always exist in the dental office.

In 1982 we initiated a patient compliance study that taught us a great deal.[3] We were aware of the important role that maintenance plays in periodontal therapy and wanted to find out what percentage of patients complied with suggested recall intervals. We had always assumed that (with the exception of those who moved away) most patients returned for maintenance. The study included all the patients treated for periodontitis during the first 8 years of practice. These patients, who numbered almost 1,000, had been referred for treatment and cared enough about keeping their teeth to follow through with suggested active therapy. We were astounded to find that of this highly educated and motivated group, only about 16% adhered to suggested maintenance intervals. To our further chagrin, we saw that almost 35% of these patients *never* came back! Our first thought was that our office was unusual and failed to inform and motivate our patients properly. Because little was written in the dental literature on this subject, we went to medical publications. We were surprised to learn that our findings were in the average range for patients with chronic problems.[4–7] To generalize, about one third of patients will comply completely, one third will not comply at all, and the remainder will occasionally do what the therapist requests. Also in general terms, patients who are concerned about their problem and whose problems are acute are more likely to comply than those with chronic, nonthreatening problems. These generalizations can be broadly applied to most practices; while some may do better and some not as well, we all can improve. To that end, we devote an entire chapter to improving compliance (chapter 14).

Properly motivating our patients to stay on maintenance is essential, but it also behooves us to know what to do once they come back. If the teeth are cleaned by a dental hygienist who doesn't understand how to root plane and are then examined by a dentist who has no understanding of periodontal conditions, the patient will suffer. The remainder of our book deals with information you can use to make your patients healthier and your practices more enjoyable. It will also include information on how other areas of dentistry interact with the periodontium.

——— *At a glance* ———

- In general, inflammatory periodontal diseases recur if not maintained.
- Our knowledge about maintenance procedures has grown dramatically.
- An essential aspect of successful maintenance is patient compliance.
- Most patients don't comply to long-term behavioral changes, especially for conditions that are not threatening.
- An essential aspect of proper maintenance is an informed dental professional, who then informs patients of their maintenance responsibilities.
- This book shows the reader how to successfully maintain those patients who have periodontal diseases and describes in detail the interrelation of periodontics with other areas of dentistry.

References

1. Waerhaug J: The interdental brush and its place in operative and crown and bridge dentistry. *J Oral Rehabil* 1976;3:107.
2. Axelsson P, Lindhe J: Effect of controlled oral hygiene procedures on caries and periodontal disease in adults. Results after six years. *J Clin Periodontol* 1981;8:239–248.
3. Wilson TG, Glover ME, Schoen J, Baus C, Jacobs T: Compliance with maintenance therapy in a private periodontal practice. *J Periodontol* 1984;55:468.
4. Eraker SA, Kirscht JP, Becker MH: Understanding and improving patient compliance. *Ann Intern Med* 1984;100:258.
5. Ice R: Long-term compliance. *Phys Ther* 1985;65:1832.
6. Haynes RB, Taylor DW, Sackett DL: *Compliance in Health Care.* Baltimore, Johns Hopkins University Press, 1979.
7. Gerber KE, Nehenkis AM: *Compliance—The Dilemma of the Chronically Ill.* New York, Springer Publ Co, 1986.

Chapter 2

Examination, Diagnosis, Classification, and Disease Activity for Patients with Periodontal Diseases*

Thomas G. Wilson, Jr

Examination

In order to make a proper diagnosis, the clinician must gather certain data. These data become an integral part of both active and maintenance therapy. Without a pretreatment and posttreatment baseline against which we can measure, it is impossible to define success. In addition, in our increasingly litigious society, proper documentation is essential. This chapter deals with practical approaches to documentation.

Health histories

Health information can be gathered in various ways, but the initial dental examination should start with a questionnaire that is filled out by the patient. This should contain information on the patient's vital statistics (age, weight, etc), current address, job, and marital status, and a review of current and past medical and dental histories as well as the patient's dental goals. Questions concerning present and past compliance to oral hygiene and dental maintenance can be of great help in formulating a treatment plan. The document should be signed and dated by the patient, reviewed with him or her, then signed and dated by the dentist and updated periodically. As a rule, the patient's current medication and vital signs should be taken and documented before any parenteral medications for anesthesia are given. An example of a long-form health history is given in Fig 2-1.

Radiographic examination

A set of appropriate radiographs should be included in the patient's original documentation. Although each case may require additional radiography, the baseline radiographic data needed for most adult patients with teeth is a full-mouth series of periapical radiographs accompanied by vertical bite-wing radiographs. The most accurate views are obtained using a parallel (right-angle) technique. This is preferred over a panographic radiograph and bite-wings for viewing the periodontium.[1] A full set of these radiographs should be taken every 2 years for the average periodontal patient and more frequently in patients with rapidly advancing disease. Bite-wing films usually provide the best views of the coronal portions of the teeth and can be used as a screening tool between full-mouth films. A set of seven vertical bite-wings is preferred over four horizontal films in adults because this allows a view of the coronal portions of the alveolar bone in both the maxilla and the mandible (Figs 2-2a and b). Mounts are available that allow placement of several series of bite-wings in the same mount. These devices permit us to follow bone patterns over time (Fig 2-3).

Radiographs for patients with dental implants

Pretreatment films are dictated by the technique and site of proposed placement, but for maintenance, panographic and right-angle periapical radiographs and computerized tomography are helpful in assessing the status of the implant. The right-angle films provide a more accurate view of the implant-bone relation than the panographic film and are preferred for root form implants. Panographic films provide helpful data on larger implants. (For a further discussion, see chapter 11.)

Charting

For the periodontal patient

Recent materials on dental risk management from the

*Portions of this chapter originally appeared in the *Texas Dental Journal* and have been reproduced with their kind permission.

PLEASE PRINT AND ANSWER ALL QUESTIONS, INITIAL THE BOTTOM OF EACH PAGE
AND SIGN THE LAST PAGE. ALL INFORMATION PROVIDED IS CONFIDENTIAL.

Name_____ Age_____ Birthdate_____ Height _____ Weight_____

☐ Single ☐ Married ☐ Separated ☐ Divorced ☐ Widowed

Residence Address_____ City_____ Zip_____ Phone_____
Business Address_____ City_____ Zip_____ Phone_____
Occupation_____ Position_____ Employer_____
Name of Spouse_____
Occupation_____ Position_____ Employer_____
Business Address_____ City_____ Zip_____ Phone_____
Party Responsible for Payment of Account_____
Referred by_____ City_____ Purpose_____
Your Dentist_____ City_____ How long?_____ Frequency?_____
Previous Dentist_____ City_____ How long?_____ Frequency?_____
Your Physician_____ How long?_____
Physician's Address_____ City_____
Date of Last Complete Physical Examination_____Purpose of Exam_____
Findings_____
Do you have Dental Insurance? ☐ Yes ☐ No Name of Insurance Carrier_____ SS#_____

GENERAL HEALTH: (Please check "yes" or "no"; if in doubt, check "U" for uncertain, and fill in other information asked for.)

Yes No U
☐ ☐ ☐ 1. Do you have any type of health problem? If so, what?_____
☐ ☐ ☐ 2. Do you have any type of heart problem? If so, what?_____
☐ ☐ ☐ 3. Do you have high or low blood pressure? If so, which?_____
☐ ☐ ☐ 4. Do you have shortness of breath after climbing one flight of stairs?
☐ ☐ ☐ 5. Do you bleed for more than 30 minutes after a minor cut or have any other minor bleeding problems? If so, what?_____
☐ ☐ ☐ 6. Are you taking any medication or drugs including aspirin, vitamins, recreational drugs? List each drug, reason, and who prescribed the drug. (Use back of this page for more space if needed.)
_____
☐ ☐ ☐ 7. Have you been hospitalized in the last 10 years? If so, for what? _____
☐ ☐ ☐ 8. Do you faint easily?
☐ ☐ ☐ 9. Have you taken cortisone or steroids in the last 6 months?
☐ ☐ ☐ 10. Have you been under the care of a physician in the last 2 years other than for a routine physical? If so, for what?_____
☐ ☐ ☐ 11. Have you had any major illness or serious operation in the last 10 years? If so, describe_____
☐ ☐ ☐ 12. Do you have kidney or liver problems? If so, describe _____
☐ ☐ ☐ 13. Have you had rheumatic fever? If so, when was it first diagnosed?_____
☐ ☐ ☐ 14. Do you have any type of artificial valve, joint pin, prosthetic hip, etc, now in place?
☐ ☐ ☐ 15. Do you have a heart murmur, mitral valve prolapse, or heart click? If so, which? (Please circle)
☐ ☐ ☐ 16. Have you ever received psychiatric care or psychotherapy? If so, which? (Please circle)

(Please circle each of the following medications to which you are allergic):

Penicillin	Doxycycline	Aspirin	Tylenol	Stadol	Halcion
Erythromycin	Carbocaine	Phenaphen	Valium	Versed	Acetaminophen
Tetracycline	Xylocaine	Codeine	Demerol	Phenergan	
Keflex/Keflin	Duranest	Novacaine	Percodan	Morphine	

List All Others:_____

Patient's Initials_____ Date_____

FOR OFFICE USE ONLY: ASA Class   I   II   III   IV

Fig 2-1 Example of a long-form health history with a separate area for periodic updates. It should be modified to include medications used by the individual dentist. The written form should be followed by an interview between dentist and patient and should be signed by both dentist and patient.

DENTAL HISTORY:

Yes No U

1. How would you describe your dental health? EXCELLENT GOOD FAIR POOR
2. What do you do to clean your teeth at home? ☐ Brush How Often?_____
   ☐ Dental Floss How Often?_____ ☐ Other (Bridge Cleaners, Stimudents, Rubber Tip, etc)
   List and Describe Frequency_____

☐ ☐ ☐ 3. Type of toothbrush used: HARD MEDIUM SOFT
☐ ☐ ☐ 4. Have you had personal instructions on proper oral hygiene? Who and when?_____
☐ ☐ ☐ 5. Do you feel your present oral hygiene is effective in cleaning your mouth?
☐ ☐ ☐ 6. Have you ever had orthodontic treatment (braces)?
☐ ☐ ☐ 7. Are you satisfied with the way your teeth and gums look?
      8. If unsatisfied, what would you wish to change?_____
☐ ☐ ☐ 9. Can you chew satisfactorily?
☐ ☐ ☐ 10. Have you noticed spaces developing between your teeth? When did this begin?_____
☐ ☐ ☐ 11. Are any of your gums receded? If so, where? _____
☐ ☐ ☐ 12. Are your teeth sensitive to hot? If so, which teeth?_____
☐ ☐ ☐ 13. Are your teeth sensitive to cold? If so, which teeth?_____
☐ ☐ ☐ 14. Are you aware that sensitivity of the teeth to cold can be caused by grinding?
☐ ☐ ☐ 15. Do you clench your teeth? If so, when?_____
☐ ☐ ☐ 16. Do you grind your teeth? If so, when?_____
☐ ☐ ☐ 17. Have you noticed your bite changing? If so, how and when?_____
☐ ☐ ☐ 18. Do you awaken with sore jaws? If so, how often?_____
☐ ☐ ☐ 19. Do you notice popping, clicking, grating, or soreness in the joints just in front of your ears? If so, describe.
      _____
☐ ☐ ☐ 20. Have you ever been treated for TMJ (temporomandibular joint) problems? If so, describe.
      _____
☐ ☐ ☐ 21. Do you get headaches? If so, where and how frequent?_____
      22. When was your last dental cleaning?_____
      23. Date of last full-mouth dental X-rays. _____
☐ ☐ ☐ 24. Have you ever had a frightening experience in a dental office?
☐ ☐ ☐ 25. Have you had previous gum trouble? If so, describe. _____
☐ ☐ ☐ 26. Have you had a previous gum abscess or gum boil? If so, when and which area?_____
      27. If you have had previous gum treatment, who performed the treatment and what type of treatment
      was performed?_____
☐ ☐ ☐ 28. Would the loss of a tooth (or teeth) disturb you?
☐ ☐ ☐ 29. Would wearing a partial denture or false teeth bother you? If so, how much?_____
☐ ☐ ☐ 30. Are any of your teeth loose? If so, which teeth?_____
      31. What concerns you most about your mouth?_____
☐ ☐ ☐ 32. Do you suck mints, lifesavers, etc, regularly?
      33. Estimate the number of cups, glasses, etc, you consume each day on the average:
         coffee_____ tea_____ soft drinks_____ alcoholic beverages_____

FAMILY HISTORY:

☐ ☐ ☐ 1. Have any of your blood relatives had heart disease or high blood pressure?
☐ ☐ ☐ 2. Have any of your blood relatives had diabetes?
☐ ☐ ☐ 3. Have any of your blood relatives lost teeth as a result of gum disease? If so, who? _____
☐ ☐ ☐ 4. Have we treated any of your relatives? If so, who?_____

MEDICAL HISTORY: Do you now have or have you ever had:

☐ ☐ ☐ 1. Anemia?
☐ ☐ ☐ 2. Frequently swollen ankles?
☐ ☐ ☐ 3. Stomach ulcers, diverticulitis, or ulcerative colitis?
☐ ☐ ☐ 4. Excessive thirst or hunger over an extended period of time?

Patient's Initials_____ Date_____

Fig 2-1 Continued.

Yes	No	U		
☐	☐	☐	5.	The need to get up nightly to urinate?
☐	☐	☐	6.	Cuts that tend to heal slowly?
☐	☐	☐	7.	Diabetes? If so, how treated?_____
☐	☐	☐	8.	Hemophilia?
☐	☐	☐	9.	Implant or transplant? Describe:_____
☐	☐	☐	10.	Thyroid disturbance or taken thyroid tablets?
☐	☐	☐	11.	Tuberculosis or emphysema?
☐	☐	☐	12.	Hepatitis?
☐	☐	☐	13.	AIDS or AIDS-related complex (ARC) or ever tested positive for AIDS virus?
☐	☐	☐	14.	Kidney or bladder disease?
☐	☐	☐	15.	Arthritis or rheumatism?
☐	☐	☐	16.	Venereal disease (syphilis; gonorrhea; herpes II)?
☐	☐	☐	17.	Epilepsy, convulsions, or seizures?
☐	☐	☐	18.	Cancer or radiation therapy?
☐	☐	☐	19.	Smoke or use tobacco in any form? If so, frequency._____
☐	☐	☐	20.	Do you wear contact lenses?
☐	☐	☐	21.	Are you taking any sort of tranquilizers?
☐	☐	☐	22.	Are you taking anticoagulants (blood thinners)?
☐	☐	☐	23.	Are you taking antacids regularly? If so, what?_____
☐	☐	☐	24.	Are you taking mood elevators such as: (Please circle)

> Parnate   Adapin   Sinequan   Elavil   Norpramin
> Marplan   Nardil   Tofranil   Aventyl   Pertofrane
> Vivactyl

Yes	No	U		
☐	☐	☐	25.	Do you have glaucoma?
☐	☐	☐	26.	Do you have asthma, hay fever, or eczema?
☐	☐	☐	27.	Do you have liver problems?
☐	☐	☐	28.	Do you have prostate problems (males only)?

MEDICAL HISTORY (FEMALES ONLY):

Yes	No	U		
☐	☐	☐	1.	Are you pregnant?
☐	☐	☐	2.	Have you had a hysterectomy or ovariectomy?
☐	☐	☐	3.	Are you taking birth control pills?
☐	☐	☐	4.	Have you been through menopause?
☐	☐	☐	5.	Had a miscarriage?

** Do you have any disease, medical condition, or health problem not listed above that you think we should know about or that you believe might affect treatment in any way?_____

Do you have any questions before the examination? If so, what? (Use back of this page if you need it.)_____

Date_____   Patient's Signature_____
                             (or that of parent or guardian if patient is younger than 18)

Date First Reviewed_____   Periodontist's Signature_____

                                        Patient's Initials_____   Date_____

Fig 2-1   Continued.

MEDICAL HISTORY UPDATE: (Choose either 1 or 2 for each date of review)

Date_____   1. I have reviewed all three pages of my health history and certify that no change has
occurred.

_____
Patient's Signature

2. Changes in my health history are:_____

_____
Patient's Signature

Date_____   1. I have reviewed all three pages of my health history and certify that no change has
occurred.

_____
Patient's Signature

2. Changes in my health history are:_____

_____
Patient's Signature

Date_____   1. I have reviewed all three pages of my health history and certify that no change has
occurred.

_____
Patient's Signature

2. Changes in my health history are:_____

_____
Patient's Signature

Date_____   1. I have reviewed all three pages of my health history and certify that no change has
occurred.

_____
Patient's Signature

2. Changes in my health history are:_____

_____
Patient's Signature

Fig 2-1 Continued.

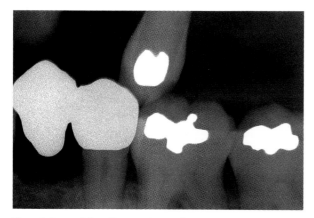

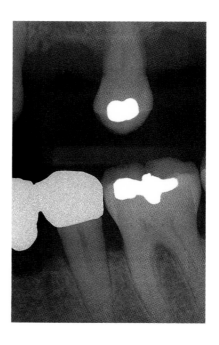

Figs 2-2a and b Comparison of horizontal and vertical bite-wing radiographs. Vertical bite-wings can give the therapist an accurate view of the tooth-related problems normally seen on horizontal films along with valuable and accurate information on the position and topography of the alveolar bone.

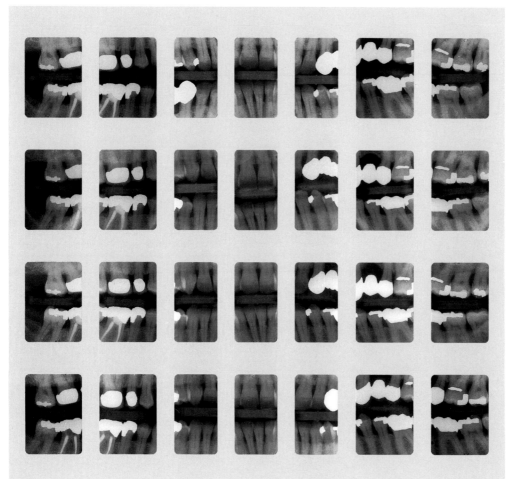

Fig 2-3 A series of vertical bite-wing radiographs taken over 4 years. This arrangement allows the therapist to follow the radiographic changes over time.

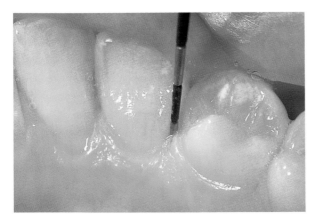

Fig 2-4 A thin periodontal probe is dragged through the sulcus (pocket) and the probing depths on the mesial facial, midfacial, and distal facial surfaces are recorded, as is any bleeding seen after probing. These are recorded for each tooth, then repeated on the lingual (palatal) surfaces. The probe should be positioned as nearly parallel to the long axis of the tooth as possible, then tilted slightly to obtain the reading under the contact.

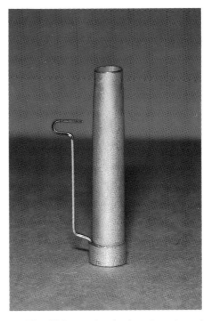

Figs 2-5a and b This mechanical probe when depressed gives a known force, ensuring more accurate and standardized readings. The sleeve fits over a standard probe *(above)*. The spring is pressed until it touches the body of the probe *(below)*, delivering a predetermined force.

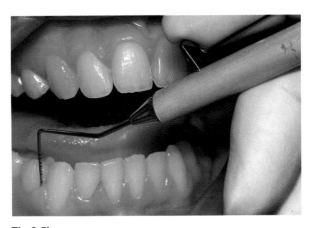

Fig 2-5b

American Dental Association strongly suggest that a number of clinical parameters be recorded on patients with teeth.[2] This section will present a view based on current information, but the reader should be aware that new material is appearing daily and is encouraged to keep abreast of the changes.

Probing depths

The basic instrument for diagnosing periodontal diseases remains the periodontal probe. This device can give more information about the status of the periodontium than any other tool currently available for everyday clinical use. But even this instrument has its limitations. We have learned that probing depths can vary greatly depending on probe angulation, pressure applied, health of the tissue, and even diameter of the probe. In inflamed tissue the probe passes through the junctional epithelium (epithelial attachment) and into the connective tissue.[3] This means that we are not measuring the true histologic depth of the pocket.[4] Consequently, the term "probing depth" has begun to replace the more traditional term "pocket depth," and probing remains an art and not a science. Great diligence is needed to standardize one's technique and thereby ensure reproducible readings.[5]

You should use a thin probe positioned as parallel to the long axis of the tooth as possible and drag it through the sulcus (pocket) (Fig 2-4). Proper force is important because the harder you push, the farther the probe tip penetrates into the tissues. Various forces have been suggested,[6] but at present a prob-

ing force of 50 g has been suggested.[7] Some patients will find this amount of force uncomfortable, but forces in the range of 25 g seem to be light and some deeper areas in tight tissue may be missed. In the author's practice it seems that the ideal force may lie between these two extremes and probing with the same force consistently makes sense. To standardize your probing force, a standard periodontal probe can be pushed against a metric scale, then this amount of force can be reproduced in the mouth. Electronic probes that deliver either a 25-g force (used to detect bleeding upon probing) or 50-g force are available (Vine Valley Research). Also available are computer-

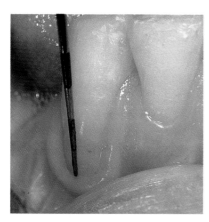

Fig 2-6 Gingival recession as measured from the cementoenamel junction reads 4 mm. Assuming that the probing depth is 3 mm, this would mean that a total of 7 mm of attachment loss had occurred on the facial surface of the canine.

ized probes that give more accurate readings than other methods,[8,9] and automated probes that detect the distance from the base of the pocket to the cementoenamel junction.[10] The standard probe has the advantage of being readily available and significantly less expensive than the other probes described. When a disposable, pressure-sensitive probe (Dental Designs of Dallas, 10246 Midway Road, Dallas, Texas 75229) is used, obtaining consistent probing forces becomes more predictable and is not expensive (Figs 2-5a and b).

Probing tells us whether the soft tissue is clinically healthy and gives an indication of bone loss, tissue tone, subgingival calculus deposits, and furcation invasions and other variations in root anatomy.

Probing depths can be misleading in the presence of excessively tight or excessively flaccid tissue, when there are large deposits of calculus, or when visibility or placement is hindered. A great deal of effort is required to standardize probing depth readings among the dental professionals in an office, but it is well worth the time.

Gingival recession

This parameter is measured from a set point on the tooth, usually the cementoenamel junction at the margin of a restoration. It is important because of the perspective it provides for probing depth. A 4-mm probing depth with no recession would be viewed with less alarm than the same probing depth with 7 mm of recession (which would equal 11 mm of attachment loss) (Fig 2-6). In most cases the midbuccal and midlingual (palatal) recessions are recorded.

Bleeding upon probing and bacterial plaque

Bleeding upon probing is found by dragging the tip of a thin periodontal probe through the gingival sulcus. Alternatively, it can be observed after the probing depth of a particular site has been taken. This reading is usually recorded as being either present or absent. There are two convenient ways to record this parameter (Figs 2-7 and 2-8). At the same time that the clinician scores bleeding upon probing, any visible dental plaque can be recorded on the same chart.

Tooth mobility

Tooth mobility has two divisions: that found when the examiner places pressure on the teeth while the jaws are apart (bidigital mobility) (Fig 2-9), and that seen when the teeth are in function (fremitus) (Figs 2-10a and b).

At present there is no simple, reproducible system for documenting bidigital mobility. In our office we use a modification of the Miller scale[11] made by the Ramfjord group.[12]

Class I: Slightly increased mobility
Class II: Definite to considerable increase in mobility, but no impairment of function
Class III: Extreme mobility; a "loose" tooth that would be uncomfortable in function
(A " + " can be used for intermediate values, eg, 1 +)

This system obviously has a great deal of individual variation. However, by using the blunt ends of two instruments and working on standardization, some degree of reproducibility is possible within your own office.

Fremitus is also called functional mobility. It is found when the patient closes into centric occlusion and then is asked to grind his or her teeth together in working, balancing, and protrusive movements. Any movement seen or felt is fremitus. Fremitus is often found earlier than tooth mobility and has been associated with increased bone and attachment loss (pocket formation) when compared to teeth without fremitus.[13]

Furcations

There are a number of good classifications for furcas, but the most helpful is the horizontal probing depth in millimeters (Fig 2-11). When combined with vertical probing depths, this is the best way to quantify bone loss in these areas. This form of analysis is difficult to apply to some palatal furcas of maxillary molars and is usually inapplicable on the mesial surfaces of maxillary first premolars. In these areas the following classification can be of assistance.

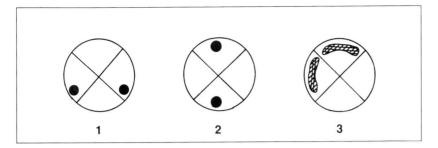

Fig 2-7 One way to record bleeding upon probing is to have a series of circles with x's denoting each tooth. Bleeding areas (or plaque) can be recorded on a separate sheet of paper or by using a rubber stamp on the patient's record. In this example, bleeding was seen after probing on the distolingual and mesiolingual surfaces of tooth 1 and on the midfacial and midlingual surface of tooth 2. Plaque was seen covering the facial and distal surfaces of tooth 3.

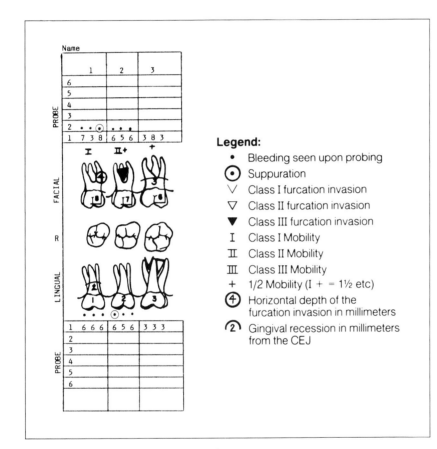

Legend:

- •   Bleeding seen upon probing
- ⊙   Suppuration
- ∨   Class I furcation invasion
- ∇   Class II furcation invasion
- ▼   Class III furcation invasion
- I   Class I Mobility
- II   Class II Mobility
- III   Class III Mobility
- +   1/2 Mobility (I + = 1½ etc)
- ④   Horizontal depth of the furcation invasion in millimeters
- ② Gingival recession in millimeters from the CEJ

Fig 2-8 Records of probing depth, bleeding upon probing, suppuration, mobility, gingival recession, and furca invasion can be kept on a single chart. The six rows for probing depth and bleeding allow easy comparison from visit to visit.

Class I: A furca that does not catch a thin Gracey 13–14 curette

Class II: A furca deep enough to catch the curette but not contiguous with other furcas on the same tooth

Class III: Bone loss through and through

Attached/keratinized gingiva

Keratinized tissue runs from the mucogingival junction coronally to the midfacial or midlingual surface of the free gingival margin. Attached gingiva is found by subtracting the midfacial or lingual probing depth from the width of keratinized gingiva (Figs 2-12a to c). A synopsis of its significance is found in chapter 7 and its relation to orthodontic care is discussed in chapter 8.

Charting for patients with dental implants

See chapter 11, p 191.

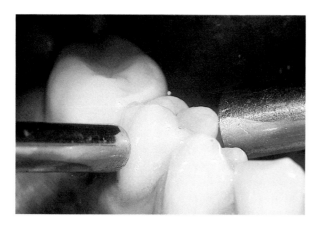

Fig 2-9 The most convenient test for tooth mobility is obtained by using the blunt ends of two instruments. Pressure is applied to first the facial then the lingual surface. Any mobility is recorded.

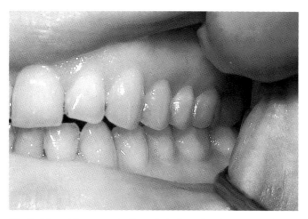

Fig 2-10a Movement of teeth in function is termed fremitus or functional mobility. Fremitus can be found by visual or digital inspection and is noted as being present or absent. Fremitus can be seen in centric relation, centric occlusion, or in any movement of the jaws where the teeth meet. To check for this parameter, the patient is first instructed to close in centric occlusion.

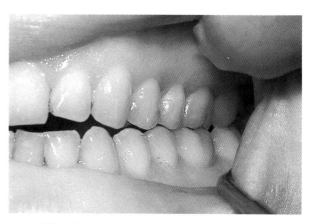

Fig 2-10b The patient is then asked to grind the teeth together in a side-to-side motion. Protrusive movement is also checked.

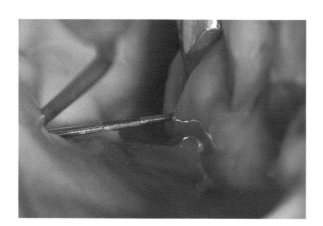

Fig 2-11 Horizontal probing of accessible furcas gives more accurate information about bone loss than the use of a curette.

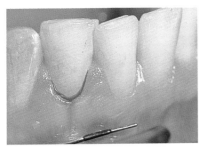 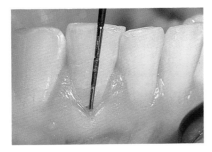 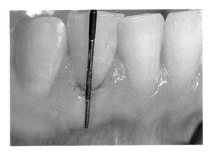

Fig 2-12a The amount of attached gingiva can be found by first locating the mucogingival junction either by sight or where the tissue is immobile.

Figs 2-12b and c The probing depth at the midfacial (or lingual) surface is then subtracted from the total width of keratinized gingiva (mucogingival junction to the margin of the free gingiva). In this example, there are 3 mm of attached gingiva.

─────── *At a glance* ───────────────────────────

Charting

- For the dentist who shares responsibility for periodontal treatment with a periodontist, the following data should be collected at the initial visit and updated at each maintenance visit.
  - Six probing depth readings per tooth—updated at least once a year
  - Gingival recession on the midfacial and midlingual surface of each tooth (from a fixed point) updated yearly
  - A set of right-angle periapical radiographs showing all the teeth and vertical bite-wings of the posterior teeth
  - Presence or absence of fremitus checked at each maintenance visit
  - Presence or absence of bleeding upon probing (six sites per tooth)
- For the dentist who wishes to take responsibility for the patient's periodontal therapy, the following data should be gathered.
  - Six probing depth readings per tooth—updated at least once a year
  - Gingival recession on the midfacial and midlingual surface of each tooth (from a fixed point) updated yearly
  - A complete set of right-angle periapical radiographs and vertical bite-wings of the posterior teeth
  - Bleeding upon probing (six potential sites per tooth) and sites of dental plaque accumulation (updated at each visit)
  - Tooth mobility
  - Presence or absence of fremitus checked at each maintenance visit
  - Areas deficient in attached gingiva
  - Recordings of furcation invasions
- A sample chart is shown in Fig 2-8.

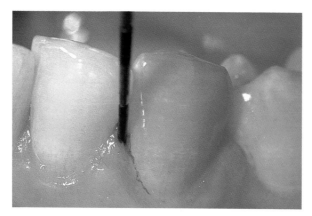

Fig 2-13 The probe penetrates approximately 3 mm and sulcular bleeding is seen after light pressure. The clinical diagnosis would be chronic gingivitis.

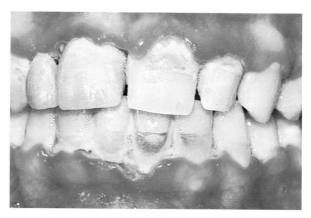

Fig 2-14 This patient presented with acute pain, cratered interdental papillae, and extreme halitosis. She was diagnosed as having acute necrotizing gingivitis.

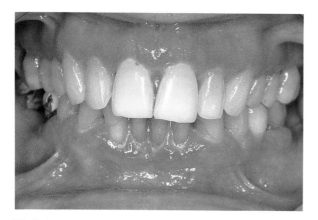

Fig 2-15 This patient was unaware that he was HIV positive when he presented to have his gingival lesion treated. (Courtesy of Dr Terry D. Rees.)

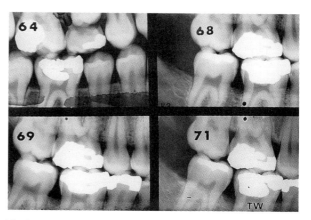

Fig 2-16 The radiographic changes occurring in chronic periodontitis can be seen on the distal surface of the mandibular first molar. In the radiograph taken in 1964 the patient was approximately 13 years old and no bone loss can be detected radiographically. When the patient was seen 7 years later (1971), there was a slight radiographic change on the distal surface of tooth 30, which clinically probed 7 mm.

Diagnosis of periodontal diseases and conditions

In years past, diagnosis for periodontal problems was reasonably simple. With increased knowledge, this is no longer true. There has been a move away from seeing periodontal disease as a monolith caused by a conglomerate of bacteria called plaque. We are becoming increasingly aware that we are dealing with a number of disease processes, some (or all) of which could very well be caused by different and perhaps disease-specific bacteria. Our knowledge is not yet complete, but we can now categorize a number of distinct diseases. These categories have recently changed and could well change again.

Gingivitis

Patients with probing depths of 3 mm or less and bleeding seen after probing have gingivitis.

Chronic gingivitis

This is the most common periodontal disease, and it is generally agreed that this stage is a precursor to periodontitis and that this problem is reversible (Fig 2-13). The major unanswered question is when and why the process shifts from gingivitis to periodontitis. Periodontitis is preceded by gingivitis but not all gingivitis later invades the bone.

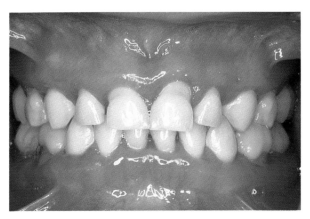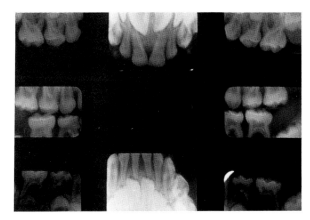

Figs 2-17a and b The gingival and radiographic changes seen in a 5½-year-old child with generalized prepubertal periodontitis. (Courtesy of Drs Kenneth S. Kornman and Jayne Delaney.)

Acute necrotizing ulcerative gingivitis (ANUG)

The diagnosis of this problem is usually simple: the acute form is accompanied by pain, bleeding, and halitosis (Fig 2-14). The histologic lesion is typified by invasion of the soft tissues with spirochetes. A clinical feature is the presence of interdental gingival craters in advanced cases. Therapy consists of gentle debridement for several consecutive days and encouraging improved oral hygiene and maintenance compliance. Antibiotics are given only if the patient is febrile.

HIV gingivitis

HIV gingivitis occurs in patients who have contracted the AIDS virus. It is characterized by severe marginal inflammation of the gingival tissues. Other oral manifestations commonly seen in HIV-positive patients can accompany the gingival lesions, but often the patient is not aware that he or she is serologically positive (Fig 2-15).

Periodontitis

Patients with periodontitis have probing depths of 4 mm or greater, seen when tissues are at or near the cementoenamel junction. Bleeding upon probing is often seen. At present there are six categories of this disease.

Chronic adult

This is the most common type of periodontitis. It is seen in adults and progresses slowly in most cases (Fig 2-16). Recent studies have suggested that the progression occurs not in a linear fashion but in bursts of attachment loss.[14] It is usually associated with accumulation of visible amounts of supra- and subgingival bacterial plaque where the patient does not (or cannot) clean. Calculus is present in varying degrees but is usually seen.

Prepubertal

This form of periodontitis is seen around the time of eruption of the primary teeth. There are generalized and localized forms. The localized form features little or no inflammation of the gingival tissues and is amenable to standard periodontal therapy along with appropriate antibiotics. Extreme gingival inflammation and rapid destruction of alveolar bone are the clinical hallmarks of the generalized form. This latter type is accompanied by severe functional defects of the neutrophils and monocytes. Otitis media and upper respiratory infections are often found in these patients. In some cases the more severe lesions are refractory to antibiotics[15] (Figs 2-17a and b).

Localized juvenile

This disease is identified by vertical bony defects around the 6-year molars and the maxillary incisors. This process is usually associated with minimal amounts of observable bacterial plaque and systemic defect of the immune system. Overt clinical inflammation of the gingival tissues is not usually present. The problem is found in circumpubertal patients and is often associated with specific bacterial species, especially *Actinobacillus actinomycetemcomitans* (Figs 2-18a to c).

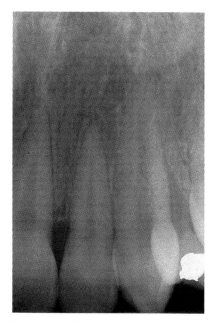

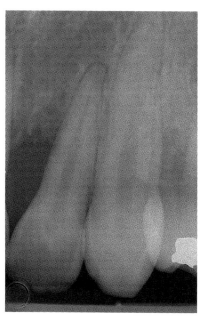

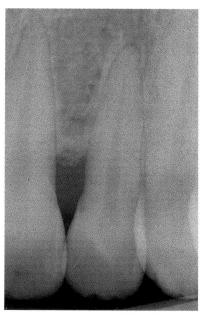

Fig 2-18a Radiograph taken when the patient was 13.

Fig 2-18b By age 15, a 10-mm vertical defect had occurred on the mesial surface of the lateral incisor.

Fig 2-18c The defect was successfully repaired with a bone graft and is seen 10 years later. The diagnosis was localized juvenile periodontitis.

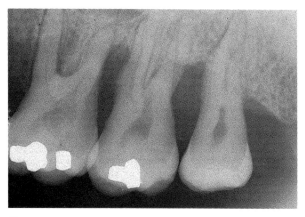

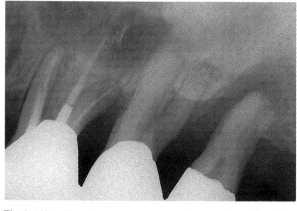

Fig 2-19a This patient presented with generalized 10- to 12-mm probing depths. The diagnosis was rapidly progressive periodontitis.

Fig 2-19b The disease was controlled and stabilized for approximately 8 years, then rapid breakdown occurred when the patient's compliance to maintenance therapy dropped off.

Rapidly progressive (also called generalized juvenile or early)

Rapidly progressive periodontitis may be a group of diseases or a single disease characterized by generalized rapid bone loss. It is seen in patients ranging from around puberty to age 35. In many cases systemic abnormalities including malaise, depression, and lower immune competency are seen during the acute stages of the disease. The oral manifestations of the active phase are red, swollen gingival tissues that bleed easily, often accompanied by mobile or drifting teeth (Figs 2-19a and b). Several distinct bacterial species have been implicated as etiologic factors of this problem.

Refractory adult

Refractory adult periodontitis may be a mixture of several diseases or the same disease manifestation with different bacterial etiologies. This disease de-

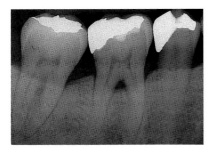

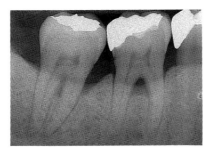

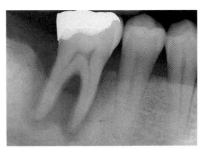

Fig 2-20a This patient, with refractory adult periodontitis, remained stable for approximately 8 years with conventional periodontal therapy and maintenance.

Fig 2-20b The patient's dental health then broke down rapidly, as seen 1 1/2 years after the radiograph in Fig 2-20a.

Fig 2-20c A great deal of bone loss was seen around the first molar, and the second molar had been lost 3 years after the view in Fig 2-20a.

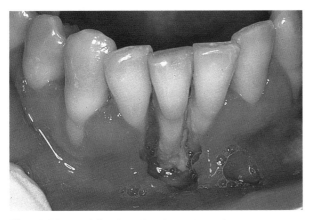

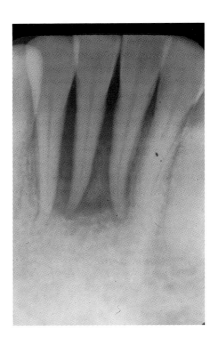

Figs 2-21a and b Localized erosion of alveolar bone associated with HIV periodontitis.

velops in adult patients who have been well treated previously for periodontitis and who experience breakdown during maintenance therapy (Figs 2-20a to c). Care should be taken to include in this group only those patients whose oral hygiene is quite good and in whom the active phase of periodontal therapy has removed local factors such as subgingival calculus and faulty restorative margins. Fortunately these patients are in the minority, because the disease is often difficult to control.

HIV periodontitis

Patients with HIV periodontitis are serologically positive for the AIDS virus. The bone loss that accompanies this problem is usually horizontal and rapid. Treatment includes palliative procedures. Systemic antibiotics should be avoided (Figs 2-21a to c).

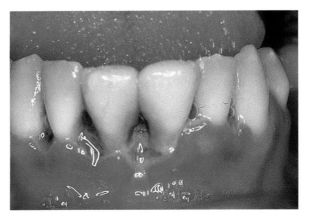

Fig 2-21c Generalized erosion of alveolar bone associated with HIV periodontitis. (Figs 2-21a to c courtesy of Dr Terry D. Rees.)

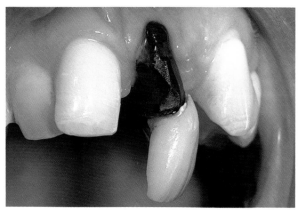

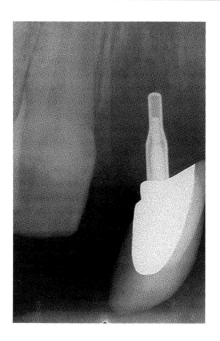

Figs 2-22a and b In this example of peri-implantitis, the exfoliation of this vitreous carbon implant was accompanied by deepened probing depths and inflammation.

Peri-implantitis

This inflammatory problem is found around dental implants and mimics periodontitis (Figs 2-22a and b). Information at this point is sketchy, but early evidence suggests the bacterial flora seen around these entities is similar to that seen around natural teeth with chronic adult periodontitis. It is also true that osseointegrated implants suffer this condition to a lesser degree than implants surrounded by thick connective tissues (the so-called fibro-osseous integrated implants).

Periodontal conditions

Gingival hyperplasia

Hyperplasia is an increase in size of an organ or its parts. It is characterized by an increase in the numbers of cellular elements and does not serve a functional purpose.[16]

There are three medications in fairly common use that cause most of these overgrowths. They are phenytoin (Dilantin®, Parke-Davis and other manufacturers), cyclosporine (Sandimmune®, Sandoz), and nifedipine (Adalat®, Miles; Procardia®, Pfizer). In general, the better the patient's oral hygiene, the smaller the problem. For an excellent review see Butler et al.[17]

──────── *At a glance* ────────

Diagnosis of periodontal diseases and conditions

- The clinician most often encounters chronic gingivitis and chronic adult periodontitis. They make up a very large majority of the periodontal diseases seen in the typical office.
- A number of new disease categories now exist for patients with periodontitis. These diseases often require more than traditional therapy for successful treatment.
- Dental implants suffer from inflammatory diseases similar to those seen around teeth.

Disease activity

Traditionally, probing depth has been used as the primary indicator of disease in periodontics; if a pocket was found, this was justification enough for therapy. Although probing depths still play a major role in decisions concerning treatment, there is also concern for determining the disease activity of the pocket. Goodson and co-workers have shown that these diseases may come in bursts, and that breakdown may occur at only a few sites at a time.[14] Assuming that this theory is correct, we must assess the activity of the disease within a pocket and know its depth. The search for the best indicator of disease activity continues.

Probing depth

Probing is the classic method for diagnosing periodontal diseases and still the most universally practiced. If sequential records of probing depths are kept, then changes can be seen. As discussed earlier, the drawback to this measurement is that it varies with the health of the tissue, force exerted upon probing, position of the margin of the gingiva, probe angulation, and other local factors. Consequently, every attempt should be made to standardize probing technique. In addition, it is a retrospective measure and doesn't accurately predict further bone loss.

Bleeding upon probing

How is bleeding measured?

Probing involves gently dragging a periodontal probe within the gingival sulcus (pocket).[18] Other methods to obtain this measure have been suggested,[19] but we prefer dragging the probe. Start with the probe in the deepest part of the interproximal sulcus (pocket) and then slowly move it toward the opposite interproximal space on the same tooth, staying within the gingival crevice at all times. Any bleeding seen within 30 seconds is counted as positive. For the average clinician, simply the presence or absence of the parameter is sufficient. The information is recorded on a site-specific chart (see Fig 2-7). With this method there are six potential bleeding points per tooth, which correspond to the points where probing depths are recorded. Ideally, a known reproducible force is used. The force most often suggested is 25 g.[7] This force can be provided by various mechanical or electronic probes. Although it is difficult,[5,20] we have found it possible to achieve a relative degree of standardization among those within our office with repetitive

practice. The use of an ordinary scale can give a relative idea of what force should be employed. We prefer to use a probe that delivers a known force (see Figs 2-5a and b, Dental Designs of Dallas). Even with such a device, this parameter is not readily reproducible.[21,22]

What does bleeding seen upon probing mean?

1. Is bleeding on probing a sign of gingivitis? Yes. The amount of inflamed connective tissue increases as bleeding upon probing increases.[23] The same is true of plasma cells in deeper probing depths[24] and lymphocytes in shallow probing depths.[25] It also is an earlier manifestation of gingival inflammation than are color changes in the gingiva.[18]

2. Does bleeding on probing mean changes in microbiota? Yes, at least of spirochetes. Armitage et al[26] showed that as the percentage of spirochetes increased, so did bleeding upon probing. This may be significant because increases in the percentage of those organisms have been associated with periodontitis.[27]

Does bleeding on probing predict attachment loss?

At present, most authors would answer in the negative.[28–31] However, some of these and other studies indicate that bleeding upon probing can be of some use for predicting attachment loss. Badersten et al[30] found that 20% of the areas that lost attachment in one of their studies had shown bleeding upon probing. Other studies showed a one in four chance of bleeding upon probing predicting breakdown and an 80% chance of not having breakdown when there was no bleeding.[28] Lang et al[32] studied 55 patients for four consecutive maintenance visits. They found that sites that bled after probing at each visit had a 30% chance of losing attachment. This diminished to a 14% chance when bleeding was seen three of four times. In addition, they found that patients who had 16% (or greater) total bleeding had a higher chance for attachment loss than those below 16%.

Should the clinician use site-specific bleeding or whole-mouth bleeding?

You should use both. In our practice, bleeding seen in one site at two consecutive maintenance visits at present is cause for concern. The patient is warned that attachment loss may follow and is instructed to concentrate oral hygiene efforts in that spot. If a large percentage of change occurs,[32] then the length of time between maintenance visits should be modified appropriately. For an in-depth discussion of this approach, see chapter 6.

─────── *At a glance* ───────

■ Bleeding upon probing should be measured by drawing a periodontal probe from interproximal sulcus to interproximal sulcus without withdrawing the tip. Any bleeding is a positive sign, and there are six potential sites per tooth that should be recorded (the same as probing).

■ In order to ensure as much accuracy as possible, a standard force should be used. There are two ways to accomplish this: *(1)* standardize everyone in the office, using about 25 g of force (this can be approximated using a metric scale for practice), and *(2)* use a mechanical or electronic probe that delivers a known force.

■ Bleeding upon probing means that gingivitis is probably present and that microorganisms associated with attachment loss may well be present. Absence of bleeding means that there is a very good probability that attachment loss will not occur.

■ Attachment loss occurs in about 20% of the areas where bleeding upon probing is seen. The following generalizations can be made.
   1. The more times an area bleeds (at different visits), the more likely breakdown is to occur.
   2. The greater the total number of bleeding sites at any one visit, the greater the likelihood of breakdown.

■ Bleeding upon probing should be measured and recorded at each maintenance visit, and some manner of comparing visit to visit should be provided (see Fig 2-7).

Attachment loss

Attachment loss gives a more accurate picture of what is happening to the junctional epithelium (epithelial attachment) than probing depth because it is measured from a fixed reference point on the tooth to the base of the clinical pocket. However, it is very difficult to do in daily clinical practice. It has the same drawbacks as probing depths (except that the gingival margin is not used as a reference point). Also, if the landmark you measure from changes (a new crown, etc), then the relationship is lost.

Radiographs

Radiographs record only gross changes in bone. Therefore, they should serve only as an adjunct for assessing disease activity. As previously suggested, films exposed with a right-angle technique and vertical bite-wings are preferred. Panographic radiographs provide little useful information concerning bone loss and should not be used. Sequential vertical bite-wings on a single mount provide the most accurate method for radiographic assessment of bone loss available for routine clinical use (see Fig 2-3).

Gingival sulcular fluid flow

The gingival sulcular fluid is a transudate that originates in the vascular complex subadjacent to the junctional epithelium, then passes between the epithelial cells and into the gingival sulcus (periodontal pocket).[33,34] It then empties into the mouth at a rate of 0.5 to 2.4 mL per day.[35]

The rate of flow may[36] or may not[37] be affected by time of day; it is increased by hormonal changes during the menstrual cycle[38] and pregnancy when the gingivae are diseased,[39] but not when they are healthy.[40] In health there is little or no exudate[41] or a minimal amount,[42] depending on the sampling technique used. As inflammation of the gingival tissues increases, so does gingival sulcular fluid flow, but this does not occur in a linear fashion.[35]

There are several methods for collecting sulcular fluid for analysis. These include absorbent paper strips, micropipettes, and gingival washings. A unit for analyzing fluid collected on filter paper strips is available (Periotron, Harco Electronics Dental Products Division). This machine is highly accurate if used correctly and calibrated daily.[43]

This method of measuring disease showed early promise. At present, however, in the words of a leading authority on the subject, "Up to now . . . none of the multiple components analyzed in the fluid has improved clinical judgment of the rate of progress of gingivitis and periodontitis or of the rate of repair of these conditions."[35]

Identification of specific bacterial species

At present there is a debate about whether individual bacterial species are responsible for causing periodontal diseases or whether these problems are caused by nonspecific masses of microbes.

The nonspecific theory maintains that most periodontal diseases are caused by a conglomeration of bacteria. In this scenario these bacteria organize above the gingival tissues and set up an environment that favors the formation of anaerobic species that colonize the crevicular areas.[44] It is this matured aggregation of bacteria and their by-products that cause disease. Masses may differ from tooth surface to tooth surface, but several combinations are capable of causing apical migration of the junctional epithelium.[45,46]

The second theory holds that at least some of the periodontal diseases have specific bacterial etiologies.[47] The bacteria most often mentioned include *Actinobacillus actinomycetemcomitans,* which has been found closely associated with localized juvenile periodontitis and other periodontal lesions[48–52] but is not found in all of these lesions.[53] *Bacteroides gingivalis* has also been implicated in advancing periodontal disease,[54,55] as has to a lesser extent *Bacteroides intermedius.*[56] *Bacteroides intermedius* seems to be less specific because it is found in gingivitis, periodontitis, endodontic infections, and odontogenic abscesses.[55] Other bacteria that have been implicated in advancing periodontitis include "fusiform" *Bacteroides, Fusobacterium nucleatum, Eikenella corrodens, Wolinella recta,* and spirochetes.[45] If a specific bacterial species (or groups of bacteria)[57] is implicated in these diseases, then it is essential for the clinician to identify the organisms involved. Traditional methods of identification included Gram stains[58] and dark-field microscopy.[27] Recent developments have increased the accuracy of identification of these bacteria using DNA probes and sophisticated bacterial growth media.

The DNA probe

Samples are collected with sterile absorbent paper points that are placed in a pocket following removal of supragingival plaque.[59] The DNA from all the bacteria in the sample is split to yield single-stranded DNA. This material is then spotted onto filter paper and the DNA probe is made in the laboratory. This process involves splitting the complementary DNA strands from stock cultures. A control DNA strand from this species tagged with a marker or label is introduced to the filter containing all DNA from the submitted sample. If binding of the test and labeled DNA probe strands occurs, this can be detected with the marker and the test organism is thus identified. At present these probes are commercially available for *A actinomycetemcomitans, B gingivalis,* and *B intermedius.*[60,61] This technique has the advantage over culture techniques in that the organisms do not have to be alive after transport to ensure an accurate test.

Culture technique

Culturing involves growing the test bacteria on selective culture media for identification. This may be followed by testing for susceptibility to selected antibiotics. This method is highly technique sensitive. Problem areas include proper selection of sample site, method of sample collection, transport and dispersion, choice of incubation system and atmosphere, selection of media for primary isolation, bacterial identification criteria, and interpretation of obtained data.[62]

Clinical concerns

Before one of these tests is ordered, the clinician must accept that the specific etiology theory is viable. At present this represents acceptance of the most recent research findings.[47] While one of these organisms *(B gingivalis)* has been shown to be the etiologic agent in periodontitis in one study using monkeys as an animal model,[63] and this and other anaerobes are often found in progressing pockets, the evidence is compelling but inconclusive. The organisms named are also found as part of normal flora when no disease is present.

Clinical applications

The DNA probe. At present, we see no reason for the routine application of DNA probes for the pretherapeutic case. It may, however, serve as a predictive test for breakdown in maintenance cases. In one study, *A actinomycetemcomitans, B gingivalis,* and *B intermedius* were found in 20% of the areas that broke down after therapy (about the same percentage of predictability seen with bleeding upon probing), whereas uninfected sites showed no breakdown.[64] Because of the cost, the limited number of microbes assayed, and the lack of antibiotic sensitivity testing, DNA probes are not recommended for routine use.

Culture techniques. In the final result we may find a common middle ground in our use of culture techniques. At present there is much evidence that *A actinomycetemcomitans* is associated with most cases of localized juvenile periodontitis. The specific theory also may apply to rapidly progressive and refractory periodontitis. It seems now that gingivitis is caused by a nonspecific group of bacteria. This is probably also true of chronic adult periodontitis.

If you have a patient who is suspected of having rapidly progressive periodontitis, a culture before therapy is reasonable. This would be followed by retesting during maintenance. Refractory cases can also benefit, but because of the definition of the disease, this would be done only during maintenance care or before re-treatment. In addition, culturing after therapy for localized juvenile periodontitis to make sure that levels of A actinomycetemcomitans are low or absent is reasonable.

The samples should be taken as suggested by the laboratory and great care should be taken in site selection (an active one), site preparation (carefully remove any supragingival plaque), and time of collection (usually late in the day for overnight transport to the laboratory). You should specify selective and non-selective media to avoid suppressing some potential pathogens.[62] Because a recent course of antibiotics can alter the microflora, these medications should be avoided for at least 30 days before testing.

It should be clearly understood when these methods are used that they serve as an adjunct to traditional care, which must include at least thorough scaling and root planing. In addition, you must be aware that we have yet to identify all the organisms in the subgingival pocket in humans, or prove beyond a doubt that these organisms cause the periodontal diseases. Therefore, these methods should not be used for the treatment of chronic gingivitis or periodontitis, but only when specific information concerning bacteria and antibiotic specificity is needed.

At a glance

Identification of specific bacterial species

- There are at present three theories of etiology of periodontal diseases.
    1. Nonspecific theory—that many microorganisms and different combinations of bacteria working together are responsible for disease
    2. Specific theory—that for some periodontal diseases a few (or in some cases a single) microorganism species may be responsible for disease production
    3. A combination of 1 and 2 with some diseases associated with specific organisms and some not
- If one accepts the specific theory or the combination theory, there are two ways to determine which specific organisms may be present: *(1)* DNA probes and *(2)* bacterial culturing and antibiotic sensitivity testing.
- At present if one is dealing with localized juvenile, rapidly progressive, or refractory periodontitis, then bacterial culturing is often helpful as an adjunct to traditional care.
- How to use culture techniques:
    1. Culture
    2. Consult with patient
    3. Scale and root plane (open or closed as needed). Either start appropriate antibiotics (usually run for 3 weeks), start chlorhexidine mouthrinses (usually run for 6 weeks), or both where indicated.
    4. Reculture in 6 months to 1 year or sooner if clinical parameters do not improve.

Immunologic assays

Immunologic assays involve reaction of bacterial antigens with antibodies. Several tests are available, including enzyme-linked immunosorbent assay (ELISA), immunofluorescent microscopy, latex agglutination, and others.[65] At present, these remain research tools and clinical applications are not yet available.

Antibody titers

When oral infection occurs, the body often produces antibodies to the various organisms involved and these levels can be measured. Enzyme-linked immunosorbent assay is often used because of its sensitivity.[66] However, some organisms may actually suppress immune reactions,[67] thus blocking any humoral response. At present there is no test that will give enough data to warrant its routine clinical use.

Enzymes

Some microbial enzymes are capable of periodontal destruction. These can be detected in the saliva[68] or in the gingival sulcular fluid.[69] One drawback to these sampling methods is that you need a large sample of the individual bacteria in order to elicit an accurate response.[70] At present these tests must undergo extensive review before they are recommended for clinical practice.

Microscopic examination of bacteria

There is evidence that increased motile rods and spirochetes occur when diseased sites are compared with healthy pockets (for a review see Greenstein and Polson[71]). These organisms can be readily seen using dark-field or phase-contrast microscopy. Unfortunately, many of the organisms associated with periodontal disease are not motile and are not rods or spirochetes. We think there is little justification for the routine use of this test in the diagnosis of disease activity at this stage.

--- *At a glance* ---

Disease activity

- At present we do not know how to predict breakdown from periodontal diseases accurately. Until this issue is resolved, the practitioner should keep an updated set of six probings per tooth.
- Bleeding upon probing is a simple, inexpensive parameter that may predict breakdown in some cases, and the absence of this finding usually indicates that breakdown will not occur.
- Other tests and measures discussed give additional information that can be useful in selected cases, and the more responsibility the practitioner takes for the treatment and maintenance of the periodontal patient, the more of these parameters that should be recorded.
- See chapter 6 for a practical approach to integrating information about disease activity into daily practice.

References

1. National Center for Health Care Technology. Current conferences—Dental radiology: A summary of recommendations from the Technology Assessment Forum. *J Am Dent Assoc* 1981;103:423.
2. American Dental Association Risk Management Series. *Diagnosing and Managing the Periodontal Patient.* Chicago, American Dental Association, 1986.
3. Listgarten MA, Mao R, Robinson PJ: Periodontal probing and the relationship of the probe tip to periodontal tissues. *J Periodontol* 1976;47:511.
4. Hancock EB, Wirthlin MR: The location of the periodontal probe tip in health and disease. *J Periodontol* 1981;52:124.
5. Hassell TM, Germann MA, Saxer UP: Periodontal probing: Inter-investigator discrepancies and correlations between probing force and recorded depth. *Helv Odontol Acta* 1973;17:38.
6. Gabathuler H, Hassell TM: A pressure-sensitive periodontal probe. *Helv Odontol Acta* 1971;15:114.
7. Proye M, Caton J, Polson A: Initial healing of periodontal pockets after a single episode of root planing monitored by controlled probing forces. *J Periodontol* 1982;53:296.
8. Magnusson I, Fuller WW, Heins PJ, Rau CF, Gibbs CH, Marks RG, Clark WB: Correlation between electronic and visual readings of pocket depths with a newly developed constant force probe. *J Clin Periodontol* 1988;15:180.
9. Magnusson I, Clark WB, Marks RG, Gibbs CH, Manouchehr-Pour M, Low SB: Attachment level measurements with a constant force electronic probe. *J Clin Periodontol* 1988;15:185.
10. Jeffcoat MK, Jeffcoat RL, Jens SC, Captain K: A new periodontal probe with automated cemento-enamel junction detection. *J Clin Periodontol* 1986;13:276.
11. Miller SC: *Textbook of Periodontia,* 2nd ed. Philadelphia, Blakiston, 1943, p 103.
12. Fleszar TJ, Knowles JW, Morrison EC, Burgett FG, Nissle RR, Ramfjord SP: Tooth mobility and periodontal therapy. *J Clin Periodontol* 1980;7:495.
13. Pihlstrom BL, Anderson KA, Aeppli D, Schaffer EM: Association between signs of trauma from occlusion and periodontitis. *J Periodontol* 1986;57:1.
14. Goodson JM, Tanner ACR, Haffajee AD, Sornberger GC, Socransky SS: Patterns of progression and regression of advanced destructive periodontal disease. *J Clin Periodontol* 1982;9:472.
15. Page RC, Bowen T, Altman L, Vandersteen E, Ochs H, Mackenzie P, Osterberg S, Engel LD, Williams BL: Prepubertal periodontitis. I. Definition of a clinical disease entity. *J Periodontol* 1983;54:257.

16. Grant DA, Stern IB, Everett FG: *Periodontics in the Tradition of Orban and Gottleib*. St. Louis, CV Mosby Co, 1979, p 389.

17. Butler RT, Kalkwarf KL, Kaldahl WB: Drug-induced gingival hyperplasia: Phenytoin, cyclosporine, and nifedipine. *J Am Dent Assoc* 1987;114:56.

18. Mühlemann HR, Son S: Gingival sulcus bleeding—a leading symptom in initial gingivitis. *Helv Odontol Acta* 1971;15:107.

19. Mühlemann HR: Psychological and chemical mediators of gingival health. *J Prev Dent* 1977;4:6.

20. Freed HK, Gapper RL, Kalkwarf KL: Evaluation of periodontal probing forces. *J Periodontol* 1983;54:488.

21. Janssen PTM, Faber JAJ, van Palenstein Helderman WH: Reproducibility of bleeding tendency measurements and the reproducibility of mouth bleeding scores for the individual patient. *J Periodont Res* 1986;21:653.

22. Van Der Velden U: Influence of probing force on the reproducibility of bleeding tendency measurements. *J Clin Periodontol* 1980;7:421.

23. Greenstein G, Caton J, Polson AM: Histologic characteristics associated with bleeding after probing and visual signs of inflammation. *J Periodontol* 1981;52:420.

24. Davenport RH, Simpson DM, Hassell TM: Histometric comparison of active and inactive lesions of advanced periodontitis. *J Periodontol* 1982;53:285.

25. Cooper PG, Caton JG, Polson AM: Cell populations associated with gingival bleeding. *J Periodontol* 1983;54:497.

26. Armitage GC, Dickinson WR, Jenderseck RS, Levine SM, Chambers DW: Relationship between the percentage of subgingival spirochetes and the severity of periodontal disease. *J Periodontol* 1982;53:550.

27. Listgarten MA, Hellden L: Relative distribution of bacteria at clinically healthy and periodontally diseased sites in humans. *J Clin Periodontol* 1978;5:115.

28. Haffajee AD, Socransky SS, Goodson JM: Clinical parameters as predictors of destructive periodontal disease activity. *J Clin Periodontol* 1983;10:257.

29. Harley A, Floyd P, Watts T: Monitoring untreated periodontal disease. *J Clin Periodontol* 1987;14:221.

30. Badersten A, Nilveus R, Egelberg J: Effect of nonsurgical periodontal therapy. VII. Bleeding, suppuration and probing depth in sites with probing attachment loss. *J Clin Periodontol* 1985;12:432.

31. Vanooteghem R, Hutchens LH, Garrett S, Kiger R, Egelberg J: Bleeding on probing and probing depth as indicators of the response to plaque control and root debridement. *J Clin Periodontol* 1987;14:226.

32. Lang NP, Joss A, Orsanic T, Gusbert FA, Siegrist BE: Bleeding on probing. A predictor for the progression of periodontal disease? *J Clin Periodontol* 1986;13:590.

33. Alfano M: The origin of gingival fluid. *J Theor Biol* 1974;47:127.

34. Pashley DH: A mechanistic analysis of gingival fluid production. *J Periodont Res* 1976;11:121.

35. Cimasoni G: *Crevicular Fluid Updated*. Monographs in Oral Science, Vol. 12:3–7, Basel, Switzerland, Karger, 1983.

36. Bissada NF, Schaffer EM, Haus E: Circadian periodicity of human crevicular fluid flow. *J Periodontol* 1967;38:36.

37. Suppipat N, Johansen JR, Gjermo P: Influence of "time of day" pocket depth and scaling on gingival fluid flow. *J Clin Periodontol* 1977;4:48.

38. Lindhe J, Attstrom R: Gingival exudation during the menstrual cycle. *J Periodont Res* 1967;2:194.

39. Hugoson A: Gingival inflammation and female sex hormones. A clinical investigation of pregnant women and experimental studies in dogs. *J Periodont Res* 1970;5(Suppl):1.

40. Holm-Pedersen P, Löe H: Flow of gingival exudate as related to menstruation and pregnancy. *J Periodont Res* 1967;2:13.

41. Löe H, Holm-Pedersen P: Absence and presence of fluid from normal and inflamed gingivae. *Periodontics* 1965;3:171.

42. Egelberg J: Gingival exudate measurements for evaluation of inflammatory changes of the gingivae. *Odontol Rev* 1964;15:381.

43. Garnick JJ, Spray JR, Vernino DM, Klawitter JJ: Demonstration of probes in human periodontal pockets. *J Periodontol* 1980;51:563.

44. Ten Napel J, Theilade J, Matsson L, Attström R: Ultrastructure of developing subgingival plaque in beagle dogs. *J Clin Periodontol* 1985;12:507.

45. Theilade E: The non-specific theory in microbial etiology of inflammatory periodontal diseases. *J Clin Periodontol* 1986;13:905.

46. Moore WEC, Holdeman LV, Cato EP, Suibert RM, Burmeister JA, Ranney RR: Bacteriology of moderate (chronic) periodontitis in mature adult humans. *Infect Immun* 1983;42:510.

47. Slots J: Bacterial specificity in adult periodontitis. A summary of recent work. *J Clin Periodontol* 1986;13:912.

48. Savitt ED, Socransky SS: Distribution of certain subgingival microbial species in selected periodontal conditions. *J Periodont Res* 1984;19:111.

49. Ebersole JL, Taubman MA, Smith IJ, Genco RJ, Frey DE: Human immune responses to oral micro-organisms. I. Association of localized juvenile periodontitis (LJP) with serum antibody responses to *Actinobacillus actinomycetemcomitans*. *Clin Exp Immunol* 1982;47:43.

50. Listgarten MA, Lai CH, Evian CI: Comparative antibody titers to *Actinobacillus actinomycetemcomitans* in juvenile periodontitis, chronic periodontitis and periodontally healthy subjects. *J Clin Periodontol* 1981;8:155.

51. Mandell RL: A longitudinal microbiological investigation of *Actinobacillus actinomycetemcomitans* and *Eikenella corrodens* in juvenile periodontitis. *Infect Immun* 1984;45:778.

52. Slots J, Reynolds HS, Genco RJ: *Actinobacillus actinomycetemcomitans* in human periodontal disease: A cross sectional microbiological investigation. *Infect Immun* 1980;29:1013.

53. Genco RJ, Zambon JJ, Christersson LA: Use and interpretation of microbiological assays in periodontal diseases. *Oral Microbiol Immunol* 1986;1:73.

54. Slots J: The predominant cultivable microflora of advanced periodontitis. *Scand J Dent Res* 1977;85:114.

55. Van Winkelhoff AJ, Van Steenbergen TJM, De Graaff J: The role of black-pigmented *Bacteroides* in human oral infections. *J Clin Periodontol* 1988;15:145.

56. Tanner ACR, Haffer C, Bratthall GT, Viscenti RA, Socransky SS: A study of the bacteria associated with advancing periodontitis in man. *J Clin Periodontol* 1979;6:278.

57. Socransky SS, Haffajee AD, Dzink JL: Relationship of subgingival microbial complexes to clinical features at sampled sites. *J Clin Periodontol* 1988;15:440.

58. Theilade E, Wright WH, Jensen SB, Löe H: Experimental gingivitis in man. II. A longitudinal clinical and bacteriological investigation. *J Periodont Res* 1966;1:1.

59. Savitt ED, Strzempko MN, Vaccaro KK, Peros WJ, French CK: Comparison of cultural methods and DNA probe analyses for the detection of *Actinobacillus actinomycetemcomitans*, *Bacteroides gingivalis* and *Bacteroides intermedius* in subgingival plaque samples. *J Periodontol* 1988;59:431.

60. French CK, Savitt ED, Simon SL, Eklund SM, Chen MC, Klotz LC, Vaccaro KK: DNA probe detection of periodontal pathogens. *Oral Microbiol Immunol* 1986;1:58.

61. Strzempko MN, Simon SL, French CK, Lippke JA, Raia FF, Savitt ED, Vaccaro KK: A cross-reactivity study of whole genomic DNA probes for *Haemophilus actinomycetemcomitans*, *Bacteroides intermedius* and *Bacteroides gingivalis*. *J Dent Res* 1987;66:1543.

62. Slots J: Rapid identification of important periodontal microorganisms by cultivation. *Oral Microbiol Immunol* 1986;1:48.

63. Holt SC, Ebersole J, Felten J, Brunsvold M, Kornman KS: Implantation of *Bacteroides gingivalis* in nonhuman primates initiates progression of periodontitis. *Science* 1988;239:55.

64. Wennström JL, Dahlen G, Svensson J, Nyman S: *Actinobacillus actinomycetemcomitans*, *Bacteroides gingivalis* and *Bacteroides intermedius*: Predictors of attachment loss? *Oral Microbiol Immunol* 1987;2:158.

65. Zambon JJ, Bochacki V, Genco RJ: Immunological assays

for putative periodontal pathogens. *Oral Microbiol Immunol* 1986;1:39.

66. Genco RJ, Zambon JJ, Murray PA: Serum and gingival fluid antibodies as adjuncts in the diagnosis of *Actinobacillus actinomycetemcomitans* associated periodontal diseases. *J Periodontol* 1985;56(Suppl):41

67. Tew JG, Smibert RM, Scott EA, Burmeister JA, Ranney RR: Serum antibodies in young adult humans with periodontitis associated treponemes. *J Periodont Res* 1985;20:580.

68. Nakamura M, Slots J: Salivary enzymes. Origin and relation-ship to periodontal diseases. *J Periodont Res* 1983;18:559.

69. Loesche WL: The identification of bacteria associated with periodontal disease and dental caries by enzymatic method. *Oral Microbiol Immunol* 1986;1:65.

70. Tanner ACR: Reaction: The identification of bacteria associ-ated with periodontal disease and dental caries by enzy-matic methods. *Oral Microbiol Immunol* 1986;1:71.

71. Greenstein G, Polson A: Microscopic monitoring of patho-gens associated with periodontal diseases. A review. *J Peri-odontol* 1985;56:740.

Chapter 3

Treatment Sequencing

I. Traditional Treatment Sequencing

Thomas G. Wilson, Jr / Mark E. Glover

This section of the chapter covers treatment sequencing for the periodontal patient. Therapy is broken down into three stages: data gathering and treatment planning, active therapy, and maintenance. An outline of this approach, which was developed some years ago,[1] can be seen in Fig 3-1. Frequent evaluations of the patient's progress are used to modify the treatment plan as therapy progresses (Fig 3-2).

Examination and treatment planning

Because of their insidious onset, most cases of periodontal diseases are first detected in the office of the general dentist. Following examination (see chapter 2) and relief of pain, a treatment outline is presented to the patient. Treatment of early cases of chronic adult periodontitis and gingivitis (see chapter 2) should be performed in the generalist's office. For more advanced cases of chronic adult periodontitis and for more aggressive periodontal diseases, other health practitioners should be involved. This group may include an orthodontist, oral surgeon, prosthodontist, endodontist, physicians, and psychologist in addition to a periodontist. After examinations by the therapy team, different approaches to the patient's problems are outlined. These ideas should range from no treatment to the most advanced therapy and should include the pros and cons of each approach with one of the plans being designated optimal for the patient. These treatment plans are presented with the recommendations of the team. After the patient accepts one of the plans, therapy begins.

Initial (basic) therapy

Initial (basic) therapy begins after the patient accepts a treatment plan and ends with a reevaluation. The goal of this stage of active therapy is to control the clinical signs and symptoms of active disease and provide an environment for healing. There are three objectives of initial therapy: to control clinical signs of inflammation, to control caries, and to control occlusion.

Control of inflammation

The first stage of initial therapy is controlling the clinical features of inflammation of the periodontal and pulpal tissues. Educating patients about the harmful effects of oral bacteria and teaching them to remove bacterial plaque is an important step in this process (see chapter 4). The therapist can then begin to remove subgingival calculus and plaque by scaling and root planing (see chapter 5). Ideally these procedures will result in biocompatibility between soft tissues and the root surface (Figs 3-3a and b). Patients with chronic gingivitis, acute necrotizing ulcerative gingivitis (ANUG), and mild to moderate chronic periodontitis (up to and including 5-mm probing depths seen after initial attempts at scaling and root planing) should be treated in the office of the generalist. In most cases, patients with more advanced chronic periodontitis or those classified as having prepubertal, refractory, rapidly progressive, or localized juvenile periodontitis should be treated by a periodontist or other practitioner with a great deal of advanced periodontal training.

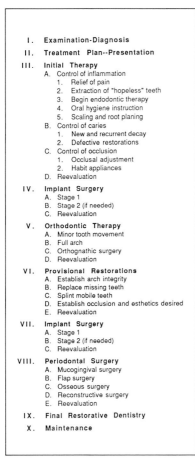

I. Examination-Diagnosis

II. Treatment Plan--Presentation

III. Initial Therapy
   A. Control of inflammation
      1. Relief of pain
      2. Extraction of "hopeless" teeth
      3. Begin endodontic therapy
      4. Oral hygiene instruction
      5. Scaling and root planing
   B. Control of caries
      1. New and recurrent decay
      2. Defective restorations
   C. Control of occlusion
      1. Occlusal adjustment
      2. Habit appliances
   D. Reevaluation

IV. Implant Surgery
   A. Stage 1
   B. Stage 2 (if needed)
   C. Reevaluation

V. Orthodontic Therapy
   A. Minor tooth movement
   B. Full arch
   C. Orthognathic surgery
   D. Reevaluation

VI. Provisional Restorations
   A. Establish arch integrity
   B. Replace missing teeth
   C. Splint mobile teeth
   D. Establish occlusion and esthetics desired
   E. Reevaluation

VII. Implant Surgery
   A. Stage 1
   B. Stage 2 (if needed)
   C. Reevaluation

VIII. Periodontal Surgery
   A. Mucogingival surgery
   B. Flap surgery
   C. Osseous surgery
   D. Reconstructive surgery
   E. Reevaluation

IX. Final Restorative Dentistry

X. Maintenance

Fig 3-1 A general guide to treatment sequencing for the patient with a periodontal disease.

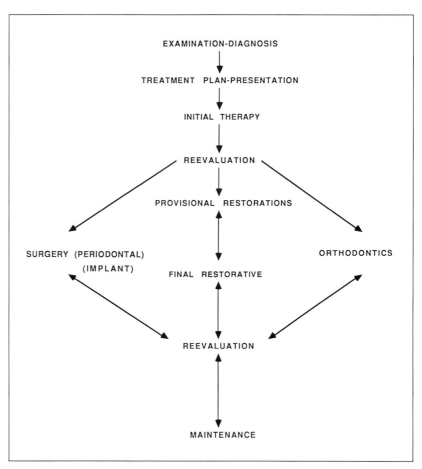

Fig 3-2 Flow diagram showing the interrelationship of the various forms of therapy.

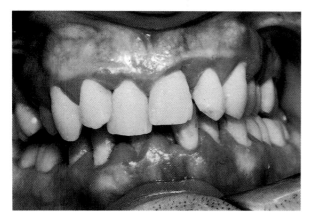

Fig 3-3a An initial photograph of a 29-year-old patient with probing depths ranging from 5 to 11 mm and advanced tooth mobility.

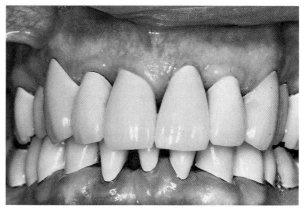

Fig 3-3b The same patient after closed scaling and root planing, orthodontics, and final restorative dentistry. The probing depths shrank significantly because of the extremely edematous nature of the gingival tissues when treatment started. (Orthodontics courtesy of Dr Gene Lamberth; restorative dentistry by Dr Frank Higginbottom.)

During this stage it is appropriate to begin any indicated endodontic therapy (see chapter 9). In addition, teeth with a truly hopeless prognosis that won't be used as anchorage for orthodontics or transitional abutments during two-stage implant therapy should be removed at this stage. Patients receiving head and neck radiation should be started on daily topical fluoride at this time (see chapter 10).

Control of caries

Two to 4 weeks after initial control of inflammation is an ideal time to place restorations needed to control active caries or replace any defective restorations. The gingival tissues should now be healed to the point that bleeding is reduced or eliminated and there is minimal gingival sulcular fluid flow, making placement of restorations and any necessary impressions of prepared teeth much easier. In instances where crown lengthening is needed or where subgingival caries exists, surgical lengthening of the clinical crown or orthodontic eruption[2] may be indicated to expose the caries and facilitate restorative procedures (see chapter 7).

Control of occlusion

A third area of concern during initial therapy is the occlusion. Occlusal trauma is a common finding in the general population[3] and in patients with periodontal disease.[4] Lindhe and Svanberg[5] have reported in dogs that trauma from occlusion in the presence of inflammation will result in more rapid periodontal pocket formation than when inflammation alone is present, and that this lesion continues when inflammation continues. When this is coupled with the finding of a study done in our office that most of our patients have some inflammation, as evidenced by bleeding upon probing,[6] it becomes apparent that occlusal therapy can be beneficial to many periodontal patients. In fact, Kegel et al[7] reported that after initial therapy, when both inflammation and occlusion were brought under control, mobility was reduced by 30%. Recent studies have shown that tooth mobility, fremitus (functional mobility), and widened periodontal ligament spaces seen on radiographs are the hallmarks of trauma from occlusion. When these signs are present, more loss of clinical attachment and less radiographic support is present than that seen around teeth without these findings.[8,9] In patients who admit to nocturnal bruxing or in whom these signs exist, a bite guard can be helpful. If fremitus or tooth mobility of I or greater on the Miller scale is found

in patients with inflammation 30 days after nocturnal bite-guard therapy, then occlusal adjustment is indicated. This adjustment should also be performed if the occlusal relationships are uncomfortable to the patient and where improved relationships can be obtained. Most periodontal patients respond best to a maxillary hard acrylic resin bite guard[10] with freedom from centric relation to centric occlusion and the maximum closure possible in both positions. In these devices the canines usually provide slight disarticulation in lateral movements; posterior disarticulation in protrusive movements is provided by the canines, sometimes in combination with the mandibular incisor teeth.[11] This design improves symptoms in most patients but reduces bruxing only in about half of them.[12] This reduction in symptoms is probably due to redistribution of forces.[13]

A reevaluation is performed 30 to 90 days following the completion of this initial therapy. This is done to determine progress in controlling inflammation, caries, and occlusion. The data collected at reevaluation are similar to those gathered at the initial examination. They cover areas of plaque retention, bleeding upon probing, probing depths, gingival recession, any remaining carious lesions, tooth mobilities, and fremitus. The information gathered at reevaluation dictates the course of the remaining therapy. The patient is consulted about any changes in the original treatment plan and questioned as to his or her desire to continue with therapy. If any probing depths greater than 5 mm that bleed when probed still exist, then the patient should have a consultation with a therapist trained in all forms of periodontal surgery.

Orthodontic therapy

For patients whose clinical inflammation and caries are controlled and who need improved tooth alignment, orthodontics is often the next step. For those with no preexisting periodontal problems, 3-month tooth cleanings will usually suffice when combined with good oral hygiene by the patient and minimal orthodontic forces as well as attention to removing interarch trauma. In years past, orthodontists hesitated to move teeth in patients with periodontal diseases, fearing that it would exacerbate existing bone loss. Their fear was justified (Figs 3-4a and b). However, in 1973 Brown[14] demonstrated that if inflammation and occlusal trauma are controlled during tooth movement, bone loss can also be controlled. In many patients treated in this manner, positive bone remodeling can be seen (Figs 3-5a and b). To keep the bone in a steady or improving state it is essential that the clinical signs and symptoms of inflammatory peri-

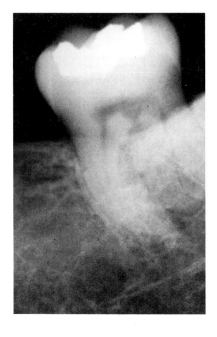

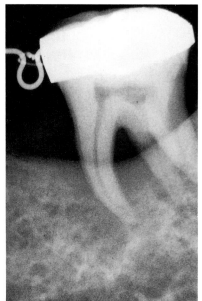

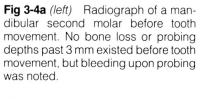

Fig 3-4a (left) Radiograph of a mandibular second molar before tooth movement. No bone loss or probing depths past 3 mm existed before tooth movement, but bleeding upon probing was noted.

Fig 3-4b (right) The same molar after approximately 6 months of orthodontics where occlusal forces and periodontal inflammation were not controlled.

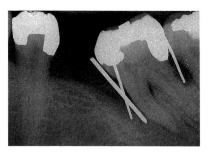

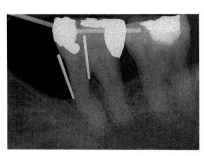

Fig 3-5a (left) Mandibular second molar before tooth movement. Severe bone loss associated with 11 mm of probing depth was found on the mesial aspect of the tooth.

Fig 3-5b (right) The same molar after tooth movement, where inflammation and trauma from occlusion were controlled. Seven years after orthodontic therapy the probing depth on the mesial aspect of the molar is 3 mm and no bleeding is noted.

odontal diseases be controlled before tooth movement is begun, and that tooth-bound accretions be continuously removed while orthodontics continues. In some advanced cases with deep probing depths, periodontal surgery using a flap approach without removal of bone may be warranted before orthodontics. This will increase the chances that all subgingival deposits are removed. At each visit the occlusion should be checked and adjusted to remove fremitus (functional mobility), and subgingival scaling and root planing should be performed. The interval between visits should be determined by clinical parameters including changes in probing depths and bleeding upon probing (see chapter 6).

Molar uprighting and extrusion of teeth

There are special situations in the periodontal patient where it is possible to level vertical bone defects using orthodontics. This can be accomplished when uprighting (and extruding) tipped mandibular molars[15] and by extruding teeth.[2] Molar uprighting can

achieve proper tooth position and improve the bone contour and probing depth mesial to the molar (see Figs 3-5a and b).

In many of these cases, placement of a Hawley bite plane with an anterior disarticulating ramp can reduce trauma from the occlusion during tooth movement.[4]

Full-mouth orthodontics

Full-mouth orthodontics is necessary when dental skeletal problems exist, multiple malaligned teeth are seen, or when realignment of a number of teeth will facilitate restorative dentistry. Light orthodontic forces should be used to reduce trauma to the periodontium.

During any type of tooth movement, patients should clean interproximally with dental floss or interproximal brushes if at all possible. They should be seen for short periods of subgingival cleanings at frequent intervals. The goal is to keep the gingival tissues free from the clinical signs of inflammation during the tooth movement. Success means no bleeding upon gentle

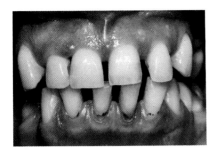

Fig 3-6a An initial photograph of a 35-year-old woman with probing depths ranging from 6 to 11 mm interproximally and advanced tooth mobility and drifting.

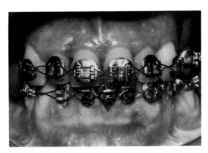

Fig 3-6b Treatment consisted of full-mouth orthodontics and orthognathic surgery.

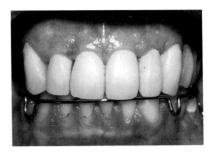

Fig 3-6c The patient's periodontal condition was stabilized and provisional restorations were placed. (Orthodontics by Dr Gene Lamberth; orthognathic surgery by Dr Arlet Dunsworth; restorative dentistry by Dr Frank Higginbottom.)

probing and no negative changes in probing depths. In practice, this maintenance interval varies from 2 weeks to 3 months.

Orthognathic surgery

When malocclusion is extreme or root resorption during orthodontic therapy is thought to be a significant risk, orthognathic surgery may be employed. Patients having rigid interarch fixation after this surgery present a real challenge if gingival inflammation is to be kept to a minimum; however, recent techniques that minimize or eliminate interarch fixation have reduced this problem. These patients should be seen just before their surgery for a thorough prophylaxis and as frequently as possible after surgery for root planing and reinforcement of plaque control. At reevaluation the next step in therapy is determined.

Provisional restorations

The step that often follows orthodontics and frequently precedes periodontal or implant surgery is stabilization of mobile teeth and replacement of missing teeth with provisional restorations (Figs 3-6a to c). If substantial bone loss has occurred, the teeth may need this type of stabilization immediately upon removal of the orthodontic bands. For less involved cases, 3 to 6 months should elapse after orthodontics before assessing the need for provisional restorations. If the teeth are mobile to the degree that the patient is uncomfortable, if a Miller Class II mobility or greater is present, if stability may increase the chance for success of a surgical procedure (as with bone grafting), or when tooth drifting is a problem, teeth should be splinted with provisional restorations at this stage. This step can also be used to replace missing teeth temporarily or to replace soft tissue-borne devices to facilitate healing after stage I placement of osseointegrated implants. The minimal amount of splinting possible should be done in the provisional phase. This phase can be used to evaluate teeth considered questionable; to check esthetics, phonetics, and function; and to make sure the patient has access for oral hygiene. It also provides a continuation of the healing period for the periodontium. In many cases this is the first time that the teeth have been stable and clean for some years. Stabilization should last at least 3 months. If this stage lasts longer, the provision restorations should be checked regularly (about every 2 months) for needed repair, recementation, or underlying caries (see chapter 7). Ideally, stabilization is done with provisional crowns, though in many cases wire and composite resin splints are used for economic reasons. At this stage endodontic therapy is usually completed, the exception being teeth that may need root removal during periodontal surgery.

Another reevaluation is performed after provisional restorations have been in place for an adequate time to permit healing of the periodontium. The therapist now assesses control of inflammation, caries, and the occlusion. If *(1)* there is no bleeding upon probing; *(2)* no caries exists; *(3)* the therapists are satisfied with the probing depths and occlusion; and *(4)* the patient is comfortable with the esthetics and masticatory efficiency of the provisional restorations, then the final restorative phase may be initiated. If the periodontium is not stable, surgery is often required. This lack of stability usually manifests as bleeding after probing in deepened pockets, or by continued probing depth increases seen at reevaluation or at maintenance visits.

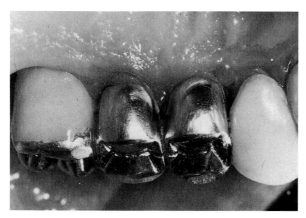

Fig 3-7a The initial view of a patient who presented with a fixed partial denture and interproximal probing depths of 5 to 8 mm. Crown contours and closed interproximal embrasure spaces made proper cleaning difficult.

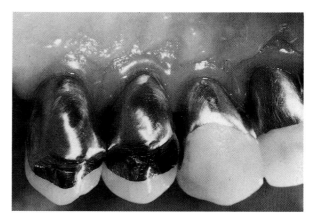

Fig 3-7b Fourteen years after initial therapy, provisional restorations, periodontal surgery, and final restorative dentistry, the periodontium is free of clinical inflammation. Probing depths are 3 mm or less. (Restorative dentistry by Dr Frank Higginbottom.)

Implant surgery

The timing of implant placement can vary from patient to patient. Osseointegrated implants can be placed in conjunction with initial therapy for those patients who will require extensive scaling and root planing. When the implants are uncovered, periodontal surgery (if needed) can be performed, thus reducing the number of surgical visits for the patient. Implants can be placed and uncovered before orthodontics in partially edentulous cases and then used for anchorage.

Periodontal surgery

The type of periodontal surgery that best serves the patient is a subject of great debate, and the definitive answer is not yet known. Common sense and clinical experience suggest that the type of surgery used should reduce probing depths as much as possible. In fact, most periodontists acknowledge the importance of obtaining a shallow crevice; they simply disagree on the best way to achieve this goal. For the purposes of this chapter, a surgical procedure that uses an apically positioned flap in the posterior areas is recommended, because the residual pockets generally are shallower than those found after replaced or coronally positioned flaps. In our opinion, judicious removal of bone in shallow bony pockets facilitates pocket reduction. Deeper pockets should be treated with fill procedures where possible. Approximately 3 months after surgery, another reevaluation is done to determine the next step in therapy. Any mucogingival defects are also corrected at this stage.

Final restorative dentistry

Three months after the completion of periodontal surgery, the average patient is ready for the final restorative phase. Exceptions are teeth that have had periodontal bone grafts placed around them; these usually should not be restored until at least 6 months after surgery. In this phase, permanent crowns and removable partial dentures are placed, using the knowledge gained during the provisional restorative phase concerning occlusion, function, mobility, phonetics, and esthetics.

Access for oral hygiene by the patient and for maintenance by the therapist achieved during the initial and surgical phases of therapy *must be maintained during the restorative phase*[16] (Figs 3-7a and b). Supragingival margins and open embrasure spaces contribute to maintaining a healthy environment.[17] Chapter 7 contains more information on these subjects.

Maintenance

The most important phase of periodontal therapy is maintenance. If the maintenance phase is not properly carried through by both patient and therapist, even the most expertly treated case is often doomed. The average periodontal cases should be followed by the therapist and hygienist on at least a 3-month basis.[18] Probing and measurement of gingival recession should be performed at each visit and other appropriate indices recorded (see chapter 2). In addition, oral hygiene should be monitored by some organized method and documented. We have found bleeding upon probing and changes in probing depths to be useful indices for determining maintenance intervals. Recall intervals may vary for different patients and for the same patient at different times (see chapter 6). For nonperiodontically involved cases, a 6-month interval is most appropriate (except for radiation patients, who need to be checked at least every 3 months). See chapter 10 for a further discussion of this topic.

Conclusion

The outline of therapy presented in this section can be applied to most patients. It must be understood that this material should serve as a guide and that it can and should be modified to meet the needs of the individual.

Some of the advanced therapy described in this section is for a select group of patients: those who have significant periodontal, restorative, and skeletal problems and who will go to great lengths to maintain their dentitions. Many patients who have opted for less involved therapy have also responded well. Each patient should be given a choice of treatment electives ranging from the most advanced therapy to no treatment. The patient should be presented with all the possible options and each option explained in as much detail as the patient requires. After all, ultimate failure or success depends upon the patient's understanding and cooperation.

This form of treatment represents a rational approach to therapy that has been shown over the years to be successful.

At a glance

Treatment sequencing

- ■ This chapter presents a conservative approach to treatment sequencing for periodontal patients.
- ■ The outline of this approach can be seen in Table 3-1 and Fig 3-1.
- ■ This approach can be used for any patient but should be adapted to individual patient needs.

II. Periodontal Therapy Based on Patient Compliance

Thomas G. Wilson, Jr

After the patient's problem has been diagnosed (see chapter 2), a treatment plan should be formulated. Traditionally, we have decided on the form of treatment based on anatomic findings (probing depth, tooth mobility, etc), disease type (debridement for ANUG and gingivitis, surgery for moderate to severe chronic periodontitis, etc), and other factors including the patient's health or economic circumstances. Recently we have added another factor: compliance. A study in our office found that only 16% of our patients comply with suggested maintenance intervals, 35% never return for care, and the rest are erratic in their compliance.[19] When tooth loss in the erratic and the complete compliers of this group was compared, it was found that complete compliers lost no teeth whereas erratic compliers lost 0.06 teeth per patient per year.[20] In a separate study, Becker et al[21] found that patients who never return for treatment lost 0.6 teeth per year per patient. So therapy, when combined with even erratic compliance to suggested maintenance, can improve the periodontal prognosis tenfold. Other studies have shown that patients who do not clean their teeth do poorly after surgery.[22] With these ideas in mind, we shall discuss therapy for different periodontal diseases based on correct diagnosis using the customary parameters (probing depths, tooth mobility, disease type) and the degree of predicted compliance with suggested oral hygiene and maintenance procedures. The latter parameters become particularly important in selecting candidates for surgical intervention.

Determining compliance

If we are to determine treatment based on compliance, we must first predict compliance. Initial information on compliance can be found from the patient's written history (chapter 2). Additional data can be gleaned as the therapist reviews the history with the patient and from past (or present) dentists. Standardized tests of compliance may serve as an adjunct. At present, determining compliance in dentistry is an art, not a science, and therapists must continue to improve their skills. In our work we recognized three categories of compliance: complete, erratic, and none (noncompliers). Complete compliers present for at least three fourths of their suggested maintenance visits. This group of people had less bleeding after probing and lost fewer teeth than the other groups.[6,20] Noncompliers never returned after active therapy, and erratic compliers returned at least once.

Choosing the appropriate therapy based on patient compliance

Patients with ANUG

Initial therapy of improved oral hygiene and repeated scaling and root planing usually suffices for the initial bouts of ANUG. Sometimes a 2-week course of chlorhexidine mouth rinse will help more advanced cases, as will antibiotics in febrile patients. In patients with recurring episodes, interproximal soft-tissue craters tend to remain, and bone involvement is often a feature. Gingivoplasty is helpful in the former, and surgery using a flap approach in the latter. Maintenance is helpful in preventing recurrences, but classically these patients do not return for maintenance care. Work needing extensive maintenance should usually be avoided until these patients prove to be good compliers.

Patients with chronic gingivitis

Patients with chronic gingivitis (up to 3-mm probing

depths that bleed) usually respond well to initial therapy (improved oral hygiene combined with subgingival scaling and root planing) followed by maintenance care. The therapy is the same for all categories of compliance.

Patients with mild periodontitis

For patients with relatively shallow probing depths (4-mm pockets and most anterior 5-mm areas, assuming normal root length) and bleeding seen after probing, initial therapy of improved oral hygiene and subgingival scaling and root planing should suffice. The objective of subgingival scaling and root planing is to remove tooth-borne subgingival deposits. This goal is very difficult to achieve.[23] In most cases the procedure in these patients will take several hours to accomplish and often requires the use of local anesthetic. Surgery is usually not necessary for this group. Maintenance care should follow. All compliance groups receive the same therapy. Complete compliers usually stay stable after this therapy, erratic compliers tend to have recurrent pocket depths, and noncompliers occasionally reappear years after therapy. This last group almost always presents with more advanced bone loss than that seen on initial examination.

Patients with moderate or severe periodontitis

For these two groups, choosing the proper periodontal therapy can be perplexing. These patients have probing depths that are 5 or 6 mm or greater. In all three compliance groups oral hygiene instructions should be given, and subgingival scaling and root planing should be performed in most of these cases before any surgery is done. If surgery is considered, its effect can be based on predicted compliance to suggested maintenance intervals and oral hygiene performance.

For compliers with suggested oral hygiene and/or maintenance

Reinforcing good oral hygiene habits and scaling and root planing will often suffice for this group. Closed scaling and root planing in these patients will take many hours and almost always requires local anesthetic. Many times an apically positioned flap is used to save time and expense to the patient, to increase the chances for removing calculus,[24] and to reduce the soft-tissue aspect of the pocket. Once the soft-tissue aspect of the pocket is reduced, the pocket will be shallower, giving both patient and therapist better access for maintenance. This group of patients tends to respond well to whatever is done once the calculus and other subgingival deposits are removed. When advanced procedures such as root removal and bone grafts are needed, this group does well.

For erratic compliers with suggested oral hygiene and/or maintenance

When it comes to formulating a treatment plan, this is the most challenging group. Erratic compliers usually brush well and floss occasionally, and although they do not adhere exactly to their maintenance schedules, they do present for care. We know that the more often they come in for cleaning, the fewer teeth they will lose.[20]

One way of managing these patients is to do initial (nonsurgical) treatment only. The rationale is that without perfect cleaning and maintenance, our best efforts are doomed.

A second approach involves reducing the pocket depths surgically. The surgery most often used in shallow bony pockets is an apically positioned flap with removal of enough supporting bone to reduce postoperative probing depths significantly but not enough to compromise tooth support. In deeper pockets regenerative procedures work well initially.

In my first years of practice I used a nonsurgical approach. In cases with pockets 6 mm or deeper (especially around furcated teeth), I could not predictably remove all the subgingival deposits and these patients' probing depths got deeper over time. This lack of access has been substantiated in the periodontal literature.[23-25] Recently I have been using a surgical approach more often, and these patients seem to be doing better. It is unclear whether this is because of the ease of removal of the deposits during surgery, the improved capability of the hygienist to remove deposits at maintenance visits, or the fact that apically positioned flaps enable the routine use of an interproximal brush. Whatever the reason, this group of patients seems to do better than those with the same type of problem treated nonsurgically. As a group, these patients tend to comply to immediate posttreatment care. Consequently, advanced procedures such as bone grafts, extensive periodontal prosthodontics, and root removals do well initially but tend to give problems directly related to how often the patient returns for follow-up care.

For noncompliers with oral hygiene and/or maintenance

This group should have their oral hygiene reinforced, and their subgingival deposits should be removed using closed subgingival scaling and root planing, because surgery has been shown to be detrimental to their periodontal status.[22]

――――――― *At a glance* ―――――――

Periodontal therapy based on patient compliance

- Traditionally, the type of periodontal therapy rendered has been based on considerations of anatomic defects and disease type and activity.
- Recent studies have shown that degree of compliance to suggested maintenance and oral hygiene procedures can have a major effect on the outcome of therapy.
- The degree of patient compliance can be estimated by determining past compliance or in some cases by testing.
- Different approaches to therapy can be employed in different groups of compliers. In general, anything that removes subgingival deposits works for complete compliers and almost nothing works for noncompliers; the large group that falls between the two extremes is the problem. This last group, when they have moderate to severe periodontitis, often responds well to surgery.

References

1. Corn H, Marks MH: Strategic extractions in periodontal therapy. *Dent Clin North Am* 1969;13:817.

2. Ingber JS: Forced eruptions: Part I. A method of treating isolated one and two wall infrabony osseous defects—Rationale and case report. *J Periodontol* 1974;45:199.

3. Glaros AG: Incidence of diurnal and nocturnal bruxism. *J Prosthet Dent* 1981;45:545.

4. Amsterdam M, Vanarsdall RL: Periodontal prosthesis—Twenty-five years in retrospect. *Alpha Omegan* December, 1974.

5. Lindhe J, Svanberg G: Influence of trauma from occlusion on progression of experimental periodontitis in the beagle dog. *J Clin Periodontol* 1974;1:3.

6. Wilson TG, Glover ME, Barraque B, Schoen JA, Dorsett D: Bleeding upon probing in maintenance patients in a private periodontal practice. Unpublished data.

7. Kegel W, Selipsky H, Phillips C: The effect of splinting on tooth mobility. I. During initial therapy. *J Clin Periodontol* 1979;6:45.

8. Pihlstrom BL, Andersen KA, Aeppli D, Schaffer EM: Association between signs of trauma from occlusion and periodontitis. *J Periodontol* 1986;57:1.

9. Fleszar TJ, Knowles JW, Morrison EC, Burgett FG, Nissle RR, Ramfjord SP: Tooth mobility and periodontal therapy. *J Clin Periodontol* 1980;7:495.

10. Zarb GA, Steck JE: The treatment of temporomandibular joint dysfunction: A retrospective study. *J Prosthet Dent* 1977;38:420.

11. Becker CM, Kaiser DA, Lemm RB: A simplified technique for fabrication of night guards. *J Prosthet Dent* 1974;32:582.

12. Clark GT, Beemsterboer PL, Solberg WK, Rugh JO: Nocturnal electromyographic evaluation of myofascial pain dysfunction in patients undergoing occlusal splint therapy. *J Am Dent Assoc* 1979;99:607.

13. Rugh JO, Harlan J: Nocturnal bruxism and temporomandibular disorders, in Jankovic J, Tolosa E (eds): *Advances in Neurology.* New York, Raven Press, 1988, Vol. 49, p 329.

14. Brown IS: The effect of orthodontic therapy on certain types of periodontal defects. I—Clinical findings. *J Periodontol* 1973;44:742.

15. Kramer GM, Reiser GM: The tipped lower molar—Therapeutic considerations. *Alpha Omegan* December, 1973, p 33.

16. Yuodelis RA, Weaver JD, Sapkos S: Facial and lingual contours of artificial complete crown restorations and their effects on the periodontium. *J Prosthet Dent* 1973;29:61.

17. Eissman HF, Radke RA, Noble WH: Physiologic design criteria for fixed dental restorations. *Dent Clin North Am* 1971;15:543.

18. Ramfjord SP, Morrison PC, Burget FG, Nissle RR, Schick RA, Zann GJ, Knowles JW: Oral hygiene and maintenance of periodontal support. *J Periodontol* 1982;53:26.

19. Wilson TG, Glover ME, Schoen JA, Baus C, Jacobs T: Compliance with maintenance therapy in a private periodontal practice. *J Periodontol* 1984;55:468.

20. Wilson TG, Glover ME, Malik AK, Schoen JA, Dorsett D: Tooth loss in maintenance patients in a private periodontal practice. *J Periodontol* 1987;58:231.

21. Becker W, Berg L, Becker BE: Untreated periodontal disease: A longitudinal study. *J Periodontol* 1979;50:234.

22. Nyman S, Lindhe J, Rosling B: Periodontal surgery in plaque infected dentitions. *J Clin Periodontol* 1977;4:240.

23. Waerhaug J: Healing of the dentoepithelial junction following subgingival plaque control. II. As observed on extracted teeth. *J Periodontol* 1978;49:119.

24. Caffesse RG, Sweeney PL, Smith BA: Scaling and root planing with and without periodontal flap surgery. *J Clin Periodontol* 1986;13:205.

25. Stambaugh RV, Dragoo M, Smith DM, Carasal L: The limits of subgingival scaling. *Int J Periodont Restorat Dent* 1981;1:30.

Chapter 4

Disruption or Reduction of Bacterial Populations in the Oral Cavity

Bacteria are normal residents of the oral cavity. Certain species or aggregations cause inflammatory periodontal diseases and caries, the two most common diseases encountered by dental professionals. Removal or disruption of noxious oral bacteria and their products assumes a major role in both active and maintenance therapy.

Bacteria found above and below the gingiva differ greatly. Supragingival plaque is usually aerobic or facultatively aerobic, is responsible for caries, and has a role in the initiation of gingivitis (Figs 4-1a to c). Subgingival bacteria associated with periodontal diseases are usually gram negative and are either anaerobic or facultatively anaerobic. With current concepts, both groups of bacteria must be disturbed, changed, or removed on a routine basis to halt disease progression. This chapter will discuss professional and personal methods for achieving this goal.

I. Approaches for the Patient

Thomas G. Wilson, Jr

Mechanical methods

The toothbrush

The toothbrush is the classic instrument for removing bacteria and their products. Most of us grew up with the idea that the toothbrush was the most important tool for personal oral hygiene. We still consider the brush important, but it has come to light that this instrument has severe limitations. It does not clean interproximally when no gingival recession exists and can clean only about 3 mm into the gingival crevice.[1] Because periodontal diseases and carious lesions begin where bacteria are left undisturbed, other aids must be used to clean the tooth completely.

Selection of manual brush

A soft-bristle brush does the least damage to the tooth and periodontium.[2] This is especially true when the individual bristle ends are rounded.[3] For maximum efficiency, these bristles need to be arranged in a multituft, multirow design. The brush should be used with a pen grip, not a palm grip, to reduce the chance for soft-tissue damage.[4] The more aggressively and often the patient uses the brush, the more frequently the brush should be changed.[5] Brushes should be replaced monthly or as soon as the bristles begin to splay. Brushes and toothpaste containers can house significant numbers of *Streptococcus mutans* (and possibly other microbes) for at least 24 hours,[6] which makes it reasonable to suggest the use of individual brushes and toothpaste containers within families. The size and shape of the brush should be dictated by the patient. The average patient needs to brush at least every 48 hours to prevent the clinical signs of gingivitis,[7] but because of the possibility of caries formation, more frequent brushing should be stan-

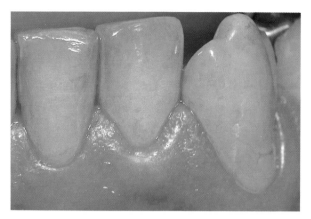

Fig 4-1a The growth of supragingival plaque. On day 0 the teeth were professionally cleaned then stained.

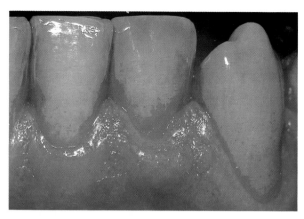

Fig 4-1b The subject refrained from oral hygiene and after 3 days plaque aggregations are seen interproximally and just coronal to the gingival sulcus.

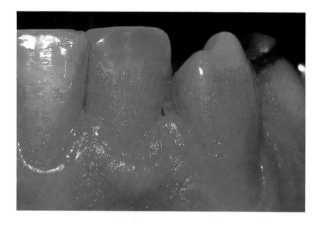

Fig 4-1c After a week of no oral hygiene, the plaque covers most of the facial, lingual, and interproximal surfaces. (From the collection of the 1974 Graduate Periodontal Class, University of Washington.)

dard. Ideally, food and bacterial products should be removed as soon as possible after eating.[8]

Method of brushing with a manual brush

Bass[9] suggested that the head of the brush be aligned parallel to the occlusal plane with the bristles placed on the occlusal surface and into the gingival sulcus. The brush is then moved anteroposteriorly in short strokes or in small circles. This is the preferred approach when the interproximal embrasure spaces are filled with gingival tissues. When interproximal recession occurs, the use of the Charters method,[10] which suggests putting slight pressure on the head of the brush toward the tooth and moving the brush in a tight circle while forcing the bristles into the interdental spaces, is preferred.

In practice, the patient should develop the method

that most effectively removes bacteria and food debris in the mouth. This usually requires continued instruction from the dental professional as well as use of disclosing agents at home. Patients should be encouraged to gently but thoroughly brush their tongues as well.[11]

Mechanical brushes

Conventional electric toothbrushes with back-and-forth or side-to-side motion have no advantage over manual brushes for the average patient[12] but can be useful for the handicapped.[13] A brush with rotating bristle groups has been suggested.[14,15] Clinical experience with this latter brush with patients who refuse to floss has been good, but this product should be used selectively because of the high expense.

The toothbrush

- Use a soft-bristle, rounded-end, multituft, multirow brush with a shape that is comfortable and effective for the patient.
- Discard the brush as soon as the bristles splay or once a month, whichever comes first.
- Suggest separate brushes and dentifrice tubes for each person.
- Brush after each meal (or three times per day).
- Patients must develop a brushing style that is effective for their oral condition. General rules include:
  - Aim the toothbrush bristles into the gingival sulcus.
  - Move the brush anteroposteriorly in short strokes or in tight circles.
  - If the interproximal areas are open, the bristles should be forced into these spaces.
- For the patient who flosses regularly, mechanical brushes offer little advantage over manual brushes. For nonflossers, a newly developed brush with rotating bristle groups has proven helpful.

Dental floss and related aids

Flossing is an effective way to remove bacterial plaque in interproximal areas where attachment loss has not occurred[16,17]; however, most patients do not use this aid routinely.[18,19] Waxed and unwaxed floss seem to be equally effective in removing plaque[20] and in reducing gingival inflammation.[21] Even though Super Floss® (Oral B Laboratories) was shown in one study to be preferred by patients to waxed dental floss, it did not clean any more efficiently.[22]

Dental floss cleans approximately 3.5 mm into the gingival crevice.[23] Floss comes in various widths and with various agents impregnated into it, but the type of floss is not as important[24] as getting the patient to use it. In practice we suggest dental floss only to those patients who do not have interproximal access for other mechanical cleaning methods, especially the interproximal brush. We suggest unwaxed floss when contact areas do not shred this material and lightly waxed floss where shredding occurs.

Floss can be wrapped around the fingers or used in mechanical devices to facilitate placement. The material is introduced into each contact area, carried gently apically until the facial and lingual gingival tissues are encountered, then brought coronally with short (5 mm or so) side-to-side strokes.

Interproximal brushes

Interproximal brushes are very effective for interproximal cleaning because they spread into the grooves and furcations found in the interdental regions after gingival recession occurs. They are the best cleaning aid available for the interproximal areas,[25] but their major drawback is that they can be used only in areas where bone loss and subsequent interproximal gingival recession have occurred.

Toothpicks

In general, dental floss works better than toothpicks interproximally[26] when the interproximal spaces are filled with gingiva. In one study, a toothpick was found to be as effective for removing plaque from lingual surfaces of teeth as a toothbrush,[27] but this is not suggested routinely because of potential tissue damage. Many patients prefer the use of toothpicks over dental floss[28]; these patients should be steered toward interproximal brushes where interdental gingival recession exists. Because several thousand medical injuries are reported yearly due to inadvertent ingestion and trauma from toothpicks, patients should be cautioned about their use. The injury rate was highest in young children.[29] Use of interdental stimulators has been suggested for both diagnostic and therapeutic reasons, especially for gingivitis and early periodontitis.[30]

For the average patient these aids offer no advantage over other cleaning aids.[31] They are too large to fit into most gingival crevices, and toothpicks can splinter and cause gingival irritation. Toothpicks placed in a plastic holder can be helpful in areas that a toothbrush or interproximal brush cannot reach.

Pulsating oral irrigators for delivery of water

Pulsating oral water irrigators are popular with some patients and a few professionals, but at present there is no evidence that oral irrigators delivering water have any significant positive effect on stainable supragingival plaque[32] or periodontal health for those patients who also use a toothbrush.[33] In addition, these devices have been implicated in causing bacteremias in patients with periodontitis[34] and have been implicated in cases of bacterial endocarditis.[35] Because they don't seem to have positive effects and may cause harm, their routine use is not recommended.

Rubber tip stimulators

Rubber tip stimulators can be useful for limiting interproximal gingival rebound seen after periodontal surgery, but other aids such as the interproximal brush will help control the problem and clean better. The concept of using these or other aids to provide gingival stimulation, which in turn improves gingival health, is no longer accepted.[36]

--------- *At a glance* ---------

Dental floss/interproximal brushes/toothpicks/ pulsating oral irrigators/rubber tip stimulators

■ It doesn't matter whether patients use waxed or unwaxed floss, just that they use it.
■ When the interdental tissues recede, interproximal brushes clean best; until that occurs, floss is recommended.
■ Use of toothpicks is not recommended for the average patient.
■ Pulsating oral irrigators delivering water are not effective for the average patient.
■ Rubber tip stimulators are not helpful for the average patient.
■ The average patient should use the chosen cleaning device at least daily.

Chemotherapeutic methods

The use of antiseptics for treating dental diseases was proposed by Miller in 1890,[37] and the subject has been debated ever since. The premise has remained the same—to find a substance that will eradicate or control the bacteria that cause dental diseases without damaging the host. With caries we are dealing with fairly specific causal organisms, so the antimicrobial can be specific, but periodontal diseases seem to be caused by a number of bacterial species. This means that a broad spectrum of antimicrobial activity is needed. The search for this agent has been extensive. As the rate of caries has declined and the knowledge of and interest in periodontal diseases have increased, more and more commercial enterprises have entered the scene. This has led to increased knowledge on the part of the lay and dental communities about periodontal diseases. However, in their haste to bring new products to the market, basic research has often been forthcoming only long after the product is being used by the public. This has led to the formation of guidelines for these products by the American Dental Association Council on Dental Therapeutics. In order to be approved, these products must show that they not only reduce dental plaque but also reduce the clinical signs of gingivitis.[38] At this writing, only two antimicrobials have been approved: chlorhexidine, marketed in the United States as Peridex® (Procter & Gamble Co), and Listerine® (Warner-Lambert Co), which contains a combination of essential oils.[39]

These products have been approved for use as *mouthrinses*. When used in this manner they affect supragingival, not subgingival, plaque and therefore have no effect on periodontitis. They are not a "magic bullet"; at present, one does not exist. The best answers are still mechanical plaque removal by the patient and the therapist with these chemicals used as adjuncts.

The following is a review of current knowledge on the subject.

Chemical agents for bacterial control

Chlorhexidine (Peridex®)

Chlorhexidine is presently the overwhelming choice for an adjunct to supragingival plaque control. The class of compounds in chlorhexidine was introduced to periodontics in 1969[40] and has been available as an over-the-counter product in Europe for many years. The recommended strength was a 0.2% oral rinse used twice daily. Lower dosages or less frequent use was thought to be ineffective.[41] Used in this manner, the compound can reduce or eliminate supragingival plaque[42] but may not stop the progress of established gingivitis.[43] The drug is not particularly powerful but works for a prolonged period because it is absorbed into the tooth surfaces and oral soft tissues and then is slowly released. This characteristic is called *substantivity*. The disadvantages of the 0.2% concentration can include *(1)* bad taste that remains for some time, *(2)* discoloration of the teeth, *(3)* sloughing of the oral mucosa, *(4)* the need for patient compliance (because the preparation must be used twice daily to be effective), *(5)* lack of effect on subgingival plaque when used as a mouthrinse, *(6)* little or no long-term effect on dental caries except in mouths with high caries incidence, *(7)* dry mouth, and *(8)* burning tongue.[44]

Chlorhexidine has been made available in the United States in a 0.12% concentration to try to decrease the undesirable side effects. At least one short-term study has indicated that this concentration is as effective as the 0.2% concentration when used twice a day.[45]

Chlorhexidine is very useful for short periods after periodontal or oral surgery. It may also have applications in treating denture stomatitis (to rinse and also soak the dentures) and for treating aphthous ulcers. It may have applications in the mentally or physically handicapped (as long as it is not swallowed), in orthodontic patients who won't use traditional cleaning methods (staining is a problem here), and in dental implant cases or large reconstructions where plaque removal is not optimal. It has also proven useful for patients after scaling and root planing and for those with poor oral hygiene. The staining is the major complaint from patients, and we have found that it requires extra office time to remove.

Fluorides

Stannous fluoride has greater antimicrobial properties than sodium fluoride. The antimicrobial action of these compounds has some positive effect in the short term but this diminishes over time.[46] The preferred concentration of stannous fluoride in gels is 0.4% for use supragingivally. It appears that fluoride is not nearly as effective in its antimicrobial action as chlorhexidine.[47]

Essential oils

In initially healthy individuals, essential oils have been shown to reduce supragingival plaque and gingivitis in persons who stayed in the studies and had no preexisting periodontal disease.[48] They also reduce the gross amount of plaque when compared with water rinses.[49] This compound is contained in a mouthrinse now available over the counter (Listerine). It has gained CDT approval but has not proven useful in my practice.

Folate mouthwash

There have been conflicting reports concerning the efficacy of folate mouthwash. A 0.1% solution is used twice daily. One report found no apparent effect on established gingivitis,[50] whereas others found that there was a positive effect.[51] Clinical and experimental gingivitis may respond differently and therefore findings would differ. At present not enough information is available on the subject to clinically judge its efficacy.

Quaternary ammonium compounds

These compounds are moderately effective as antiplaque agents. Their action is short lived. They may be useful in reducing plaque along with all the usual home care methods when used as suggested.[52]

Antibiotics

Most commercially available antibiotics have been tested for efficacy on chronic periodontal diseases. In the long term all have been found lacking. This is because each of these compounds suppresses some part of the microbial spectrum, which allows overgrowth of the unaffected strains. This can result in exacerbation of the problem. In addition, the development of resistant microbes is often seen.[53]

Against most aggressive forms of periodontal disease, these drugs can be useful adjuncts to traditional clinical methods. Tetracycline and metronidazole have been most tested. Tetracycline is often administered in conjunction with scaling and root planing (open or closed) for patients with localized juvenile periodontitis and it, as well as metronidazole, has been advocated for adjunctive use for patients with rapidly progressive periodontitis and refractory periodontitis. Tests are currently available that can identify specific bacterial strains and determine their susceptibility to specific antibiotics (see chapter 2).

Sanguinarine

Sanguinarine has been extensively advertised to dentistry and the general public. A number of studies have been performed on the efficacy of the material. The studies performed in-house by the manufacturer have been laudatory,[54–56] whereas studies done in other laboratories find almost universally that the compound is not effective.[57–59]

Sodium benzoate

At present there is one widely advertised, poorly documented product on the market that appears to use sodium benzoate as its active ingredient. It is touted as a "prebrushing" rinse and supposedly makes brushing more effective.[60] It cannot be recommended until further testing is done.

Microbiologically monitored and modulated periodontal therapy

This mode of therapy is placed under chemical agents because it proposes the use of hydrogen peroxide and sodium bicarbonate as a dentifrice, salt solutions in an oral irrigator, and tetracycline.[61] It has the appeal of common sense, but it failed the test of scientific relevancy and is now held in disrepute[62-67] and is not recommended.

Other agents

Many other agents have been suggested, including aloe vera, chlorine, copper sulfate, iodine solutions, and others. At present none have proven effective for the long-term control of bacterial plaque and its products.

──────── *At a glance* ────────

Chemotherapeutic methods

- ■ If a chemotherapeutic agent is needed, chlorhexidine is the chemical of choice, with stannous fluoride a distant second.
- ■ Chlorhexidine in the form of Peridex mouthwash can be helpful following:
  - • Periodontal surgery
  - • Implant surgery
  - • In patients who don't comply well to suggested oral hygiene but who will rinse
- ■ Drawbacks to chlorhexidine:
  - • Staining
  - • Taste
  - • Expense
  - • Must be used twice a day

Chemical delivery systems for patient use at home

What is the best way for the patient to deliver a chemotherapeutic agent? The choice of system is influenced by the area we are trying to affect—supragingival or subgingival—and by which agent you choose to deliver. This section will deal only with the delivery of chlorhexidine and stannous fluoride.

Dentifrices

In times past the purpose of a dentifrice was to clean stains from the teeth. This was accomplished with a combination of abrasives, soaps, humectants, and thickening agents. However, the mechanical action of most dentifrices is of little help in removing bacteria,[68] and if their abrasiveness is increased, tooth or gingival injury may occur.

Chlorhexidine has been incorporated into dentifrices and studied with mixed results.[69,70] At this point a dentifrice containing 0.4% stannous fluoride is not available, but the gel can be used for this purpose.

Because most of our patients brush, a dentifrice would be an ideal delivery system. Unfortunately, the evidence so far is that a dentifrice is not an efficient way to deliver chemicals to affect supragingival plaque and appears to have little if any effect on subgingival bacteria.

Mouthrinses

The concept of using a mouthrinse to control periodontal disease is attractive because compliance to use of this delivery system can be good. The reality is that this approach is limited to the control of gingivitis. One of the main reasons for failure of these systems is the difficulty in gaining access to the pocket environment. It seems that anatomy, along with factors such as the gingival sulcular fluid flow, tend to exclude materials used as rinses.

The most effective mouthrinse now available is chlorhexidine.[71] Many compounds will inactivate chlorhexidine (including stannous fluoride); therefore, patients should be instructed to eat breakfast, clean their teeth, rinse thoroughly with water, then rinse with the chemical. This must be repeated 12 hours later to be maximally effective.

Pulsating oral irrigators for delivery of chemicals

Having the patient use chlorhexidine in a pulsating oral irrigator has real appeal since this chemical is so effective against supragingival bacteria. While some short-term work has shown positive results,[72] the majority of studies indicate that this approach has no overall long-term benefit.[73–75] The use of fluoride by the patient in an oral irrigator has recently been suggested,[76] but further studies are needed to prove its effectiveness. Tooth staining and unpleasant taste have frequently been reported with the use of these products. Patients with heart murmurs or heart prostheses should not use these devices because of potential bacterial showering.[34,35,77]

Irrigation with a syringe by the patient

Frequent (usually daily) irrigation of deepened pockets has been suggested by some. To deliver the medication to the subgingival area, a blunt or canulated needle must be inserted approximately 3 mm into the crevice, then the solution (usually chlorhexidine) is delivered. Where no interproximal oral hygiene is performed by the patient, this method proved helpful in one series of studies.[78–81] This method has the following drawbacks (see section II in this chapter for further discussion):

1. Most patients do not have the dexterity to deliver the material properly.
2. This approach has not been approved by appropriate governing bodies, making it a possible medico-legal question.
3. Most of the studies on the subject show little or no long-term benefit.[82–85]

At a glance

Chemical delivery systems for patient use at home

- Chlorhexidine mouthrinses are effective supragingivally but do not have much effect on subgingival plaque.
- Pulsating oral irrigators delivering chlorhexidine (Peridex) appear to have little or no long-term effect on adult periodontitis but may be of benefit in more aggressive periodontal problems.
- Delivery of chemicals into the sulcus with a syringe by the patient is rarely indicated and then the only possibility should be in the pocket maintenance patient who did not respond to traditional therapy.

II. Subgingival Irrigation by the Professional

Thomas G. Wilson, Jr / Reta Carlson

The professional use of chemicals to remove bacteria and their products from the peridontal pocket has a long history, and this approach has recently enjoyed a revival. The first question should be, "Do these agents reach the bottom of the pocket?" The answer seems to lie in the delivery system and the placement of the tip for delivery. In general, medications delivered in mouthrinses do not penetrate the sulcus to any appreciable depth.[86] Some dye reaches the subgingival plaque when the solution is delivered supragingivally using a syringe,[87] but it is more effective to place the tip of the needle subgingivally.[88] The question then becomes, "Is there an agent that is effective when delivered in this manner?" This section will cover the two most effective topical medications: chlorhexidine and stannous fluoride.

Chlorhexidine

Subgingival irrigation with chlorhexidine has been tested extensively. Most of the studies have been on the 0.2% solution and may not apply to the 0.12% concentration. While some short-term studies have shown reduction of bleeding upon probing,[89,90] other studies indicate little or no long-term positive results with this method.[91-94] It can therefore be concluded that if the professional wishes to see the patients every 2 to 4 weeks for irrigations, these methods can be a helpful adjunct to traditional care in areas where breakdown continues. In clinical practice this method has not proven routinely beneficial.

Stannous fluoride

Stannous fluoride has been tested for its effects on subgingival bacteria. In one study there was a substantial drop in the number of spirochetes,[95] but in another only a transient effect on black-pigmented *Bacteroides*.[96] This compound is most effective when the 1.64% concentration is used. Data on the clinical effects of this compound when used subgingivally are still scanty, and judgment must be withheld until more definitive studies are produced.

Antibiotics

Most forms of antibiotics have been used at one time or another in irrigating solutions. They have proven ineffective in the long run when used in this method because of their transient effect.

While the placement of fibers impregnated with tetracycline,[97] chlorhexidine,[98] and metronidazole[81] has shown some positive short-term results, it is too early to judge the long-term efficacy of this delivery system.

A warning

At present some individuals are recommending the routine use of various materials for subgingival irrigation using a variety of delivery devices. Some advocate in-office use, others support having these chemicals delivered at home by the patient. Although these ideas may have merit, there is a paucity of information supporting this approach. The practitioner using chemicals for in-office or especially at-home use by the patient needs to make sure that the patient understands that the approach must be monitored closely.

Chemical curettage

A popular type of chemical curettage involves the use of a sodium hypochlorite solution.[99] There are those who support the use of this material,[100] yet it seems to have little positive effect on long-term healing,[101] and if the dentist uses this material it should only be in recalcitrant areas found during maintenance.

Other aids

Various other chemicals have been used in an attempt to reduce the amount of subgingival plaque and improve clinical parameters. The chemicals include iodine, Chloramine T, peroxide, and various antibiotics. While each has shown some efficacy, the consensus is that their effect is short-term and adds little to conventional periodontal therapy. However, recent findings that bacteria may be found in dentinal tubules adjacent to periodontal pockets may lead to a renewed desire to "detoxify" the root surface.

- Although some studies have indicated that the use of chlorhexidine (Peridex) irrigation by the professional is helpful in reducing bacterial populations, others have shown no benefit.
- Those studies that yielded positive results called for professional irrigation every 2 to 4 weeks. In most practices and for most patients, this is highly impractical, and home use by the patient may be indicated in some conditions that do not respond to traditional care.
- Introduction of these medications by the professional or by the patient has not been approved by the appropriate governing bodies and therefore cannot be recommended for routine use.
- Impregnation of various agents into strips that are implanted into the pocket is appealing but is not adequately tested at present.

III. Individual Professional Approaches to Oral Hygiene

This section contains short discussions of individual approaches to oral hygiene. These professionals have worked to revise and refine their approach until it fits their needs and the needs of their patients.

Fred E. Aurbach

Successful dental maintenance is like success in any area of life; it is a journey, not a destination. The journey to successful dental maintenance cannot be accomplished without the proper preparation. The educational preparation of the patient should focus on two areas: the how and the why of personal oral hygiene. The patient will not be motivated to perform routine daily procedures until he or she can manipulate the device(s) necessary for proper maintenance. These may range from simple floss and toothbrush to interproximal brushes or the rotary toothbrushes. Once the patient can use the device in the office, the only remaining step is to get the patient to do the procedures at home, correctly and consistently. The key to this step is motivation. I have found that most of my patients know that they should be flossing and brushing, and that quite a few are familiar with the proper techniques, but very few of them know why. The explanation of "why" *must* be in terms the patient can understand. I have found that comparing the organization of the bacterial plaque and its ramifications to something the patient can visualize has been

helpful in achieving understanding. For example: "Mrs Jones, I'm sure that sometime in your life, either you or someone you were with, deliberately stepped in a red ant bed just to watch the ants. What did the ants do?" The usual answer is that the ants scattered, there was total confusion, etc. "Now, Mrs Jones, if you went back once a day and stepped in the ant bed, the ants wouldn't move, but they'd never get their house built, either. It's much the same in your mouth. Think of having a miniature ant bed between your teeth. We know through research that it usually takes bacteria 24 hours to organize or build their house, and that once their house is built, they go in search for food— and that food is you. If you would step in their house just once a day with dental floss, they would never get organized. They won't go away because they're the first phase of the digestive process, but if they can't get organized, they can't do any damage."

Most patients easily relate to this illustration, and once they understand the "why" they are more likely to follow through with their home care.

The toothbrushes that we give to our patients are imprinted—not with our name and phone number, but with the two-word message "Floss First." It is my feeling that the "FBI" rule should prevail: Floss, Brush, Irrigate—in that order. I explain to my patients that I would rather see them floss than brush, the reason being that most cavities and gum diseases begin between the teeth where the toothbrush cannot reach. Also, if they floss first, chances are they will still go ahead and brush, even if sleepy or in a hurry. I further explain that by flossing first, the particles are loosened, and the sudsing agent in the toothpaste will help to float the loose particles out. Then when they irrigate, their mouths will feel fresh. I usually tell the patient that in order to develop a habit, it is best to take it one step at a time. So to encourage their flossing I tell them they do not have to floss all of their teeth—only the ones they want to keep. This touch of humor is remembered by the patient. We also encourage the patients to floss without looking in a mirror. We show them how the "jaw bone" comes forward when you open wide and prevents the head of the toothbrush from getting back far enough to brush the outside (buccal surface) of the teeth and makes it difficult to put the fingers back far enough to floss. We also suggest that our patients keep their floss in a place where it is convenient to use; next to the chair where they watch television is one possible location.

Many patients ask about oral irrigators. (Most, in fact, simply tell me that instead of flossing they have purchased an oral irrigator.) Rather than tell them that this device alone is not enough, I ask them if they have a car. If the answer is yes, I ask them to do themselves a favor. I ask them to take the time on the way home to drive into one of those do-it-yourself high-pressure car washes and to wash their car using water only. They are instructed not to touch the car with anything but the high-pressure jet, and then let the car dry and see how clean it is. They get the point very quickly. Then I emphasize that the pressure in the oral irrigator is not nearly as high as the car wash, and that the dirt on the car is not made up of live bacteria hanging on for dear life.

For those patients who, for whatever reason, have been delinquent on their recall, I do not make an issue of their neglect; instead, I apologize. "Mr Wilson, I'm sure the reason you've not been in is due to my lack of communication. I must not have spoken clearly. I said 6 months and perhaps you thought I said 6 years!" or "Your checkups are two times a year, not once every 2 years." The patients usually laugh and say that they will do better.

When a patient asks whether it is preferable to use waxed or unwaxed floss, my answer is always the same: whichever you will use.

It is truly amazing how many patients feel guilty because they have not flossed regularly or have not kept their recall appointments. Rather than badger them, I compliment them on the fact that they are in the office now. I stress that we will not look back, and that we will make a fresh start. If necessary, we change the recall period to 3 months, 4 months, or whatever interval is best for monitoring the patient's dental condition.

Michael J. Newman

The most important part of dental maintenance is helping our patients to understand the cause of dental problems and encouraging them to perform the necessary procedures. With some patients, this knowledge is enough to stimulate them to exercise immaculate home care. However, many others who possess the knowledge and home hygiene training still lack proper motivation.

We approach hygiene maintenance on an individual basis. So what if a patient does not floss? If there is minimal gingival inflammation and no Class II caries, he or she is in good shape. If whatever they do is working, good for them! We will see them every 6 months or once a year, but they still need an understanding of what is accomplished. The other side of that coin is the patient who needs the entire armamentarium of threaders, or various dental flosses, oral irrigator, interproximal brush, floss holder, rotary brushes, and a 2-month recall schedule to keep them out of trouble.

We can expect our patients to remember only about 6% of what we tell them. But allowing them to see and hear will increase their retention to about 86%. We always try to "show" our patients, with a mirror, their problems, and the necessary cleaning procedure. In every learning situation, repetition produces results. Sales research indicates that it takes five to six presentations for someone to "buy" an idea. Reinforcing the same information at subsequent visits may become boring for us, but clinical results are what we want. Repetition helps.

One motivational tool we have been using for some time, with seemingly good success, is the idea of keeping score toward the goal of "Dental Fitness." The Dental Fitness scoring method is not an original idea; it came to us through Dr Michael Schuster and Dr Dale Greer. It uses visual imagery and gives patients an idea of what category their oral health occupies relative to their life-span. This Dental Fitness program allows us to recommend necessary restorative procedures and delegate responsibilities. We use this along with a bleeding index score upon probing as a way to gauge improvement between recalls. This gives the patients a more concrete idea of how they are managing their hygiene than the doctor's verbal "everything looks good" seal of approval.

Almost every patient wants a healthy mouth. Some will do everything necessary to achieve and maintain dental health. Patience and understanding on our part are sometimes difficult to exercise. Showing anger or disappointment will not have a positive influence on our patients' desire to accomplish the objectives of health. We believe that no other office "wants" to take better care of them than we do, so if we drive them away, who has been helped? Not that patient, and certainly not our practice.

We will continue to modify our approach to motivation as newer ideas reach us. For now, individual scheduling and visual demonstrations of bleeding and of cleaning procedures, together with the Dental Fitness Report, seem to help stimulate our patients' participation.

Steven A. Levy

I agree that most patients do not do what we ask them. However, in some general dental offices nothing is asked of them, so nothing is what is received.

In my opinion, it is our responsibility to ask the patients if they would like to learn how to take care of (clean) their mouths properly. Their answer to that question will tell us how much time and energy we should spend with them. We feel it is most effective to give toothbrush and floss instruction before the cleaning procedure is done. Nothing is more dramatic than for the patient to see tartar, plaque, puffy tissue, blood, and pus. We explain about bacteria forming protective colonies in the gingival sulcus, and that if they aren't removed, they sit there and borrow the food you eat and return the favor by making waste products in your mouth. We explain that brushing without flossing is like washing your hands without cleaning between the fingers. We ask the hesitant flossers to eat ribs or corn, then brush thoroughly. If they *then* use floss, they will be shocked at how much food is still there. We explain that other foods and bacterial plaque are always between the teeth but are not as noticeable.

When the actual instruction is done, it is a "watch, then do" procedure. Telling is not teaching and listening is not learning. After the patient has watched in a mirror while brushing and flossing are reviewed, my assistant holds the mirror and observes while the patient attempts the techniques.

If areas of plaque retention are noted on future recall visits, our hygienist repeats the process of demonstrating and then observing.

We chart the amount of tartar, plaque, bleeding, pocket depth, mobility, and regularity of flossing at each recall visit. I generally ask my hygienist for some of these scores in the presence of the patient. This lets them know that we are monitoring them and seems to inspire them to improve their performance. We heap praise for the slightest bit of improvement. Everyone likes to be praised. When there is some backsliding, we try not to berate them. We appreciate their honesty and gently encourage them to get back on the program.

We feel strongly that active participation in regular recall programs is essential, and that the *most effective* recall system should be utilized. My receptionist (who has been with me for 8 years) knows how to run this system effectively. It involves using her interpersonal skills coupled with a familiarity with the idiosyncrasies of each patient. At the first of each month she telephones each patient on that month's call list. She uses whatever communication skill necessary to set each patient up with an appointment. With some, it takes several phone calls over a period of several weeks; with others, perhaps a reminder of how much tartar they get. She knows who is on the verge of a periodontal referral and gently (or maybe not so gently) urges them to face the thing they are trying to avoid—surgery, pain, expense, etc. The trick is that she keeps on trying until she makes the appointment. This method is far more costly than a postcard but is many times more effective.

We find that when we praise our patients for being conscientious about their recall regularity (as well as their punctuality), they really make an effort.

Seeing people return with improved performance and increased health is one of the most rewarding and satisfying aspects of my practice.

Leonard J. Ledet, Jr

The foundation of a preventive health–oriented dental practice is an effective hygiene department. We are responsible for delivering not only quality restorations with which patients can prevent dental disease, but also a structured program to aid them in taking care of their health and investment. It is the quality of the dentist's restorations and the effectiveness of his or her hygiene program that determine whether he or she is practicing true preventive dentistry or simply functioning in a reparative manner—always "putting out fires."

Our program is based on the philosophy that *(1)* whatever condition exists is the patient's problem and *(2)* we cannot prevent dental disease, only the individual can. Given that premise, we believe education, evaluation of the existing condition, and the results of our treatment are our major responsibilities. This is not to diminish the significance of thorough scaling and root planing, but rather to emphasize the importance of education and treatment evaluation. If we consider that the major responsibility of the hygienist is to "clean teeth," we are in essence accepting the patient's poor oral hygiene and health as our problem and not the patient's. By educating and evaluating, we are acting more as consultants and helping them with their problem. It is imperative that they understand the necessity of accepting responsibility for their own health and actual prevention of disease. Once they accept the fact that it is their problem, that we don't "clean" their teeth, they do, and that they come to us for examination and evaluation (in addition to prophylaxis in areas they missed), then they will be more inclined to maintain proper oral hygiene. Admittedly, all of this is more internal philosophy than "what to say" or what hygiene aids we use, but we think that the major factor determining patient compliance is our ability to educate and motivate. There will be a better chance of motivating a patient if the dentist and staff have developed their own philosophy of what they can and should be doing with hygiene. Patients should understand that as they return for their exams over a period of time, they will develop their own technique and dexterity to the point where they are more effective with their hygiene, thereby lengthening the time between examinations. This is presented as a slow, ongoing process that takes years to fine-tune before achieving the goal of having very little for the hygienist to remove at each examination. At that time we can determine what interval between evaluations would be best for them: 3, 4, 6, or 12 months.

For patients who do not floss regularly, we stress the importance of flossing. We tell these patients that flossing is more effective and more important than brushing, assuming they have good nutrition. We explain that it is not flossing, but rather developing the habit of flossing, that is difficult. Therefore, we divide the process into two phases: (1) developing the habit and (2) improving technique. In the first phase we have them floss only the mandibular anterior teeth. This area takes little dexterity and very little time. We stress the importance of flossing this area every day and to floss only this area. They will be more likely to develop a habit that only takes 20 seconds, and we will also be able to demonstrate to the patient the difference between the areas being flossed and the areas that are not. On subsequent recalls we progressively add a quadrant at a time. We explain that we are not interested in whether they floss for the next 6 months as we are in flossing 6 years from now.

The degree to which we, as dental professionals, are able to look at our function with recall patients as behavior modification rather than hands-on treatment will be the degree to which our recall program is a success.

Arvinder K. Malik

Removal of plaque and other soft debris from the oral cavity on a regular consistent basis is the key to practicing good preventive care. Professional dental prophylaxis and evaluation are important in the maintenance of that care.

A well-established, efficient maintenance program will only be successful if the philosophies of the dental team (ie, dentist, dental hygienist, assistant, etc) are the same. I am a practicing dental hygienist in a private periodontal office. The hygienists and periodontist have regular meetings to exchange information. At these meetings we discuss the dental literature and how it can be of help to our patients.

In our office we think that the most important assessment of gingival health is bleeding upon probing. At our maintenance visits (prophies) we examine for bleeding points along with changes in probing depths to determine periodontal health. The results of this examination are given to the patient. We also check for fremitus and correct it to minimize further periodontal breakdown. We think a general evaluation of oral hygiene is adequate as long as the same clinician sees the patient at subsequent visits. If patients exhibit no bleeding upon probing at recall appointments, we reward them with a longer interval between further recalls. Our intervals range between 2 and 6 months, with the vast majority of our patients on a 3-month interval.

I have seen that compliance is more likely to be achieved if the task is first demonstrated by the clinician then performed by the patient. We inform our patients if they can adequately use an interproximal brush interdentally then there is no need to floss. We deemphasize negative feedback. Negatives do not contribute to positive behavior change. Instead, praise the positives (ie, "Thank you for coming today!" or "You're flossing three times a week? That's great!") and reward them. This makes the patient more apt to comply.

Communication, especially terminology, should always be on a level the patient can understand. This facilitates the exchange of information. We as the clinicians can only use our experience and expertise to inform and educate the patients about their mouths, oral hygiene, and pathological findings within the oral cavity. The degree of compliance performed by the patient will actually be the determining factor of success of dental health, and our communication skills have a direct impact on the patient's compliance.

References

1. Douglass GL: Plaque control, in Schluger S, Yuodelis RA, Page RC (eds): *Periodontal Disease: Basic Phenomena, Clinical Management, and Occlusal Restorative Interrelationships.* Philadelphia, Lea & Febiger, 1977, pp 344–369.

2. Niemi ML, Sandholm L, Ainamo J: Frequency of gingival lesions after standardized brushing as related to stiffness of tooth brush and abrasiveness of dentifrice. *J Clin Periodontol* 1984;11:254.

3. Breitenmoser J, Mörmann W, Mühlemann HR: Damaging effects of tooth brush bristle end form on gingiva. *J Periodontol* 1979;50:212.

4. Niemi ML, Ainamo J, Etemadzadeh H: The effect of tooth brush grip on gingival abrasion and plaque removal during tooth brushing. *J Clin Periodontol* 1987;14:19.

5. Glaze PM, Wade AB: Toothbrush age and wear as it relates to plaque control. *J Clin Periodontol* 1986;13:52.

6. Svanberg M: Contamination of toothpaste and toothbrush by *Streptococcus mutans. Scand J Dent Res* 1978;86:412.

7. Lang NP, Cumming BR, Löe H: Toothbrushing frequency as it relates to plaque development and gingival health. *J Periodontol* 1973;44:396.

8. Goldman HM: Effect of single and multiple tooth brushing in the cleansing of the normal and periodontally involved dentition. *Oral Surg Oral Med Oral Pathol* 1956;9:203.

9. Bass CC: An effective method of personal oral hygiene. Part II. *J Louisiana Med Soc* 1954;106:100.

10. Charters WJ: Proper home care for the mouth. *J Periodontol* 1948;19:136.

11. Christen AG, Swanson BZ Jr: Oral hygiene—A history of tongue scraping and brushing. *J Am Dent Assoc* 1978;96:215.

12. McKendrick AJW, Barbenel LMH, McHugh WD: A two-year comparison of hand and electric toothbrushes. *J Periodont Res* 1968;3:224.

13. Smith JF, Blankenship J: Improving oral hygiene in handicapped children by the use of an electric toothbrush. *J Dent Child* 1964;31:198.

14. Schifter CC, Emiling RC, Seibert JS, Yankell SL: A comparison of plaque removal effectiveness of an electric versus a manual toothbrush. *Clin Prev Dent* 1983;5:15.

15. Long DE, Killoy WJ: Evaluation of the effectiveness of the Interplak™ home plaque removal instrument on plaque removal and orthodontic patients. *Compend Cont Educ Dent* 1985;6(Suppl):S156.

16. Smith BA, Collier CM, Caffesse RG: In vitro effectiveness of dental floss in plaque removal. *J Clin Periodontol* 1986;13:211.

17. Lobene RR, Soparker PM, Newman MB: Use of dental floss—Effect on plaque and gingivitis. *Clin Prev Dent* 1982;4:5.

18. Murtomaa H, Turtola L, Rytömaa I: Use of dental floss by Finnish students. *J Clin Periodontol* 1984;11:443.

19. Johansson L-Å, Öster B, Hamp S-E: Evaluation of cause-related periodontal therapy and compliance with maintenance care recommendations. *J Clin Periodontol* 1984;11:689.

20. Hill HC, Levi PA, Glickman I: The effects of waxed and unwaxed dental floss on interdental plaque accumulation and interdental gingival health. *J Periodontol* 1973;44:411.

21. Finkelstein P, Grossman E: The effectiveness of dental floss in reducing gingival inflammation. *J Dent Res* 1979;58:1034.

22. Wong CH, Wade AB: A comparative study of effectiveness in plaque removal by Super Floss® and waxed dental floss. *J Clin Periodontol* 1985;12:788.

23. Waerhaug J: Healing of the dento-epithelial junction following the use of dental floss. *J Clin Periodontol* 1981;8:144.

24. Keller SE, Manson-Hing LR: Clearance studies of proximal tooth surfaces. II. In vivo removal of interproximal plaque. *Ala J Med Sci* 1969;6:266.

25. Waerhaug J: The interdental brush and its place in operative and crown and bridge dentistry. *J Oral Rehabil* 1976;3:107.

26. Anaise JZ: Plaque-removing effect of dental floss and toothpicks in children 12–13 years of age. *Commun Dent Oral Epidemiol* 1976;4:137.

27. Schmid MO, Balmelli OP, Saxer UP: Plaque removing effect of a toothbrush, dental floss and a toothpick. *J Clin Periodontol* 1976;3:157.

28. Nixon KC: An analysis of interdental cleaning habits. *Aust Dent J* 1978;23:389.

29. Budnick LD: Toothpick-related injuries in the United States, 1979 through 1982. *J Am Med Assoc* 1984;252:796.

30. Caton J, Polson A, Bouwsma O, Blieden T, Frantz B, Espeland M: Associations between bleeding and visual signs of interdental gingival inflammation. *J Periodontol* 1988;59:722.

31. Bergenholtz A, Brithon J: Plaque removal by dental floss or toothpicks. An intra-individual comparative study. *J Clin Periodontol* 1980;7:516.

32. Fine DH, Baumhammers A: Effect of water pressure irrigation on stainable material on the teeth. *J Periodontol* 1970;41:468.

33. Hugoson A: Effect of the Water Pik device on plaque accumulation and development of gingivitis. *J Clin Periodontol* 1978;5:95.

34. Felix JE, Rosen S, App GR: Detection of bacteremia after the use of an oral irrigation device in subjects with periodontitis. *J Periodontol* 1971;42:785.

35. Drapkin MS: Endocarditis after the use of an oral irrigation device. *Ann Intern Med* 1977;87:455.

36. Bonfil JJ, Fourel J, Falabregues R: The influence of gingival stimulation on recovery from human experimental gingivitis. *J Clin Periodontol* 1985;12:828.

37. Miller, WD: *The Microorganisms of the Human Mouth.* Philadelphia, The SS White Dental Manufacturing Co, 1890. (Reprinted by S. Karger, 1973.)

38. Council on Dental Therapeutics of the American Dental Association. Guidelines for the acceptance of chemotherapeutic products for the control of supragingival dental plaque and gingivitis. *J Am Dent Assoc* 1986;112:529.

39. Council on Dental Therapeutics of the American Dental Association. Council on Dental Therapeutics accepts Listerine. *J Am Dent Assoc* 1988;117:515.

40. Löe H: Present day status and direction for future research on the etiology and prevention of periodontal diseases, in International Conference on Periodontal Research. *J Periodont Res* 1969;4(Suppl):38.

41. Gjermo P: Hibitane in periodontal disease. *J Clin Periodontol* 1977;4:94.

42. Ainamo J: Control of plaque by chemical agents. *J Clin Periodontol* 1977;4:23.

43. Flotra L, Gjermo P, Rolla G, Waerhaug J: A four-month study on the effect of chlorhexidine mouth washes on 50 soldiers. *Scan J Dent Res* 1972;80:10.

44. Emilson CG: Outlook for Hibitane in dental caries. *J Clin Periodontol* 1977;4:136.

45. Segreto VA, Collins EM, Beiswanger BB, De La Rosa M, Isaacs RL, Lang NP, Mallatt ME, Meckel AH: A comparison of mouthrinses containing two concentrations of chlorhexidine. *J Periodont Res* 1986;21(Suppl):23.

46. Nisengard RJ: *In* Giangrego E, Mitchell EW (eds): Emphasis: Chemical agents for the reduction of plaque. *J Am Dent Assoc* 1986;112:18.

47. Goodson JM: Drug delivery, in *Perspectives on Oral Antimicrobial Therapeutics.* Littleton, Mass, PSG Publ Co, 1987, p 61.

48. Gordon JM, Lamster IB, Seiger MC: Efficacy of Listerine antiseptic in inhibiting the development of plaque and gingivitis. *J Clin Periodontol* 1985;12:697.

49. Fine DH, Letizia J, Mandel ID: The effect of rinsing with Listerine antiseptic on the properties of developing dental plaque. *J Clin Periodontol* 1985;12:660.

50. Pack AR: Effects of folate mouthwash on experimental gingivitis in man. *J Clin Periodontol* 1986;13:671.

51. Vogel RI, Deasy M: Folic acid and experimentally produced gingivitis. *J Dent Res,* 1977;56 (Sp Iss A):134.

52. Ciancio SG, Mather ML, Bunnell HL: Clinical evaluation of a quaternary ammonium-containing mouthrinse. *J Periodontol* 1975;46:397.

53. Helderman WHVP: Is antibiotic therapy justified in the treatment of human chronic inflammatory periodontal disease? *J Clin Periodontol* 1986;13:932.

54. Southard GL, Parsons LG, Thomas LG Jr, Boulware RT, Woodall IR, Jones BJB: The relationship of sanguinaria extract concentration and zinc ion to plaque and gingivitis. *J Clin Periodontol* 1987;14:315.

55. Southard GL, Parsons LG, Thomas LG, Woodall IR, Jones BJB: Effect of sanguinaria extract on development of plaque and gingivitis when supragingivally delivered as a manual rinse or under pressure in an oral irrigator. *J Clin Periodontol* 1987;14:377.

56. Parsons LG, Thomas LG, Southard GL, Woodall IR, Jones BJB: Effect of sanguinaria extract on established plaque and gingivitis when supragingivally delivered as a manual rinse or under pressure in an oral irrigator. *J Clin Periodontol* 1987;14:381.

57. Mauriello SM, Bader JD: Six-month effects of a sanguinarine dentifrice on plaque and gingivitis. *J Periodontol* 1988;59:238.

58. Wennström J, Lindhe J: The effect of mouth rinses on parameters characterizing human periodontal disease. *J Clin Periodontol* 1986;13:86.

59. Etemadzadeh H, Ainamo J: Lacking anti-plaque efficacy of 2 sanguinarine mouth rinses. *J Clin Periodontol* 1987;14:176.

60. Emiling RC, Yankell SL: First clinical studies of a new pre-brushing mouthrinse. *Compend Cont Educ Dent* 1985;6:636.

61. Keyes PH: Microbiologically monitored and modulated periodontal therapy. *Gen Dent* 1985;33:105.

62. Weitzman SA, Weitberg AB, Niederman R, Stossel TP: Chronic treatment with hydrogen peroxide—Is it safe? *J Periodontol* 1984;55:510.

63. Rees TD, Orth CF: Oral ulcerations with use of hydrogen peroxide. *J Periodontol* 1986;57:689.

64. Pihlstrom BL, Wolff LF, Bakdash MB, Schaffer EM, Jensen JR, Aeppli DM, Bandt CL: Salt and peroxide compared with conventional oral hygiene. I. Clinical results. *J Periodontol* 1987;58:291.

65. Wolff LF, Pihlstrom BL, Bakdash MB, Schaffer EM, Jensen JR, Aeppli DM, Bandt CL: Salt and peroxide compared with conventional oral hygiene. II. Microbial results. *J Periodontol* 1987;58:301.

66. Bakdash MB, Wolff LF, Pihlstrom BL, Aeppli DM, Bandt CL: Salt and peroxide compared with conventional oral hygiene. III. Patient compliance and acceptance. *J Periodontol* 1987;58:308.

67. Listgarten MA, Levin S, Schifter CC, Sullivan P, Evian CI, Rosenberg ES, Laster L: Comparative longitudinal study of 2 methods of scheduling maintenance visits; 2-year data. *J Clin Periodontol* 1986;13:692.

68. Bergenholtz A, Lignell L, Öberg G: Quantitative evaluation of the plaque-removing ability of four commercial dentifrices, in Lindhe J (ed): *Textbook of Clinical Periodontology.* Copenhagen, Munksgaard, 1983, p 334.

69. Etemadzadeh H, Ainamo J, Murtomaa H: Plaque growth-inhibiting effects of an abrasive fluoride-chlorhexidine toothpaste and a fluoride toothpaste containing oxidative enzymes. *J Clin Periodontol* 1985;12:607.

70. Bain MJ, Strahan JD: The effect of a 1% chlorhexidine gel in the initial therapy of chronic periodontal disease. *J Periodontol* 1978;49:469.

71. Greenstein G, Berman C, Jaffin R: Chlorhexidine—An adjunct to periodontal therapy. *J Periodontol* 1986;57:370.

72. Macaulay WJR, Newman HN: The effect on the composition of subgingival plaque of a simplified oral hygiene system including pulsating jet subgingival irrigation. *J Periodont Res* 1986;21:375.

73. Haskel E, Esquenasi J, Yussim L: Effects of subgingival chlorhexidine irrigation in chronic moderate periodontitis. *J Periodontol* 1986;57:305.

74. Watts EA, Newman HN: Clinical effects on chronic periodontitis of a simplified system of oral hygiene including subgingival pulsated jet irrigation with chlorhexidine. *J Clin Periodontol* 1986;13:666.

75. Sanders PC, Linden GJ, Newman HN: The effects of a simplified mechanical oral hygiene regime plus supra-gingival irrigation with chlorhexidine or metronidazole on subgingival plaque. *J Clin Periodontol* 1986;13:237.

76. Boyd RL, Leggott P, Quinn R, Buchanan S, Eagle W, Chambers D: Effect of self-administered daily irrigation with 0.02% SnF$_2$ on periodontal disease activity. *J Clin Periodontol* 1985;12:420.

77. Romans AR, App GR: Bacteremia, a result from oral irrigation in subjects with gingivitis. *J Periodontol* 1971;42:757.

78. Wan Yusof WZA, Newman HN, Strahan JD, Coventry JF: Subgingival metronidazole in dialysis tubing and subgingival chlorhexidine irrigation in the control of chronic inflammatory periodontal disease. *J Clin Periodontol* 1984;11:166.

79. Pitcher GR, Newman HN, Strahan JD: Access to subgingival plaque by disclosing agents using mouthrinsing and direct irrigation. *J Clin Periodontol* 1980;7:300.

80. Yeung FIS, Newman HN, Addy M: Subgingival metronidazole in acrylic resin vs. chlorhexidine irrigation in the control of chronic periodontitis. *J Periodontol* 1983;54:651.

81. Khoo JGL, Newman HN: Subgingival plaque control by a simplified oral hygiene regime plus local chlorhexidine or metronidazole. *J Periodont Res* 1983;18:607.

82. Wennström JL, Heijl L, Dahlen G, Gröndahl K: Periodic subgingival antimicrobial irrigation of periodontal pockets. I. Clinical observations. *J Clin Periodontol* 1987;14:541.

83. Wennström JL, Dahlen G, Gröndahl K, Heijl L: Periodic subgingival antimicrobial irrigation of periodontal pockets. II. Microbiological and radiographical observations. *J Clin Periodontol* 1987;14:573.

84. MacAlpine R, Magnusson I, Kiger R, Crigger M, Garrett S, Egelberg J: Antimicrobial irrigation of deep pockets to supplement oral hygiene instruction and root debridement. I. Bi-weekly irrigation. *J Clin Periodontol* 1985;12:568.

85. Braatz L, Garrett S, Claffey N, Egelberg J: Antimicrobial irrigation of deep pockets to supplement non-surgical periodontal therapy. II. Daily irrigation. *J Clin Periodontol* 1985;12:630.

86. Wunderlich RC, Singleton M, O'Brien WJ, Caffesse RG: Subgingival penetration of an applied solution. *Int J Periodont Rest Dent* 1984;5:64.

87. Pitcher GR, Newman HN, Strahan JD: Access to subgingival plaque by disclosing agents using mouthrinsing and direct irrigation. *J Clin Periodontol* 1980;7:300.

88. Hardy JH, Newman HN, Strahan JD: Direct irrigation and subgingival plaque. *J Clin Periodontol* 1982;9:57.

89. Lander PE, Newcomb GM, Seymour GJ, Powell RN: The antimicrobial and clinical effects of a single subgingival irrigation of chlorhexidine in advanced periodontal lesions. *J Clin Periodontol* 1986;13:74.

90. Soh LL, Newman HN, Strahan JD: Effects of subgingival chlorhexidine irrigation of periodontal inflammation. *J Clin Periodontol* 1982;9:66.

91. Löe H, Schiött CR, Glavind L, Karring G: Two years' oral use of chlorhexidine in man. I. General design and clinical effects. *J Periodont Res* 1976;11:135.

92. Haskel E, Esquenasi J, Yussim L: Effects of subgingival chlorhexidine irrigation in chronic moderate periodontitis. *J Periodontol* 1986;57:305.

93. Wennström JL, Heijl L, Dahlen G, Gröndahl K: Periodic subgingival antimicrobial irrigation of periodontal pockets. I. Clinical observations. *J Clin Periodontol* 1987;14:541.

94. Wennström JL, Dahlen G, Grondahl K, Heijl L: Periodic

subgingival antimicrobial irrigation of periodontal pockets. II. Microbiological and radiographic observations. *J Clin Periodontol* 1987;14:573.

95. Mazza J, Newman M, Sims T: Clinical and antimicrobial effect of stannous fluoride in periodontitis. *J Clin Periodontol* 1981;8:203.

96. Schmid E, Kornman KS, Tinanoff N: Changes of subgingival total colony forming units and black pigmented bacteroides after a single irrigation of periodontal pockets with 1.64% SnF$_2$. *J Periodontol* 1985;56:330.

97. Goodson JM, Holborow D, Dunn RL, Hogan P, Dunham S: Monolithic tetracycline-containing fibers for controlled de-livery of periodontal pockets. *J Periodontol* 1983;54:575.

98. Coventry J, Newman HN: Experimental use of a slow release device employing chlorhexidine gluconate in areas of acute periodontal inflammation. *J Clin Periodontol* 1982;9:129.

99. Hecker F: *Pyorrhea Alveolaris*. St Louis, CV Mosby Co, 1913.

100. Kalkwarf KL, Tussing GJ, Davis MJ: Histologic evaluation of gingival curettage, facilitated by sodium hypochlorite solu-tion. *J Periodontol* 1982;53:63.

101. Viera EM, O'Leary TJ, Kafrawy AH: The effect of sodium hypochlorite and citric acid solutions on healing of peri-odontal pockets. *J Periodontol* 1982;53:71.

Chapter 5

Removing Tooth-Borne Dental Deposits: Mechanical Means by the Professional

Thomas G. Wilson, Jr / Jan Schoen / Pat Fallon

This chapter will deal with the removal of tooth-borne deposits by the dental professional. These deposits include calculus, tooth-borne bacteria, bacteria found in the pocket or soft tissues that are incidentally removed, and bacteria and their products that become embedded in the tooth surface.

The process

Tooth-borne material can be removed in two ways. Superficial soft deposits can be removed by the patient through personal oral hygiene or by the dental professional using mechanical means (scaling, root planing, polishing, etc) or chemical means (see chapter 4). Hard deposits are best removed by the professional using mechanical methods. The clinical end point of this process is a smooth root surface above and below gingiva accompanied by removal of stains. These clinical end points are desirable but may or may not accomplish the goal of therapy. It is easy for dental professionals to confuse the process of removing tooth-accumulated materials with the therapeutic goal.

The goal

As described above, many may think that the ultimate goal of cleaning the tooth surface is the removal of calculus and the production of a smooth, hard root surface. The true goal, however, is the arrest or cure of the periodontal disease. To achieve this goal we must establish and maintain a clinically healthy state. To accomplish this, the tooth surface must be made biologically compatible with the surrounding periodontal tissues and this may[1] or may not[2] occur without smoothness of the root. We shall now consider how the dental professional can approach the process of scaling and root planing and achieve the goal

of a biologically compatible root surface. This chapter will deal with closed (nonsurgical) techniques, but many of the same principles can be applied when flaps are raised.

Supragingival cleaning

Tooth polishing abrasives and rotary instruments

The purpose of professional polishing is to remove stains and to smooth the tooth surface. Traditionally, gross stains are removed with ultrasonic or hand instruments. Remaining stain was usually removed with an abrasive material carried in a rubber cup attached to a slow-speed contra-angle handpiece.

Polishing agents contain an abrasive, which can be volcanic ash, feldspar, or other components contained in a base of binding materials and coloring and flavoring agents.

Polishing reduces microorganisms[3] and slows the rate of plaque regrowth when compared with toothbrushing.[4] Frequent polishing (every 2 weeks) has been shown to drastically reduce the levels of periodontal diseases and caries in both children and adults.[5,6]

The negative effects of this procedure include the great importance placed on stain removal by some clinicians, which often results in inadequate time during maintenance visits for other more important procedures, including subgingival scaling and root planing. Other negatives include a reduced uptake of topically applied fluoride[7] and the possibility of abrading enamel, but especially dentin, if the rubber cup is not held at right angles to the tooth.[8]

An air-powder abrasive system

There is an air-powder abrasive system on the market

called Prophy Jet® (Dentsply Equipment Division). It delivers a high-speed stream of air and water at 100°F along with sodium bicarbonate particles.

It is suggested that this mixture be delivered in three or four short bursts (3 to 5 seconds each) on the enamel surfaces of the teeth 1 cm away and aimed diagonally toward the tooth surface. When used in this manner it leaves a smooth, stain-free surface when compared to polishing with an abrasive and rubber cup.[9] In addition, this instrument has been found to be faster than the traditional use of a rubber cup and abrasive.[10] It also removes less root surface than a curette when used to remove stain.[11] When used on root surfaces, it can readily remove cementum and dentin and leaves no connective tissue fibers.[9,12]

On the negative side, it can severely damage tooth surfaces if held for prolonged periods or at right angles. It can also damage soft tissues and should not be used on teeth surrounded by severely inflamed tissues because of the possibility of abscess formation or facial emphysema.[13] In addition, this system should be used judiciously (or not at all) in the patient with cardiovascular hypertension because of the possible uptake of sodium bicarbonate. This method can also damage composite resins.

At a glance

Air-powder abrasive systems/tooth polishing with abrasives

- Polishing should be secondary to root planing where the latter is needed.
- Polishing with rotary abrasives should be done at right angles to the tooth surface with a rubber cup at slow speeds.
- Air-powder abrasive systems clean better and faster than rotary abrasives.
- Air-powder abrasives can damage soft and hard tissues if they are:
  - Held stationary for more than a few seconds
  - Held at right angles to the tooth surface
  - Used on severely inflamed tissues
- At present, we prefer the air-powder abrasive systems over polishing with a rubber cup in most situations, if the abrasive system is correctly applied. This is because of the time saved, which can then be used for more important procedures.

Subgingival cleaning

Expectations and limitations

What are the clinical signs of a successfully treated periodontal case? First, the tissue is healthy, pink, stippled, does not bleed when probed, and probing depth or attachment loss does not increase with time. Second, the pocket depths are such that they can be easily cleaned by both the patient and therapist. The shallower the probing depth, the more likely both the patient and the dental health professional are to be able to clean out bacteria and their products. Because many patients do not return for routine maintenance, shallow probing depths present an ideal end point in therapy.

What factors keep us from achieving a successful result?

Two of the most important factors are the patient's oral hygiene and his or her compliance with suggested maintenance care (see chapters 4 and 14). The periodontal patient with inflammatory disease who neglects oral hygiene and professional maintenance usually has a recurrence. On the other hand, patients who do comply fare well. Our problems come with patients who fall between these extremes. The erratic compliers' success will vary with their efforts—the more they do to help themselves, the more they succeed. This group also benefits in most cases from more advanced periodontal procedures designed to reduce the remaining pockets.

Success in patients with systemic problems depends on their disease, its severity, and its effect on the periodontium. Diabetics as a group need more aggressive therapy than their nondiabetic counterparts, and the better their diabetic control, the better their outlook periodontally (see chapter 13). Systemic problems that interfere with oral hygiene can also detrimentally affect therapy. Arthritis and certain mental disorders fall in this group.

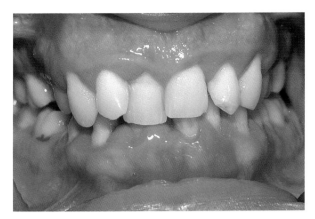

Fig 5-1a A 29-year-old man with rapidly progressive periodontitis who has very edematous tissue.

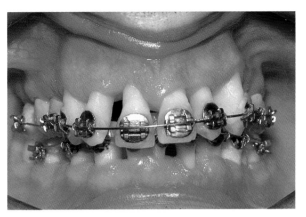

Fig 5-1b After improved oral hygiene, several hours of closed scaling and root planing, and orthodontic care, the clinical signs of inflammation subsided and the probing depths shrank to normal. The reduction of probing depth was due to reduction of inflammation and soft tissue shrinkage.

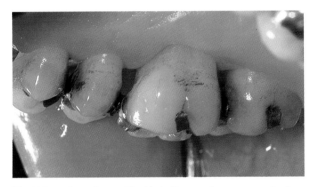

Fig 5-2a A patient with thick fibrous tissue seen before therapy.

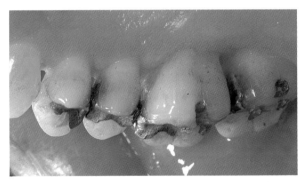

Fig 5-2b Same patient after 13 months and several rounds of closed subgingival scaling and root planing. Very little shrinkage or pocket reduction has occurred. This case typifies the average periodontal patient seen in the dental office to a greater degree than the case seen in Figs 5-1a and b.

Response after scaling and root planing can also depend on the character of the soft tissue when therapy begins. The more edematous the tissue, the greater the shrinkage of the soft tissues after inflammation is reduced (Figs 5-1a and b). So-called fibrotic tissue will shrink less and probing depths may not be reduced (Figs 5-2a and b). Also, the thinner the tissue (in a buccolingual dimension), the greater the reduction in probing depth.

The type of periodontal disease and its rapidity of onset also affect prognosis. Given similar probing depths initially, young patients generally fare worse in the long run than their older counterparts. This may be because they have a more aggressive bacterial flora or their immune system may not be as efficient, or both of these problems may exist simultaneously.

Another factor that affects success is the ability of the therapist to remove plaque and its products from the root surface. Results vary, but some general statements can be made. The more trained and experienced the therapist, the greater the chance of success. With more anterior teeth, the better the access (mouth opening, tongue pressure, etc), the more likely we are to remove dental deposits. Teeth without grooves, furcas, and depressions are easier to clean. Probing depth also has an effect. Several studies have shed light on the limitations of closed scaling and root planing.[1,14–17] They show that the deeper the pocket, the less likely we are able to remove plaque and calculus. In probing depths of 1 to 3 mm it has been shown that with diligence, all plaque and calculus can be removed from the tooth. In probing depths

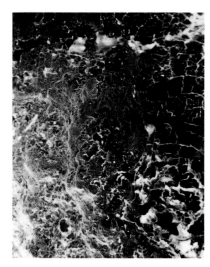

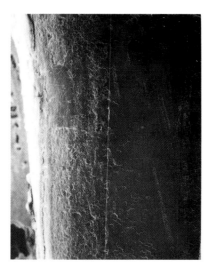

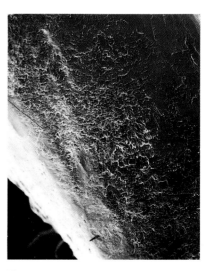

Fig 5-3 This tooth had severe chronic periodontitis surrounding it when it was extracted. The area shown is a large piece of subgingival calculus. (Original magnification × 20.)

Fig 5-4 Closed scaling and root planing was used for 20 minutes on the area shown in this figure. The area was clinically smooth. (Original magnification × 20.)

Fig 5-5 An ultrasonic cleaner was used on this area of the tooth during closed scaling. Compare the root surface with that in Fig 5-4. (Original magnification × 20.)

6 mm or deeper, failure is usually predestined, especially in posterior teeth. For pockets in the 4 to 5 mm range, the chances of failure and success are about equal. In these studies up to 45 minutes *per tooth* was necessary to obtain the desired result. We may conclude that closed scaling and root planing can be helpful but are not a panacea. If the goal is to remove all tooth-borne plaque and calculus, then surgical intervention (open scaling and root planing) in areas of deeper probing depths is frequently helpful. In addition, closed scaling and root planing can consume a great deal of time. Closed procedures are among the most difficult in periodontics, and years of effort are needed to attain clinical proficiency. In some cases surgery can save time and effort, increase the efficacy of tooth cleansing, and reduce the residual pocket.

What are the clinical end points?

When the root feels smooth and you can't see any calculus, stop. A recent study showed that large amounts of cementum may not need to be removed when root planing.[18] Blowing air into the gingival sulcus may facilitate this step, as will use of delicate root explorers described on pp 72–73.

What type of healing occurs after root planing?

Ideally, root planing would result in a new attachment of soft tissues and tooth. In this case a new attach-

ment is described as "the reunion of connective tissue with a root surface that has been deprived of its periodontal ligament. This reunion occurs by the formation of new cementum with inserting collagen fibers."[19] This would result in a shallow, healthy crevice. There have been speculations about how these tissues may reattach. Aleo et al[20] have shown that fibroblasts in tissue culture would not attach to diseased root surface but would attach once the areas of diseased cementum were removed. It has also been shown that epithelial cells were negatively affected by periodontally involved root surfaces.[21] However, in vivo new attachment does not seem to occur routinely. When thorough subgingival root planing is done, the previously pathologically altered ecosystem of the pocket is reversed. This results in at best a long junctional epithelium (epithelial attachment).[22] There seems to be little evidence that significant amounts of new connective tissue attachment occur or cementum forms. This may be a result of the finding that diseased cementum seems to contain agents with cytotoxic effects[23] and that with closed curettage, the toxic material on or in the root may not be completely removed.[22] This long epithelial attachment has proved clinically to be a tenuous one. Although there are disagreements,[24] we think that this is not the most desirable situation for most of our patients. Complete compliers to oral hygiene or maintenance tend to do well with a long junctional epithelium, whereas erratic compliers and noncompliers do not. Therefore, not treating some of the patients in these latter groups surgically should be viewed as an error.

When all of the suggestions in this chapter are followed, what really happens to the tooth root? We know that this answer changes from operator to operator, from tooth to tooth, and from patient to patient. However, we took some severely periodontally involved teeth and cleaned them in place (in the mouth), extracted them, and then examined them under a scanning electron microscope (SEM). Figure 5-3 shows an untreated tooth. The tooth in Fig 5-4 had been cleaned on one surface (the mesial surface of a maxillary lateral incisor) under anesthesia with sharp curettes. After 20 minutes' cleaning, the root felt glassy, hard, and smooth to the operator, but when examined under SEM, the tooth appeared less than smooth. The same was true for the tooth surface seen in Fig 5-5, which is a tooth that was cleaned (subgingivally) for 20 minutes with an ultrasonic scaler before extraction. The critical question here is, are the tooth and soft tissue biologically compatible? The answer cannot be seen with the microscope but must be given by the soft tissues.

What does this mean in clinical terms?

The reader should come away with the following general conclusions. Closed subgingival scaling and root planing works well in probing depths from 1 to approximately 5 mm. For deeper probing depths, if the clinician feels it necessary to remove as much of the subgingival tooth accumulated materials as possible from probing depths of 6 mm or greater, then surgery is often needed when initial therapy has failed to produce stability. Exceptions can include: complete compliers to oral hygiene or maintenance suggestions, patients with health or emotional problems that rule out surgery, and noncompliers to oral hygiene and maintenance suggestions.

At a glance

Expectations and limitations of subgingival scaling and root planing

- To achieve a healthy periodontium where bacteria and their products have attached to the tooth surface, these accretions should be removed.
- The process involves using dental instruments to achieve a smooth, hard root surface.
- The goal is to render the soft tissues of the periodontium biologically compatible with the root surface.
- There are several factors that keep us from achieving a successful result. They include:
  - Patient compliance to *(1)* oral hygiene measures and *(2)* maintenance
  - Systemic diseases, including *(1)* diabetes, *(2)* arthritis, and *(3)* immune system deficiencies
  - The tone of the soft tissue: *(1)* "fibrotic" tissue, which shrinks less, or *(2)* edematous tissue, which shrinks more
  - Type of periodontal disease
  - The clinical ability of the therapist
  - The initial probing depth
  - The shape of the root
  - The position of the tooth in the mouth
- How to know when to stop root planing—
  - The root is smooth and hard to an explorer
  - You can't see any calculus or plaque when air is blown into the sulcus
- Root planing creates a long junctional epithelium.
  - This is clinically a tenuous situation for the patient who is an erratic or noncomplier to suggested home or maintenance care.
  - To root plane properly, surgical intervention is often necessary to *(1)* save time and expense in removing tooth accumulated materials and *(2)* provide a shallow crevice, which is easier for both patient and therapist to clean.
- In general, patients with 6 mm or greater probing depths that bleed after initial therapy or whose probing depths continue to deepen are candidates for surgery.

Scaling and root planing

As described previously, of primary importance in treating inflammatory periodontal disease is the removal of calculus, bacteria, bacterial toxins, and roughened tooth surfaces. The clinical procedures used for doing this are scaling and root planing.

Scaling is the procedure designed to remove calculus by mechanically fracturing the deposit from the tooth surface. Scaling may also be the selected procedure to remove bacterial plaque by mechanical scraping. The American Academy of Periodontology defines scaling as "a treatment procedure necessary to remove hard and soft deposits from the tooth's surface. When it is performed on patients with periodontal disease, it is therapeutic, not prophylactic, in nature."[25] Root planing is defined by the American Academy of Periodontology as "a meticulous treatment procedure designed to remove the microbial flora, bacterial toxins on the root surface or in the pocket, calculus, and diseased cementum or dentin."[26]

The differences between scaling and root planing are subtle. Scaling is the procedure used to remove gross deposits; root planing is used to remove fine deposits or roughness often impregnated into the cementum. Lateral pressure, the pressure created when force is applied against the surface of a tooth with the cutting edge of the bladed instrument, is lighter in root planing than scaling. The root planing stroke is more of a scraping motion rather than the sharp removal of a definite deposit. The pressure is firm when removing the deposit and diminishes with the final root planing strokes. Instrument angulation, referring to the angle between the face of the blade and the tooth surface, is usually between 75° and 85° for a root planing procedure. The scaling strokes may be only one or two whereas numerous strokes are needed for root planing. Root planing is considered to be an extension of the scaling procedure or the final finishing and smoothing of the root surface.

Rationale for root planing

Garrett in 1977[27] set forth the rationale for root planing: *(1)* root smoothness, *(2)* removal of diseased cementum, and *(3)* preparation for new attachment. Complete removal of calculus is important to promote total gingival health. Rough root surfaces contribute to further plaque and calculus accumulation and to the continuation of inflammation and disease.[1] It has also been shown that scaling alone often does not remove all the calculus, and remnants may remain imbedded in the cementum even after the scaling procedures have been completed.[28]

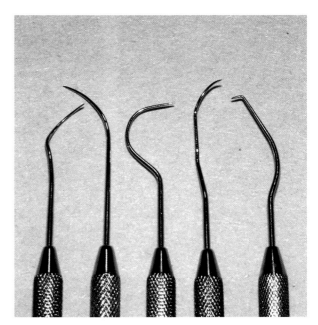

Fig 5-6 Various explorers. From left to right: No. 17, No. 11/12, No. 23 (also known as the Shepherd's Hook), No. 3A, and the pigtail explorer.

Hand scaling and root planing techniques

Some general considerations must always be taken into account before scaling and root planing procedures are begun. The patient's needs vary with the amount of inflammation and calculus present. Instrument selection will be based on the difficulty of the case, the area to be treated, the amount of inflammation, and probing depth. The instruments must always be sharp and correctly contoured. When using the instrument, the clinician must always keep the working end of the instrument against the surface of the tooth. It is most important to understand and keep in mind the root morphology so that precise adaptation can be maintained.

Instrument selection

Explorers

Deposits in periodontal pockets cannot be seen and the clinician must rely on tactile acuity to locate the deposit or roughness. The explorer is a fine, sharp instrument used to detect deposits, convolutions, or any roughness in the root surface. There are several types of explorers (Fig 5-6). The explorers are designed for a variety of uses and for various areas of the mouth. The longer shanks work well in areas of deep pockets, and the contra-angle shanks adapt

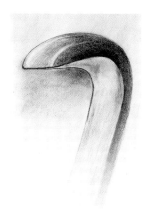

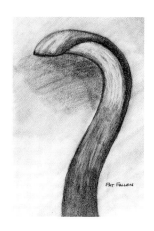

Fig 5-7 *(left)* Universal curette. Each working end has two cutting edges.

Fig 5-8 *(right)* Gracey curette. Designed to be area specific. Each working end has one cutting edge.

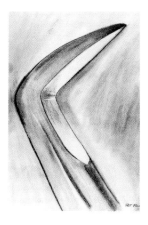

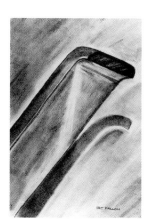

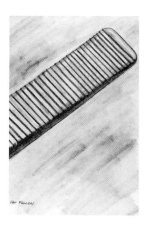

Fig 5-9 *(left)* Sickle scaler. Designed to be used for removal of supragingival calculus. It has two cutting edges.

Fig 5-10 *(middle)* Hoe instrument. Designed for removal of supragingival and subgingival calculus in easily accessible areas.

Fig 5-11 *(right)* File instrument. Note the many cutting edges. It is designed for crushing calculus.

well interproximally. The EXP 11/12 (Hu-Friedy) works well in deep interproximal pockets. The No. 17 is designed for exploring deep pockets in the anterior area, as is the No. 3a.

Curettes

Curettes are the most effective hand instruments for subgingival scaling and root planing. There are two basic groups of curettes: universal and Gracey.

Universal curettes have the following design and use characteristics:

1. The instrument face is set at a 90° angle to the shank nearest the working end.
2. The instrument has paired, mirror-image working ends, enabling it to be used in all areas of the mouth.
3. Each working end has two cutting edges.
4. The universal curettes have a rounded toe and back and are designed for subgingival use (Fig 5-7).

Gracey curettes have the following design characteristics:

1. The instrument face is set at a 60° to 70° angle to the shank nearest the working end.
2. The Gracey curettes were designed to be area-specific:

Anterior sextants:	Gracey 1/2, 3/4
Anterior and premolar:	Gracey 5/6
Posterior sextants, facial and lingual surfaces:	Gracey 7/8, 9/10
Posterior sextants, mesial, facial, and lingual surfaces:	Gracey 11/12 (Fig 5-8)
Posterior sextants, distal surfaces:	Gracey 13/14

3. Each working end has only one cutting edge.
4. Regular Gracey curettes have long flexible shanks, which makes them excellent for root planing.
5. Gracey rigid curettes have the same shank design but are more rigid and are better for removing calculus.
6. These curettes were designed to be area-specific, but can be adapted for use in other areas.

Scalers

Other instruments used for hand scaling, but not root planing, are the sickle, the hoe, and the file.

The sickle scaler (Fig 5-9) is triangular in cross section and has a pointed tip and two cutting edges. It is used to remove supragingival calculus. Because of the instrument design, it is difficult to insert this instrument into the sulcus for submarginal scaling without traumatizing the surrounding tissue (see Fig 5-9).

The hoe (Fig 5-10) is another instrument useful in special situations. It is used for removing heavy supragingival and subgingival calculus in easily accessible areas. It has a straight cutting edge that is formed by the junction of the face and the beveled toe of the blade. The hoe is used with a pull stroke.

The file (Fig 5-11) is an instrument with multiple cutting edges. Some types are bulky and difficult to use. Its primary function is to crush or fracture heavy, tenacious calculus with a pull stroke. The files were popular at one time but are not widely used today because they may gouge root surfaces. However, in certain areas (such as the mesial groove of a maxillary first premolar or the straight lingual groove of a maxillary incisor) and with a thin-headed file (such as the Hirschfeld), these instruments can be useful.

At a glance

Scaling and root planing

■ To remove calculus, bacterial toxins, and rough tooth surface successfully, the clinician must perform scaling and root planing procedures.

■ Root planing procedures are considered to be an extension of scaling.

■ The differences between scaling and root planing are subtle:
  • The instrument angulation of blade to tooth is 45° to 65° for root planing and 75° to 85° for scaling.
  • Scaling removes larger deposits whereas root planing smooths the surfaces.
  • The lateral pressure used is lighter for root planing.
  • Root planing requires more strokes than scaling.

■ The selection of the proper instrument involves considering the:
  • Amount of calculus or root roughness
  • Location of the calculus or roughness
  • Tissue tone and pocket depth
  • Specifics of instrument selection are discussed in the following section.

■ The explorer is the evaluation instrument used to detect any surface roughness on the tooth.

■ The curettes, universal and Gracey, are the most efficient instruments for scaling and root planing.

■ Instruments of differing designs used to remove deposits, but not to root plane, are the hoe, the sickle scaler, and the file.

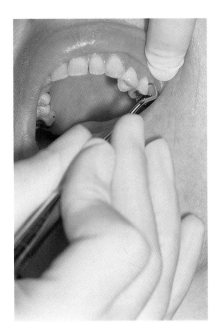
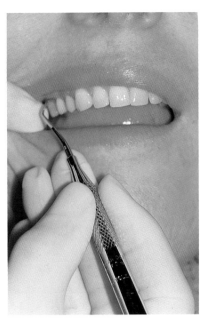

Fig 5-12 *(left)* Modified pen grasp. Extraoral fulcrum—palm down, resting on mandible for stability.

Fig 5-13 *(right)* Modified pen grasp. Extraoral fulcrum—palm up, back of hand resting on mandible for support.

Instrumentation and root morphology of selected teeth

The following is a detailed description of the morphology and instrumentation of six key teeth (teeth 3, 9, 12, 19, 25, 28) that serve as representative examples of the entire dentition.[29] The assumption is made that the junctional epithelium is 3 mm apical to the cementoenamel junction (CEJ), because of periodontal disease. This would correspond clinically to a 6-mm probing depth.

The instrument should be held with a modified pen grasp to enable the operator to move the instrument and roll it in the thumb and forefinger, keeping the proper angulation and adaptation at all times. The correct angulation of the face of the blade to the tooth should be 75° to 85° for scaling and 45° to 65° for root planing. The strokes are most often vertical and oblique. Many times an extraoral fulcrum is needed to reach an area of difficult access (Figs 5-12 and 5-13). It is necessary to be stable and secure when using any extraoral fulcrum and to make sure that the patient's lip is not being traumatized.

The maxillary central incisor, mandibular central incisor, mandibular first premolar, maxillary first premolar, and the maxillary and mandibular first molars will be represented in the review of root morphology. Each tooth will be viewed from the facial, mesial, lingual, and distal aspects and in cross section.

Maxillary anterior teeth

We will use the left maxillary central incisor to demonstrate the type of anatomy typically found in anterior teeth in this region. This tooth presents the typical anatomy of a maxillary anterior tooth.

From the facial aspect the root exhibits a gentle convex shape in a mesiodistal direction. The root tapers to a conical shape apically (Fig 5-14).

Following the facial surface to the mesial surface, there is a very convex mesiofacial line angle. The mesial surface is very much like the facial surface—slightly convex to flat (Fig 5-15).

The mesiolingual line angle is very convex as is the lingual surface. The lingual surface has a distal convergence toward the distolingual line angle (Fig 5-16).

The distal surface is similar to the mesial surface but has less surface area. The line angles are both very convex (Fig 5-17).

In cross section in the area of the middle one third, the root appears roughly triangular with a distal swing of the cingulum. The faciolingual width of the root is greater than the mesiodistal width. Progressing apically, this basic triangular shape remains (Fig 5-18).

Instrument selection: Gracey 1/2, 3/4, 13/14; Columbia 13/14.

The areas that most often cause difficulty in scaling the maxillary anterior teeth are the direct lingual surfaces and the line angles of the facial surface. In these areas the surface shape changes rapidly from a broad, flat surface to a highly convex surface. It is very important to establish the correct angulation of the blade to the tooth (45° to 90°) with the terminal one third of the instrument blade (Fig 5-19).

The terminal one third of the blade always remains in contact with the tooth surface while scaling or root planing. As the instrument moves horizontally across the broad facial surface, the handle must be rolled between the thumb and forefinger to keep the terminal portion in contact. As the line angle is reached, the amount of tooth surface scaled lessens. Hence, the more convex the surface, the more scaling strokes are needed. The lingual surface requires many strokes with the terminal one third of the blade. If the curette is not adapted correctly on the lingual surface, the gingival tissue will be traumatized.

The facial, mesial, and distal surfaces of anterior teeth are broader and allow more of the instrument to touch the tooth at a given point during scaling. It is still important to keep in mind that many strokes are necessary.

Often it is necessary to use many different instruments to smooth a tooth surface adequately. Also, it is often a good idea to change the stroke direction to ensure that the root surface is not being gouged by repeated instrumentation of the same area. A horizontal stroke may be used, but use extreme care not to traumatize tissue or break off calculus into the tissue.

─────── *At a glance* ───────

Maxillary anterior teeth

- The roots of the maxillary anterior teeth exhibit root surfaces that have a lingual convergence and very convex line angles.
- In instrumenting the described anatomy, it is necessary to use increased scaling strokes with the terminal one third of the blade.

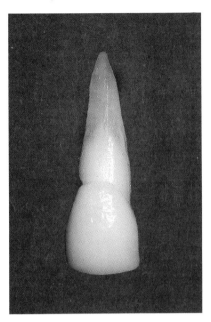

Fig 5-14 Facial view of maxillary central incisor.

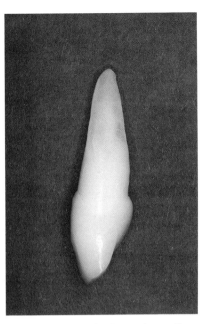

Fig 5-15 Mesial view of maxillary central incisor.

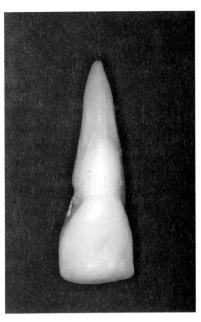

Fig 5-16 Lingual view of maxillary central incisor.

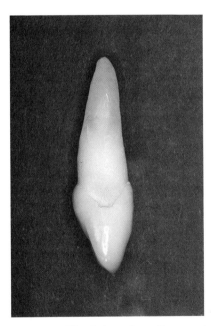

Fig 5-17 Distal view of maxillary central incisor.

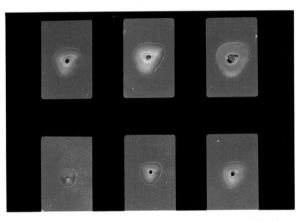

Fig 5-18 Cross-sectional view of maxillary central incisor. (Courtesy of Dr Arthur R. Vernino.)

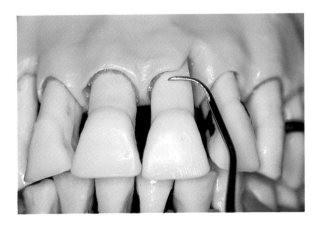

Fig 5-19 Using the Gracey 1/2 curette to root plane the facial surface of a maxillary central incisor.

Mandibular anterior teeth

The mandibular right central incisor represents the mandibular anterior group of teeth. The mandibular right lateral incisor is similar anatomically to the central incisor.

From the facial aspect, the mesiodistal width is narrow and exhibits a convex curvature. Moving toward the mesiofacial line, we encounter a very convex line angle (Fig 5-20).

The mesial surface may exhibit a longitudinal depression or root concavity on the middle one third of the root surface. Otherwise the surface is flat and tapers evenly toward the apex (Fig 5-21).

The lingual surface is similar to the facial aspect in curvature but has a slight lingual convergence. The faciolingual width is much greater than the mesiodistal width (Fig 5-22).

The distal surface is similar to the mesial surface. The longitudinal depression may be more prominent from this aspect than on the mesial surface (Fig 5-23).

In cross section through the middle one third, the outline of the root appears hourglass shaped with moderate to slight concavities on the mesial surface. The distal root surface may exhibit a deep root concavity. The line angles on the root surface are convex (Fig 5-24).

Instrument selection: Gracey 1/2, 3/4, 13/14; Columbia 13/14.

Many of the same difficulties encountered in scaling the maxillary anterior teeth appear also in the mandibular dentition.

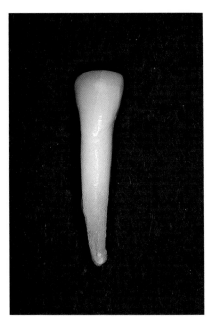

Fig 5-20 Facial view of mandibular central incisor.

The terminal one third of the instrument blade is used to scale the convex facial and lingual surfaces. Care must be taken to roll the instrument into the concavity if the calculus or plaque involved is on the middle one third of the root surface. The same approach must be taken on the distal surface (Figs 5-25 and 5-26).

──────── *At a glance* ────────

Mandibular anterior teeth

- ■ The mandibular anterior teeth are very narrow mesiodistally with extremely convex facial and lingual surfaces.
- ■ The proximal surfaces may exhibit mesial and/or distal root concavities.
- ■ Again, many strokes with the terminal one third of the blade are necessary for the convex surfaces, line angles, and root concavities.

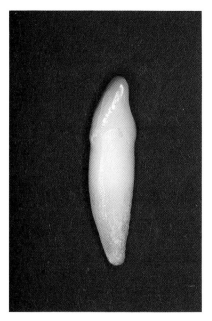

Fig 5-21 Mesial view of mandibular central incisor.

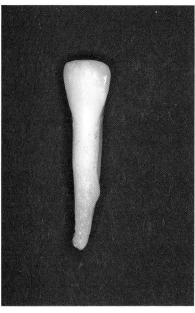

Fig 5-22 Lingual view of mandibular central incisor.

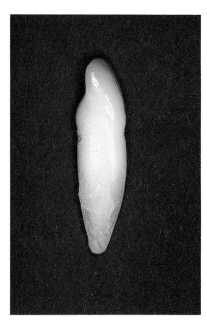

Fig 5-23 Distal view of mandibular central incisor.

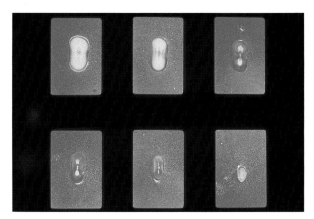

Fig 5-24 Cross-sectional view of mandibular central incisor. (Courtesy of Dr Arthur R. Vernino.)

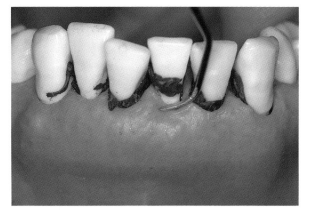

Fig 5-25 Scaling the mandibular central incisor using a Gracey 1/2 curette. Note that the tip is not correctly adapted and is gouging the tissue.

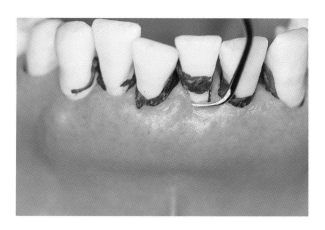

Fig 5-26 Scaling the mandibular central incisor using the Gracey 1/2 curette. The tip is correctly adapted.

Maxillary premolars

The maxillary premolar presents a transitional picture with its usually bifurcated roots. The facial and lingual roots are similar in shape and size. The facial surface of the maxillary first premolar is slightly convex (Fig 5-27).

The mesial surface exhibits a root concavity extending from 2.35 mm to 9.4 mm apical to the CEJ.[30] The deepest portion of the concavity is two thirds across the mesial surface toward the lingual aspect. A developmental depression on the furcation surface of the buccal root (buccal furcation groove) was found in 35 (78%) of the teeth. Each remaining tooth had a bifurcation located in the apical third of the root, resulting in short buccal and lingual roots without buccal furcation grooves. Most maxillary first premolars with well-formed buccal and lingual roots have buccal furcation grooves that may represent the partial formation of two separate buccal roots during development of the tooth[31] (Fig 5-28).

The lingual aspect is similar to the buccal except for the lingual convergence. The root is wider faciolingually (Fig 5-29).

The distal surface usually exhibits a concavity on the middle one third of the root. Otherwise the surface is flat (Fig 5-30).

The root cross section at the junction of the cervical and middle thirds appears kidney shaped with a deep concavity on the mesial surface and only a slight concavity on the distal surface. In the bifurcation the roots appear conical with a longitudinal depression on the furcation aspect of the buccal root (Fig 5-31).

Instrument selection: Gracey 5/6, 11/12, 13/14; Columbia 13/14, 4R/4L.

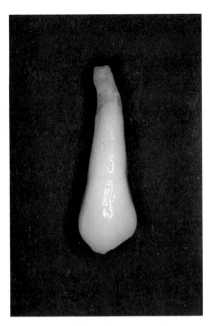

Fig 5-27 Facial view of maxillary premolar.

The most difficult area, and one that requires extreme concentration when scaling the maxillary premolar, is the mesial surface. The instrument tip must be kept in contact with the root surface and rotated into the deepest portion of the concavity that is two thirds across the mesial surface toward the lingual aspect. The handle of the instrument may need to be moved away from the tooth to ensure that the tip is in and more than halfway across the mesial surface. The depth of the concavity should be scaled from both the labial and the lingual aspects (Figs 5-32 and 5-33).

At a glance

Maxillary premolars

- The maxillary premolars present the greatest challenge in treatment.
- The mesial surface exhibits a deep root concavity, often with a groove on the furcation aspect of the buccal root.
- In instrumentation on the mesial surface the terminal tip of the instrument must be kept in contact with the root surface and rotated into the deepest portion of the concavity.

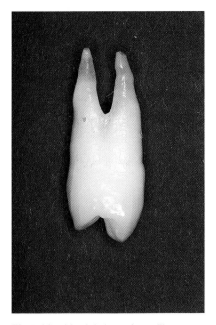

Fig 5-28 Mesial view of maxillary premolar.

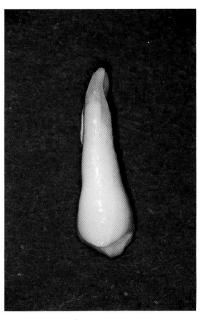

Fig 5-29 Lingual view of maxillary premolar.

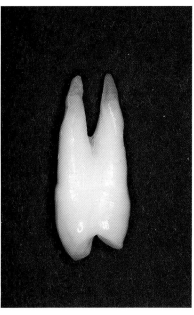

Fig 5-30 Distal view of maxillary premolar.

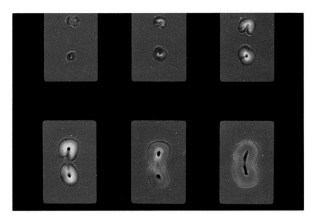

Fig 5-31 Cross-sectional view of maxillary premolar. (Courtesy of Dr Arthur R. Vernino.)

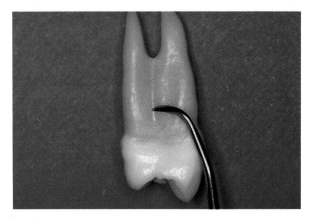

Fig 5-32 Adapting the Gracey 11/12 curette into the mesial concavity of the maxillary first premolar, entering from the buccal aspect.

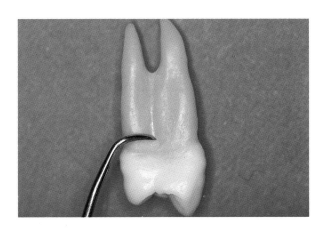

Fig 5-33 Adapting the Gracey 11/12 curette into the mesial concavity of the maxillary first premolar, entering from the lingual aspect.

Mandibular premolars

The mandibular right first premolar is a transitional tooth with characteristics of both the canine and second premolar.

The buccal root surface is broad and convex. The root is wider buccolingually than mesiodistally (Fig 5-34).

The mesial root surface is slightly convex and broad. In the apical and middle thirds of the surface there may be a longitudinal depression that becomes deeper apically (Fig 5-35).

The convex lingual surface has a lingual convergence. The cervical one third to one half has a straight profile and tapers to a blunt apex (Fig 5-36).

The distal surface has a broad convex area. The distal root surface may have a longitudinal depression that often is deeper than the mesial surface (Fig 5-37).

In cross section the root appears ovoid with a lingual convergence. The mesial surface may exhibit a deepening of the longitudinal depression in the cervical one third to one half. Otherwise the surface is slightly convex. The convex lingual surface converges lingually. The distal surface is broad and flat with an occasional longitudinal depression (Fig 5-38).

Instrument selection: Gracey 3/4, 5/6, 11/12, 13/14; Columbia 13/14.

The mandibular premolar does not have exceptionally difficult access or morphologic complications. Remember that the root is wider buccolingually than mesiodistally, hence the curette must be extended more than halfway across the root surface. When the mesial and distal surfaces are being scaled, the handle should be moved away from the tooth to ensure that the tip moves in and more than halfway across the tooth surface. It is important to keep the terminal portion of the blade in contact with the tooth.

The lingual surface is convex, and again care must be taken to use the terminal one third of the blade for scaling (Fig 5-39).

At a glance
Mandibular premolars

- The mandibular premolars exhibit no morphologic complications.
- In cross sections, the roots are ovoid with a lingual convergence and root concavities on the proximal surfaces.
- The root is wider buccolingually, requiring that the curette be extended more than halfway across the root surface.

Maxillary molars

The maxillary first molar presents a complex anatomic picture. From the buccal aspect, the buccal furcation occurs at about the junction of the cervical and middle thirds of the root surface. This is approximately 4 mm apical to the CEJ (Fig 5-40).

The mesiobuccal root, the second longest and largest root, is widest faciolingually. The root inclines mesially in the middle one third and has a distal inclination in the apical one third. There are longitudinal depressions on both the furcation and mesial aspects of the root.

The smallest and shortest distobuccal root inclines mesially and buccally in the middle one third and then curves distally in the apical one third. Frequently there is a longitudinal depression on the furcation aspects of the distobuccal root.

From the mesial aspect, the mesial furcation presents 3 mm apical to the CEJ. The furcation area is located more lingual to the midline than the distal furca (Fig 5-41).

The lingual root is the longest, largest, and strongest. In the middle one third the root leans toward the lingual aspect and then shows a buccal inclination in the apical one third. There is usually a longitudinal depression extending from the root trunk onto the root surface. Gher and Vernino[31] state that a longitudinal depression occurs on the furcation side of the lingual root in 17% of the population (Fig 5-42).

The distal furcation is located 5 mm apical to the CEJ. This aspect is similar to the mesial, except that the distobuccal root is shorter and smaller. The furcal surface of the distobuccal root is convex and extends buccally. The apical one third has a slight lingual

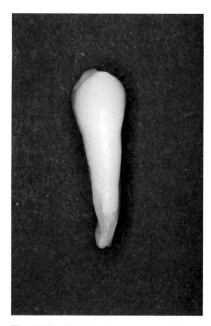

Fig 5-34 Facial view of mandibular first premolar.

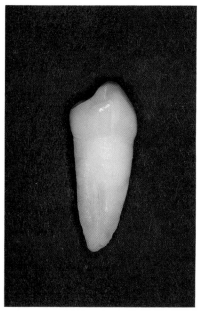

Fig 5-35 Mesial view of mandibular first premolar.

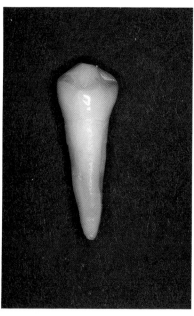

Fig 5-36 Lingual view of mandibular first premolar.

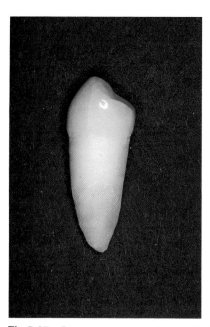

Fig 5-37 Distal view of mandibular first premolar.

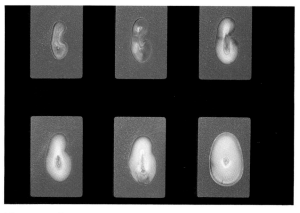

Fig 5-38 Cross-sectional view of mandibular first premolar. (Courtesy of Dr Arthur R. Vernino.)

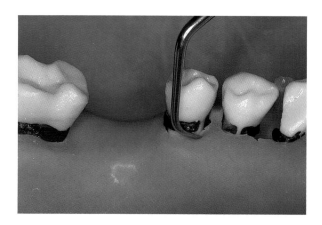

Fig 5-39 Scaling lingual mandibular premolars using a Gracey 7/8 curette.

inclination. There may be a longitudinal depression on the furcation aspect (Fig 5-43).

The cross section at the furcation areas demonstrates the three roots clearly. The kidney-shaped mesiobuccal root has a longitudinal groove on the mesial and furcation surfaces. The mesiobuccal root is very wide buccolingually (Fig 5-44).

The distobuccal root has an ovoid appearance, often with a longitudinal depression on the furcation surface. It is the smallest of the roots.

The lingual root presents an ovoid shape and is wider mesiodistally. There is a longitudinal depression on the palatal and sometimes on the furcation side of the root.

Instrument selection: Gracey 11/12, 13/14, 7/8, 9/10; universal 4R/4L; Columbia 13/14.

The furcation areas of the maxillary first molar make it difficult or impossible to scale without reflecting flaps when there has been bone loss. The buccal furcation and the groove leading to the furcation are often felt by the clinician. In scaling the buccal furcation, it is best to use two different instruments if access permits: the Gracey 11/12 to scale the mesial surface of the distal root and Gracey 13/14 to scale the distal surface of the mesial root. The Gracey instruments are recommended because of the beveled blade angle, which seems to facilitate access and adaptability (Figs 5-45 and 5-46).

The mesial furcation is often missed by the clinician because it is accessible only from the lingual or palatal side of the tooth. The instrument recommended is the Gracey 11/12 or possibly the universal

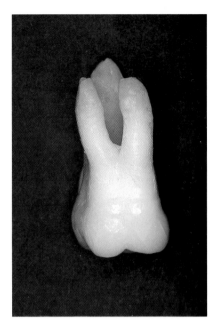

Fig 5-40　Buccal view of maxillary first molar.

4R/4L. It is important to adapt the blade to the surfaces within the furcation itself.

The distal furcation is impossible to scale unless the second molar is missing. In this case the Gracey 13/14 or possibly a universal curette may be used. This is an extremely difficult area to scale.

The broad palatal root is best scaled with the Gracey 9/10 using the oblique stroke.

_____ *At a glance* _____

Maxillary molars

- The maxillary first molar presents the most complex anatomic picture, with three furcation areas.
- The mesiobuccal root is widest buccolingually with longitudinal depression on the furcation and mesial aspects of the root.
- The smallest, shortest distobuccal root frequently has a longitudinal depression on the furcation aspect of the distobuccal root.
- The longest, largest, strongest lingual root frequently exhibits a longitudinal depression on the lingual aspect and occasionally on the furcation surface.
- If there is bone loss in the furcation areas, ideally a flap should be reflected to scale effectively.
- In the buccal furcation it is best to use the Gracey 11/12 on the mesial surface of the distal root and the Gracey 13/14 to scale the distal surface of the mesial root.
- The mesial furcation should be scaled from the lingual aspect with the Gracey 11/12 or universal 4R/4L.
- The distal furcation should be scaled with the Gracey 13/14 and only if the second molar is missing.
- The broad palatal root is best scaled with the Gracey 9/10 using the oblique stroke.

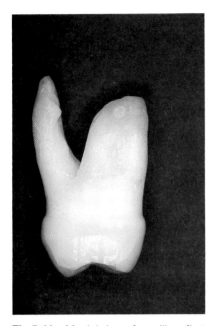

Fig 5-41 Mesial view of maxillary first molar.

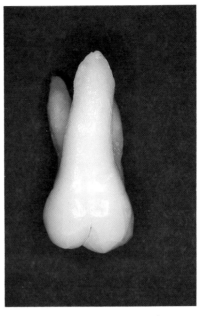

Fig 5-42 Lingual view of maxillary first molar.

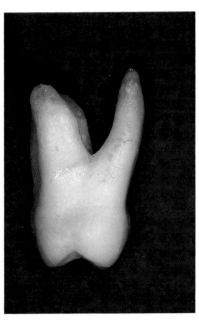

Fig 5-43 Distal view of maxillary first molar.

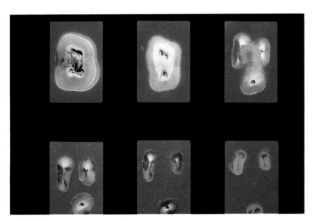

Fig 5-44 Cross-sectional view of maxillary first molar. (Courtesy of Dr Arthur R. Vernino.)

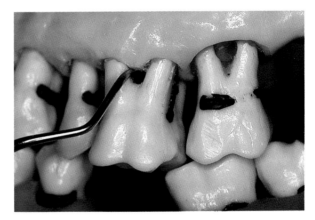

Fig 5-45 Scaling buccal furcation, adapting a Gracey 13/14 curette on the distal surface of the mesial root.

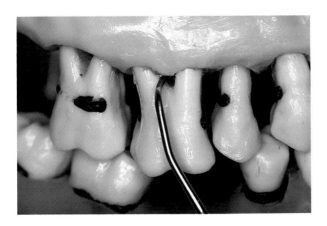

Fig 5-46 Scaling buccal furcation, adapting a Gracey 11/12 curette on the mesial surface of the distal root.

Mandibular molars

The mandibular first molar is not as complex anatomically as the maxillary first molar, yet it presents its own anatomic uniqueness.

From the buccal aspect, the buccal furcation entrance is located 3 mm from the CEJ. The buccal root trunk surface is flat with a large concavity in the middle one third of the root trunk, which begins the furcation area. The roots are not as divergent as in the maxillary molars (Fig 5-47).

From the buccal aspect the mesial root surface is convex, with a mesial rotation so that the distal surface of the mesiobuccal root is visible. The "intermediate bifurcation ridge," a furcation structure described by Everett et al,[32] is present in 73% of the mandibular first molars. This ridge crosses from the mesial to the distal root at the midpoint of the bifurcation. In addition, Everett et al have described alternative ridges buccal and lingual to the midfurcation area.

The mandibular first molar is a good example of how concavities on the furcal aspect of both the mesial and distal roots can complicate instrumentation of roots. Furcation entrances are generally narrow and lack sufficient space for instrumentation.[31]

Enamel projections may further complicate treatment of the periodontally involved furcation. Masters and Hoskins[33] reported on the prevalence of enamel projections in mandibular molars (28.6%). Projections ranging from those classified as mild to those extending into the furca were rated on a scale of 1 through 3. The prevalence of grade 3 projections was 4.3% in mandibular molars. Masters and Hoskins suggested that furcations with enamel projections have an increased potential for formation of a pocket.

The distal root is not quite as broad buccolingually or as long as the mesial root. The distobuccal root surface is very convex.

The mesial root surface is broad with a greater buccolingual width. The lingual profile is relatively straight with a convex buccal surface. A concavity is found on the mesial and furcal aspects of the mesial root. The mesial root has more pronounced flutings over a larger total surface area (Fig 5-48).

On the lingual surface the lingual furcation occurs 4 mm apical to the CEJ. The lingual surfaces of the mesial and distal roots are very convex (Fig 5-49). There may be a slight root concavity on the furcal aspect of the distal root (Fig 5-50).

In cross section at the cementoenamel junction the root trunk has a somewhat rectangular appearance. The slight concavity on the buccal and lingual surfaces is attributed to the furcation area. The mesial surface exhibits a concavity associated with the longitudinal root depression. These concavities deepen until the roots divide. In Fig 5-51 the mesial root becomes hourglass shaped because of the root concavities on the mesial and furcal aspects of the root. The distal root has a root concavity on the mesial surface. Progressing apically the distal root becomes smaller and more ovoid in shape in comparison to the mesial root (see Fig 5-51).

Instrument selection: Gracey 11/12, 13/14, 9/10.

The furcation areas of the mandibular molar are also very difficult areas to scale. As with the maxillary molar furcation, each surface of the furcation must be thought of individually. The distal surface of the mesial root is scaled with the Gracey 13/14, and the mesial surface of the distal root is scaled with the Gracey 11/12. Both the buccal and lingual furcations are scaled in a similar manner. Care should be taken to adapt the tip of the instrument to the root concavity within the furcation if possible.

The Gracey 9/10 is a good instrument to use in the developmental depression leading to the concavity of the broad lingual root.

——— *At a glance* ———

Mandibular molars

- The mandibular first molar features its own anatomical complexity.
- The buccal furcation area often presents an intermediate bifurcation ridge.
- Although the lingual furcation is less complicated, the furcation entrances are generally narrow and lack sufficient space for instrumentation.
- The mesial and distal roots are very wide buccolingually. Wide longitudinal depressions exist on all proximal root surfaces except the distal surface of the distal root.
- Each root should be scaled as an individual root, scaling the mesial surface of the distal root with the Gracey 11/12 and the distal surface of the mesial root with the Gracey 13/14.

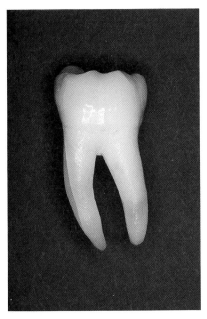

Fig 5-47 Buccal view of mandibular first molar.

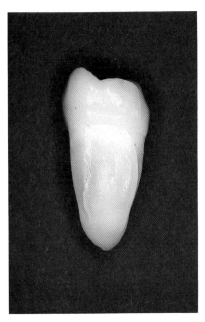

Fig 5-48 Mesial view of mandibular first molar.

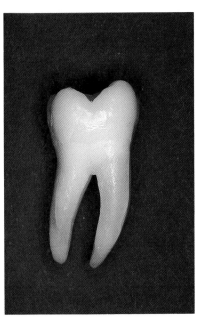

Fig 5-49 Lingual view of mandibular first molar.

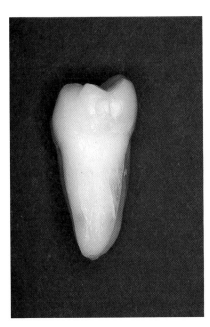

Fig 5-50 Distal view of mandibular first molar.

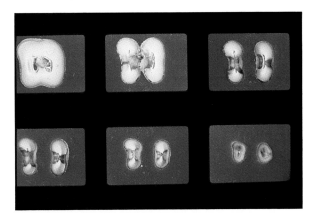

Fig 5-51 Cross-sectional view of mandibular first molar. (Courtesy of Dr Arthur R. Vernino.)

Ultrasonic cleaning devices

Ultrasonic cleaning devices have been in use for over 30 years and their place in therapy is still questioned. Their action is derived from the physical vibration of particles of matter at frequencies from 20,000 to many millions of cycles per second.

Early debate centered on which devices would most effectively smooth root surfaces. A study of papers that look at in vivo subgingival applications shows approximately equal division between those that favored hand instruments alone[2,34,35] and those that favored ultrasonic devices followed by hand instruments.[17,28,36,37] A smaller number[37,38] found ultrasonic devices alone to be superior. The entrance to furcas is often narrow,[39] and in grade II and III furcas ultrasonic devices have proved to have some advantages over hand scalers.[40] One study compared various ultrasonic scalers (Titan-S®, Syntex Dental Products; Micro-Mega®, Micro-Mega SA; Calens®, Kollega Konsult A/S; Cavitron®, Dentsply International Inc) using universal tips on extracted teeth. They found that the Titan-S scaler was superior to the other scalers.[41] However, in our practice the Cavitron has shown itself to be superior over years of use.

As discussed earlier, the emphasis has shifted from the goal of root smoothness to creating biologic compatibility between the root surface and the soft tissues of the periodontium. In this regard it has been found that fibroblasts in tissue culture will attach equally well to extracted teeth that were cleaned with either hand or ultrasonic instruments.[42] However, another study found that hand scaling removed more endotoxin than did ultrasonic cleaning.[43]

Clinically, the ultrasonic device is a time saver, and we suggest that its judicious use be followed by hand instruments where possible. It should be kept in mind that ultrasonic instruments were originally designed to cut cavity preparations and can do great damage to the root surface if applied improperly. Therefore, you should not touch the tip of the instrument to the tooth and should use it with continual movement. It is also prudent to avoid any restorative margin to reduce the possibility of damage. The exception would be the amalgam overhang that needs to be removed.

───────── *At a glance* ─────────────────────────────

Scaling and root planing—A summary

- Scaling and root planing involves removing all detectable calculus and smoothing of the root.
- The goal of scaling and root planing is to make the root and the soft tissue biologically compatible.
- To select the proper instrument you must know the amount of calculus, its location and tenacity, the probing depth, tissue tone, and instrument sharpness.
- There are a number of instruments designed to be scalers; if these are used, they generally should be followed by curettes to smooth the root surface.
- A detailed study of root anatomy is essential for improved success in removing subgingival tooth-borne deposits.
- Ultrasonic instruments can serve as adjuncts to hand scaling and may clean more effectively in deeper furcas.

References

1. Caffesse RG, Sweeney PL, Smith BA: Scaling and root planing with and without periodontal flap surgery. *J Clin Periodontol* 1986;13:205.
2. Rosenberg RM, Ash MM: The effect of root roughness on plaque accumulation and gingival inflammation. *J Periodontol* 1974;45:146.
3. Handleman SL, Hess C: Effect of dental prophylaxis on tooth-surface flora. *J Dent Res* 1970;49:340.
4. Waring MB, Newman SM, Lefcoe DL: A comparison of engine polishing and toothbrushing in minimizing dental plaque reaccumulation. *Dent Hyg* 1982;56:25.
5. Axelsson P, Lindhe J, Waseby J: The effect of various plaque control measures on gingivitis and caries in schoolchildren. *Community Dent Oral Epidemiol* 1976;4:232.
6. Axelsson P, Lindhe J: Effect of controlled oral hygiene procedures on caries and periodontal disease in adults. *J Clin Periodontol* 1978;5:133.
7. Christensen RP, Bangerter VW: Determination of rpm, time, and load used in oral prophylaxis polishing in vivo. *J Dent Res* 1984;63:1376.
8. Christensen RP, Bangerter VM: Immediate and long-term in vivo effects of polishing on enamel and dentin. *J Prosthet Dent* 1987;57:150.
9. Willman DE, Norling BK, Johnson WN: A new prophylaxis instrument: Effect on enamel alterations. *J Am Dent Assoc* 1980;101:923.
10. Weaks LM, Lescher NB, Barnes CM, Holroyd SV: Clinical evaluation of the Prophy-Jet as an instrument for routine removal of tooth stain and plaque. *J Periodontol* 1984;55:486.
11. Berkstein S, Reiff, RL, McKinney JF, Killoy WJ: Supragingival root surface removal during maintenance procedures utilizing an air-powder abrasive system or hand scaling—An in vitro study. *J Periodontol* 1987;58:327.
12. Atkinson DR, Cobb CM, Killoy WJ: The effect of an air-powder abrasive system on in vitro root surfaces. *J Periodontol* 1984;55:13.
13. Finlayson RS, Stevens FD: Subcutaneous facial emphysema secondary to use of the Cavi-Jet. *J Periodontol* 1988;59:315.
14. Waerhaug J: Healing of the dentoepithelial junction following subgingival plaque control. II. As observed on extracted teeth. *J Periodontol* 1978;49:119.
15. Stambaugh RV, Dragoo M, Smith DM, Carasal L: The limits of subgingival scaling. *Int J Periodont Rest Dent* 1981;5:31.
16. Rabbani GM, Ash MM, Caffesse RG: The effectiveness of subgingival scaling and root planing in calculus removal. *J Periodontol* 1981;52:119.
17. Thornton S, Garnick J: Comparison of ultrasonic to hand instruments in the removal of subgingival plaque. *J Periodontol* 1982;53:35.
18. Nyman S, Westfelt E, Sarhed G, Karring T: Role of "diseased" root cementum in healing following treatment of periodontal disease. A clinical study. *J Clin Periodontol* 1988;15:464.
19. American Academy of Periodontology: *Glossary of Terms.* Chicago, American Academy of Periodontology, 1986, p 19.
20. Aleo J, DeRenzis F, Farber P: In vitro attachment of human gingival fibroblasts to root surfaces. *J Periodontol* 1975;46:639.
21. Hatfield CG, Baumhammers A: Cytotoxic effect of periodontally involved surfaces of human teeth. *Arch Oral Biol* 1971;16:465.
22. Dragoo MR: *Regeneration of the Periodontal Attachment in Humans.* Philadelphia, Lea and Febiger, 1981, pp 35–48.
23. Nabik NM, Bissada NF, Simmelink JW, Goldstine SN: Endotoxin penetration into root cementum of periodontally healthy and diseased human teeth. *J Periodontol* 1982;53:368.
24. Beaumont RH, O'Leary TJ, Kafrany AH: Relative resistance of long junctional epithelial adhesions and connective tissue attachments to plaque-induced inflammation. *J Periodontol* 1984;55:213–223.
25. American Academy of Periodontology: *Current Procedural Terminology for Periodontics,* 5th ed. Chicago, American Academy of Periodontology, 1987, p 32.
26. American Academy of Periodontology: *Current Procedural Terminology for Periodontics,* 5th ed. Chicago, American Academy of Periodontology, 1987, p 31.
27. Garrett JS: Root planing: A perspective. *J Periodontol* 1977;48:553.
28. Jones SJ, Lozdan J, Boyde A: Tooth surfaces treated in situ with periodontal instruments: Scanning electron microscopic studies. *Br Dent J* 1972;132:57.
29. Ramfjord SP: Indices for prevalence and incidence of periodontal disease. *J Periodontol* 1959;30:51.
30. Booker BW: *A Morphologic Study of the Mesial Root Surface of the Adolescent Maxillary First Bicuspid,* master's thesis. The University of Texas Health Science Center, Houston, 1982.
31. Gher ME, Vernino AR: Root morphology—Clinical significance in pathogenesis and treatment of periodontal disease. *J Am Dent Assoc* 1980;101:627.
32. Everett FG, et al: The intermediate bifurcational ridge: A study of the morphology of the bifurcation of the lower first molar. *J Res Dent* 1958;37:162.
33. Masters DH, Hoskins SW: Projection of cervical enamel into molar furcations. *J Periodontol* 1964;35:49.
34. Kerry GJ: Roughness of root surfaces after use of ultrasonic instruments and hand curettes. *J Periodontol* 1967;38:340.
35. Wilkinson RF, Maybury JE: Scanning electron microscopy of the root surface following instrumentation. *J Periodontol* 1973;44:559.
36. Stende GW, Schaffer EM: A comparison of ultrasonic and hand scaling. *J Periodontol* 1961;32:312.
37. D'Silva IV, Nayak RP, Cherian KM, Mulky MJ: An evaluation of the root topography following periodontal instrumentation. A scanning electron microscopic study. *J Periodontol* 1979;50:283.
38. Ewen SJ, Gwinnett AJ: A scanning electron microscope study of teeth following periodontal instrumentation. *J Periodontol* 1977;48:92.
39. Bower RC: Furcation morphology relative to periodontal treatment. *J Periodontol* 1979;50:366.
40. Leon LE, Vogel RI: A comparison of the effectiveness of hand scaling and ultrasonic debridement in furcations as evaluated by differential dark-field microscopy. *J Periodontol* 1987;58:86.
41. Lie T, Leknes KN: Evaluation on the effect on root surfaces of air turbine scalers and ultrasonic instrumentation. *J Periodontol* 1985;56:522.
42. Checchi L, Pelliccioni GA: Hand versus ultrasonic instrumentation in the removal of endotoxins from root surfaces in vitro. *J Periodontol* 1988;59:398.
43. Nishimine D, O'Leary TJ: Hand instrumentation versus ultrasonics in the removal of endotoxins from root surfaces. *J Periodontol* 1979;50:345.

Chapter 6

A Typical Maintenance Visit*

Thomas G. Wilson, Jr

This chapter outlines a typical maintenance visit for the patient with an inflammatory periodontal disease. The topics are listed in the order of importance for the average patient. This order should be individualized from patient to patient and sometimes for the same patient over time. Proper periodontal maintenance takes time — the average patient will require about an hour. It is often the dental hygienist's responsibility to perform the listed maintenance procedures, and it is the dentist's responsibility to give the hygienist enough time to do a thorough job. If you ask yourself, which steps can I eliminate because patients (or insurance companies) won't pay enough (or often enough) to justify the time needed?, my response is that to eliminate any of these steps could jeopardize the patient's periodontal health. Once enough professionals allow adequate time and charge adequate fees, the compensation from third parties should rise accordingly. We have found that patients are willing to pay for above-average care if they are properly informed of their options.

Review of chart

Before seeing patients it is helpful to review their charts to determine any special situations. These may include previously deepened periodontal pockets, areas that are sensitive when scaled, past oral hygiene, and maintenance compliance problems. A review of any pretreatment medications that might be needed is also pertinent. Many patients now need antibiotic coverage for heart murmurs, prosthetic devices, and such (see chapter 13). The patient's treatment plan should also be reviewed.

*Portions of this chapter originally appeared in the *Texas Dental Journal* and have been reprinted with their kind permission.

Talk with patient

This may seem inconsequential, but conversation affords an opportunity to establish a rapport and to find out whether there are any problems on the patient's part. In the middle of a busy day, we may lose sight of the fact that there is a person attached to the teeth. This person has a myriad of situations to confront that may directly or indirectly affect the stomatognathic system. Notes of the patient's concern should be placed in the chart for future reference. In addition, a few notes about the patient's personal life can establish a person-to-person bond, which also increases the probability of success because increased compliance is seen after these bonds have been formed.

History update

The medical history can usually be updated by asking the following three questions:

1. Has there been any change in your health?
2. Are you taking any new medications or has there been any change in present medications?
3. Have there been any hospitalizations since your last visit?

The dental history can usually be covered with the following three questions:

1. Has there been any change in your dental health?
2. Do you have any new dental work?
3. What are you doing at home on a routine basis to clean your teeth?

An alternative is to have the patient review his or her health history, make appropriate changes, then sign an addendum (see Fig 2-1). Either way, responses should be made part of the patient's permanent record.

Head, neck, and intraoral examination

The major concerns here are lesions of the head or neck, problems with the temporomandibular joint, and any intraoral lesions of the soft or hard tissue.

Data collection

There are five areas of data collection: (1) examination for dental caries, failing restorations, and to make sure that dental devices fit properly; (2) a check for supragingival plaque as a measure of recent home care; (3) recording of probing depths and gingival recession—these should be checked at each visit but recorded only yearly unless changes have occurred since the last visit; (4) recording of bleeding upon probing—this information should be recorded at each visit; and (5) a check for fremitus. Historically, checking for tooth-related problems has been part of the routine in the dental office. Recently, because of increased knowledge in the field of periodontics and because of a more litigious atmosphere, it has become necessary to check for periodontal problems as well. In general, the more responsibility the dental office takes for the patient's periodontal condition, the more information on the subject that should be looked for and recorded. For an in-depth review on examination, refer to pp 17–27.

Plaque control

Those of us who have been in practice for a long time sometimes forget the importance of reinforcing the patient's oral hygiene. It is easy to assume that everyone has been properly instructed and practices good plaque control. However, this is not the fact. Many patients have been told that oral hygiene is important but never shown how to accomplish the task on a one-to-one basis. Oral hygiene should be checked and reinforced at every visit. The importance of plaque control cannot be overemphasized. For more information, see pp 51–62.

Removal of subgingival accretions

There is no question that this is one of the more important parts of the maintenance visit. This step should be performed before any hard supragingival accretions are removed, because subgingival materials play a far greater role in the etiology of periodontal problems than their supragingival counterparts. The goal of subgingival scaling and root planing is to make the root surface compatible with the soft tissues. The mechanics of this procedure are among the most difficult in dentistry. The expectations for success should be based on the amount of calculus and bacteria encountered, on the depth of the pocket, on the tissue tone, the skill of the operator, and on access. It should be kept in mind that most patients with probing depths of 6 mm or greater seen on maintenance will be potential candidates for periodontal surgery. This subject is covered in great detail in chapter 5.

Removal of supragingival accretions

Supragingival accretions such as calculus and stain have little or no effect on the progression of diseases of the periodontium, with the exception of helping to create the environmental changes necessary to form subgingival plaque. Consequently, much more time should be spent on removing subgingival accretions than on supragingival accretions. This area is also covered in chapter 5.

Radiographs

A full-mouth set of right-angle radiographs should be exposed every 2 years for the average periodontal patient and more frequently when rapid destruction is occurring. A yearly set of seven vertical bite-wings can be used as a screening tool between these surveys.

Selecting maintenance intervals

In times past, dental maintenance intervals were set by the calendar. The 6-month interval was assumed correct and was reinforced by the fact that many insurance companies pay for only two "cleanings" each year. Until recently there was little scientific evidence to challenge this practice. However, a number of recent articles show that twice a year is usually not adequate for patients with periodontal diseases.[1-3]

We need to set maintenance intervals according to periodontal disease activity. Patients whose disease is less severe and less active may be seen less frequently than those whose problems are more acute and active. Recent work has shown that periodontal disease activity may progress in stages.[4] In this scenario an active stage is followed by an inactive stage, and breakdown and repair may occur simultaneously in different areas of the same mouth. The difficult part of this process is deciding when the disease is active (see chapter 2). Until this question is resolved, we must rely on clinical and radiographic data to make our decision. For the present, I use a number of indices, including probing depth and bleeding upon probing, as indicators. Patients who have increased bleeding points or increased probing depth compared to their last visit should often have their maintenance interval shortened, whereas those with fewer problems than before may be seen less frequently.[5]

Adult patients having orthodontic therapy, orthognathic surgery, or who have systemic diseases that make them more prone to breakdown (diabetes, etc) should be seen more frequently than patients not in these categories. The same applies to most patients with poor oral hygiene.

In our practice, patients just completing active therapy for periodontal disease control are placed on a 3-month interval. At their first maintenance visit the interval is reviewed and modified as necessary, and so on.

Setting maintenance intervals

We have set up guidelines for specific therapy decisions that can be used for patients on periodontal recall (Figs 6-1 to 6-3). This method is based on our research with Dr Mark Glover and on a paper by Lang.[5]

Definitions

1. Complete complier — a person who presents for at least 75% of suggested maintenance visits.
2. Erratic complier — a person who attends less often than the complete complier.

Assumptions

1. Sites with bleeding seen after probing will break down faster than those with no bleeding.
2. The more bleeding, especially repeated bleeding points at successive maintenance visits, the more likely it is that bone loss will follow.
3. Data including probing depths, bleeding upon probing, and gingival recession (along with other suggested parameters, see chapter 2) are recorded for each patient at each maintenance visit.

Caveats

1. Inaccuracies in probing depths can be misleading; attachment levels are more accurate.
2. Bleeding upon probing may not be an acutely sensitive method of determining disease activity.
3. If you err, do so on the side of being too conservative.

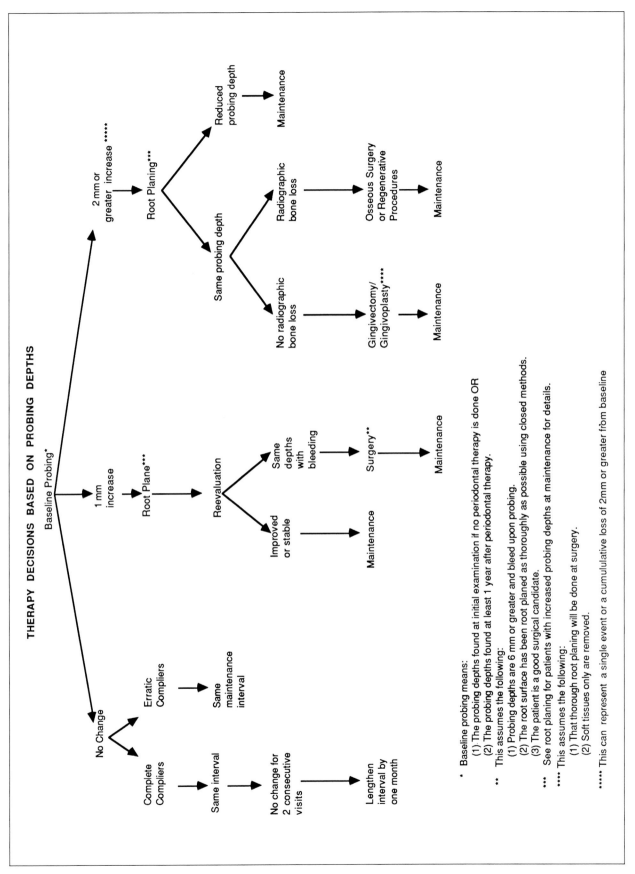

THERAPY DECISIONS BASED ON PROBING DEPTHS

Baseline Probing*

No Change
- Erratic Compliers → Same maintenance interval
- Complete Compliers → Same interval → No change for 2 consecutive visits → Lengthen interval by one month

1 mm increase → Root Plane*** → Reevaluation
- Improved or stable → Maintenance
- Same depths with bleeding → Surgery** → Maintenance

2 mm or greater increase***** → Root Planing***
- Reduced probing depth → Maintenance
- Same probing depth
  - Radiographic bone loss → Osseous Surgery or Regenerative Procedures → Maintenance
  - No radiographic bone loss → Gingivectomy/ Gingivoplasty***** → Maintenance

* Baseline probing means:
 (1) The probing depths found at initial examination if no periodontal therapy is done OR
 (2) The probing depths found at least 1 year after periodontal therapy.

** This assumes the following:
 (1) Probing depths are 6 mm or greater and bleed upon probing.
 (2) The root surface has been root planed as thoroughly as possible using closed methods.
 (3) The patient is a good surgical candidate.

*** See root planing for patients with increased probing depths at maintenance for details.

**** This assumes the following:
 (1) That thorough root planing will be done at surgery.
 (2) Soft tissues only are removed.

***** This can represent a single event or a cumulative loss of 2mm or greater from baseline

Fig 6-1

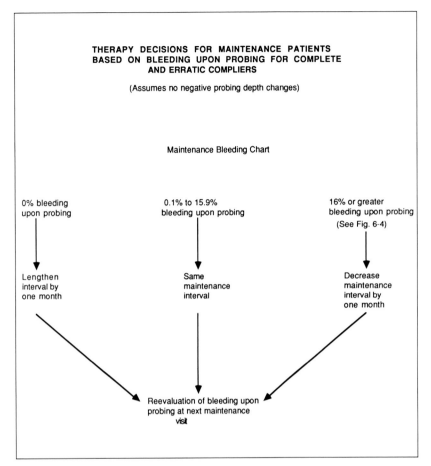

THERAPY DECISIONS FOR MAINTENANCE PATIENTS
BASED ON BLEEDING UPON PROBING FOR COMPLETE
AND ERRATIC COMPLIERS

(Assumes no negative probing depth changes)

Maintenance Bleeding Chart

0% bleeding
upon probing

0.1% to 15.9%
bleeding upon probing

16% or greater
bleeding upon probing
(See Fig. 6-4)

Lengthen
interval by
one month

Same
maintenance
interval

Decrease
maintenance
interval by
one month

Reevaluation of bleeding upon
probing at next maintenance
visit

Fig 6-2

PERCENTAGE BLEEDING TABLE

Total Number of Teeth	Total Number of Bleeding Sites Equal to 16%	Total Number of Teeth	Total Number of Bleeding Sites Equal to 16%
1	1	17	16
2	2	18	17
3	3	19	18
4	4	20	19
5	5	21	20
6	6	22	21
7	7	23	22
8	8	24	23
9	9	25	24
10	10	26	25
11	11	27	26
12	12	28	27
13	12	29	28
14	13	30	29
15	14	31	30
16	15	32	31

Fig 6-3 This table can be used to calculate 16% total bleeding. It assumes that there are six potential bleeding sites per tooth. As an example, if a patient with 32 teeth was found to have 31 or more total bleeding points, his or her maintenance interval would be shortened by 1 month (assuming that probing depths were stable).

Root planing for patients with increased probing depths at maintenance

Once the decision has been made to root plane in a setting other than at a routine prophylaxis (see Fig 6-2) this outline should be followed:

For most of these patients we provide the following:
1. Perform root planing with local anesthesia
2. Allow time for thorough cleaning (an hour per quadrant is average)
3. Reinforce oral hygiene
4. Eliminate any fremitus on the involved teeth
5. Where clinically or microbiologically appropriate, place the patient on an appropriate antibiotic(s) (for up to 3 weeks) or chlorhexidine (Peridex®) rinse (for at least 30 days)
6. Evaluate therapy at 30 days

Which dentist should take responsibility for maintenance?

The question of who should take responsibility for a patient's maintenance after a periodontist completes therapy often arises. Unfortunately, the issue is often decided on an economic basis rather than therapeutic basis. A rational solution to this problem has been suggested based on severity of disease[6]: patients with minimal disease should be seen by the referring dentist; patients with moderately active problems can be seen on an alternating basis; and patients with very severe chronic adult periodontitis can be seen by the periodontist with appropriate monitoring by the generalist. In addition, patients with localized juvenile periodontitis, rapidly progressive periodontitis, or refractory periodontitis should be seen by someone with advanced training in treating these periodontal diseases.

Responsibility for maintenance includes the necessity to monitor the disease accurately (see chapter 2), to provide adequate scaling and root planing, oral hygiene modification, elimination of fremitus, and to suggest re-treatment when appropriate.

───── *At a glance* ─────

The maintenance visit

- ■ The sequence below is for a routine maintenance visit for a patient with periodontal disease:
    - Review chart
    - Talk with patient
    - Update history
    - Examine head/neck, and mouth
    - Collect data
    - Control plaque
    - Remove subgingival accretions
    - Take radiographs
    - Remove supragingival accretions
    - Make future considerations for the patient
    - Set recall intervals by disease activity
- ■ At present, bleeding after probing and changes in probing depth offer the best indications of disease activity.
- ■ The question of who takes the responsibility for maintenance of patients after periodontal therapy can best be determined by severity and activity of disease. In general, the more active and severe the problem, the more often a therapist with advanced training should see the patient.

References

1. Rosling B, Nyman S, Lindhe J, Jorn B: The healing potential of the periodontal tissues following different techniques of periodontal surgery in plaque-free dentitions. A 2-year clinical study. *J Clin Periodontol* 1976;3:233.

2. Ramfjord SP, Morrison EC, Burgett FG, Nissle RR, Shick RA, Zann GJ, Knowles JW: Oral hygiene and maintenance of periodontal support. *J Periodontol* 1982;53:26.

3. Lindhe J, Nyman S: The effect of plaque control and surgical pocket elimination on the establishment and maintenance of periodontal health. A longitudinal study of periodontal therapy in cases of advanced disease. *J Clin Periodontol* 1975;2:67.

4. Goodson JM, Tanner ACR, Haffajee AD, Sornberger GC, Socransky SS: Patterns of progression and regression of advanced destructive periodontal disease. *J Clin Periodontol* 1982;9:472.

5. Lang NP, Joss A, Orsanic T, Gusberti FA, Siegrist BE: Bleeding on probing. A predictor for the progression of periodontal disease? *J Clin Periodontol* 1986;13:590.

6. Broline LE: Personal communication, 1987.

Chapter 7

Restorative Dentistry and Its Effect on Periodontal Maintenance

I. Periodontal-Restorative Interrelationships

Thomas G. Wilson, Jr

Knowledge of the interrelationship between periodontics and restorative dentistry is growing. The impact that dental procedures will have on the periodontium has become an important consideration in treatment planning the restorative case. It is now understood that it is difficult to perform any dental service (for a patient who has teeth) that does not affect the periodontium. The effect may be direct or indirect, short or long lasting, positive or negative, immediate or delayed, but periodontal health will be affected. The goal for the dentist should be simple—Do no harm. The integrity of a healthy periodontium should be uncompromised; the diseased state should be improved. The most sensitive indicator of the efficacy of restorations is their effect on the hard and soft tissues surrounding the tooth. The gingiva will let the professional know whether or not the contours and margin placement are biologically compatible with the soft tissues. Increased tooth mobility, fremitus (functional mobility), and widening of the periodontal ligament seen on radiographs will indicate whether undue forces have been placed on the teeth and periodontium. Monitoring probing depths before and after placement of restorations will show whether the attachment apparatus has been detrimentally affected.

The health of the periodontium also has a direct effect on restorative dentistry. Impressions for restorative procedures are more accurate and easier to take when there is minimal crevicular flow and no gingival bleeding. Patients with esthetic concerns don't appreciate gingival recession that exposes previously subgingival margins. And of course, a well-made prosthesis that must be removed because of periodontal problems benefits no one. The guidelines that follow are generalized, and they must be modified where indicated by the oral tissues. The restorative dentist makes the survival of the dentition possible or dooms it by the type, contour, and fit of the dentistry he or she delivers.

Access for personal and professional cleaning

Patients must be able to clean each tooth surface and the surrounding gingival crevice. Interproximal embrasures must be open enough for the patient (and the therapist) to get cleaning aids between the teeth and into the gingival crevice (Figs 7-1a and b and 7-2a and b). In addition, the contours replaced during restorative dentistry should at least reproduce the contours of the original tooth or, preferably, provide more access for oral hygiene than originally existed. The restoration should be flat or concave in the gingival two thirds of the restoration to facilitate plaque removal. Failure to provide access for cleaning can have far-reaching implications. In previously healthy sulci this allows a shift away from bacteria associated with health toward those found in periodontal disease (Figs 7-3a to d). This can occur within 1 or 2 weeks.[1] The implications for contours and cleaning accessibility in provisional restorations are obvious.

Emergence profile

Two major factors determine the contour of the fin-

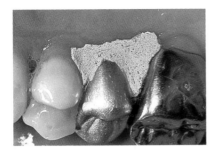

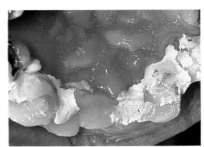

Figs 7-1a and b Two extreme examples of lack of access for oral hygiene—a preformed metal crown used as provisional restoration and an acrylic resin provisional fixed partial denture. The patients were informed that the cement was for retention and were instructed not to clean the area to avoid displacement of the restorations. This situation sets up the potential for a shift to more unfavorable bacterial populations with resulting periodontal problems.

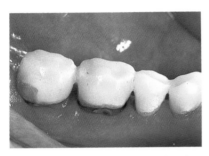

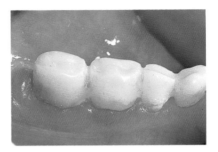

Fig 7-2a A more subtle situation than that shown in Figs 7-1a and b. In this case the contours of the provisional restoration do not allow interproximal cleaning and the thick subgingival margins aid plaque retention. The provisional restoration was intended for short-term use but was not replaced with a final prosthesis for a prolonged period. The provisional prosthesis is still in use 4 years after placement.

Fig 7-2b The tissue shrinkage resulting after improved access for cleaning, which was provided by thinning the provisional restoration, not by scaling or root planing.

Figs 7-3a to d A series of radiographs exposed over 11 years shows the problems created by overcontoured margins. The amalgam on the maxillary second premolar was placed just before the radiograph in Fig 7-3a was exposed. The bone appears healthy. Calculus could be seen (on the amalgam) 4 years later (Fig 7-3b). The restoration was replaced in 6 years but the root was not cleaned (Fig 7-3c), and bone loss continued and resulted in a 9-mm probing depth upon initial examination in our office (Fig 7-3d).

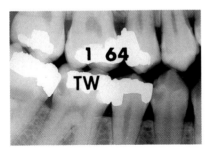

Fig 7-3a

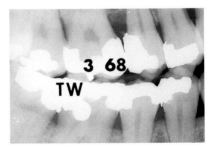

Fig 7-3b

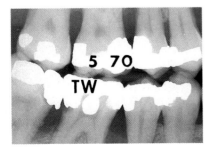

Fig 7-3c

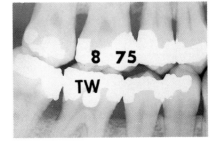

Fig 7-3d

Figs 7-4a to d Examples of various emergence profiles and their relation to gingival health in patients with optimal oral hygiene.

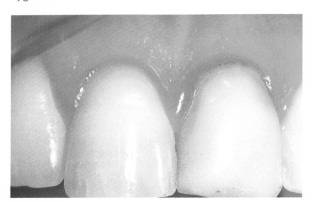

Fig 7-4a The gingival tissues have negatively responded to slightly overcontoured laminate veneers 90 days after placement.

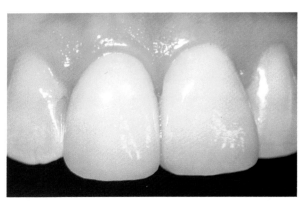

Fig 7-4b Three years after placement of similar restorations with a flatter emergence profile the gingival tissues remain healthy. (Restorative dentistry courtesy of Dr Robert L. Wasson.)

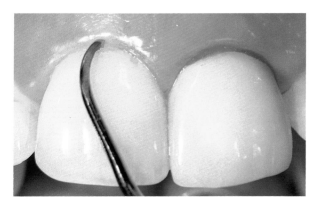

Fig 7-4c This crown on the right central incisor bleeds easily, whereas its natural counterpart remains healthy.

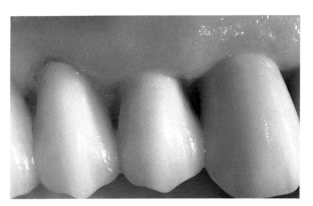

Fig 7-4d The tissues around crowns with subgingival margins remain healthy several years after placement. (Restorative dentistry courtesy of Dr Frank L. Higginbottom.)

ished restoration: adequate reduction of tooth structure and proper construction of the restoration. Overcontoured cast restorations usually result from underpreparation of the tooth in the gingival third. When the required thickness of restorative material is placed on the underprepared tooth, a bulge can occur subgingivally and at the site where the restoration emerges from the gingiva (the emergence profile). The emergence profile is flat in natural teeth, and this form should be mimicked in the restoration; otherwise, dental plaque will accumulate while the gingiva is forced into an unnatural position. These factors result in the periodontal problems so commonly seen around overcontoured crowns. Overcontours are commonly seen when the teeth are underprepared during esthetic dentistry procedures (Figs 7-4a to d).

Embrasures

To allow access for the patient to remove dental plaque, restorations should have proper embrasure form. To achieve this goal we suggest the following guidelines:

1. *Labial embrasures* should be open with the facial line angles not being placed too far interproximally. The contact area should be placed toward the facial aspect. Room must be left for the interproximal gingival tissue and to allow proper oral hygiene.
2. *Lingual embrasures* should be open for access to cleaning and to allow adequate room for the gingival tissues. With proper placement of the contact area toward the facial aspect, the lingual embra-

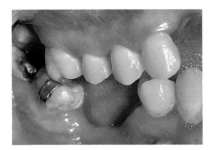

Fig 7-5a This 30-year-old patient was scheduled for full-mouth periodontal surgery and sought a second opinion.

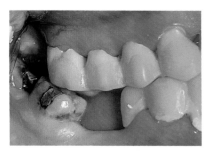

Fig 7-5b Because of poor plaque control, severe mobility, and fremitus, oral hygiene instruction, scaling and root planing, and provisional splinting were suggested. The patient was seen by her original dentist for provisional restorations.

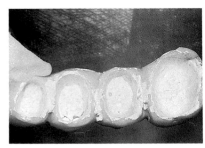

Fig 7-5c Closed embrasure spaces in the provisional restorations made interproximal oral hygiene impossible.

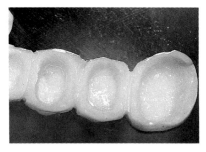

Fig 7-5d The provisional restorations were recontoured.

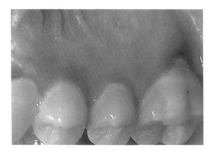

Fig 7-5e Because of inadequate tooth preparation, the embrasure spaces were still minimal, making cleaning most difficult. The interproximal tissues were still inflamed.

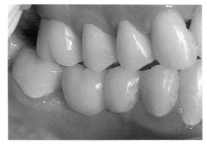

Fig 7-5f The patient opted to see another restorative dentist and had the teeth reprepared and new provisional restorations placed. The tissues responded well and periodontal surgical procedures were avoided in all but the molar areas. (Final provisional restorations courtesy of Dr Frank L. Higginbottom.)

sure will be accessible for cleaning. As with the labial embrasures, the lingual line angles should not be placed too far interproximally.

3. *Gingival embrasures* should be open for access to cleaning by placing the contact toward the occlusal or incisal aspect, leaving the gingival aspect open for access to plaque removal and sufficient space for the interproximal soft tissue.

Failure to follow these guidelines will lead to negative tissue responses (Figs 7-5a to f).

Pontic form

Pontics should have a contact with the ridge that is flat or convex while allowing complete cleaning with dental floss or other cleaning aids on the gingival surface of the pontic. A bullet-shaped pontic touching the ridge is good for mandibular posterior areas. In the maxilla a modified ridge lap design serves well.

Margin placement, fit, and the subcrevicular physiologic dimension (biologic width)

Margin placement

The best position for the margin of a restoration is 1 mm or more coronal to the free gingival margin.[2,3] The second choice is at the margin of the free gingiva.[4] Placing the margin in the gingival sulcus is always a compromise as far as the periodontium is concerned[5] in that it can lead to increased gingival crevicular fluid flow unless oral hygiene is optimal.[6] Also, the deeper the restoration is placed into the sulcus, the greater the degree of gingival inflammation caused.[7] If it is necessary to take the margin below the tissue, be sure that the gingival crevice is shallow and healthy. The finish line should then be placed about 1 mm apical to the crest of the gingival

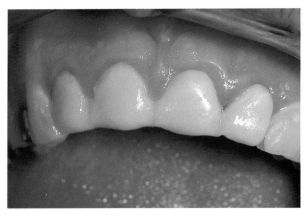
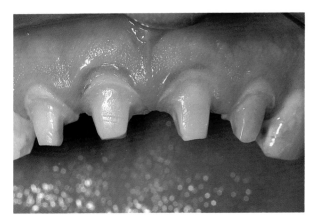

Figs 7-6a and b These provisional restorations extended past the preparation, violating the subcrevicular physiologic dimension (biologic width), resulting in gingival recession. In most cases this recession is not reversible.

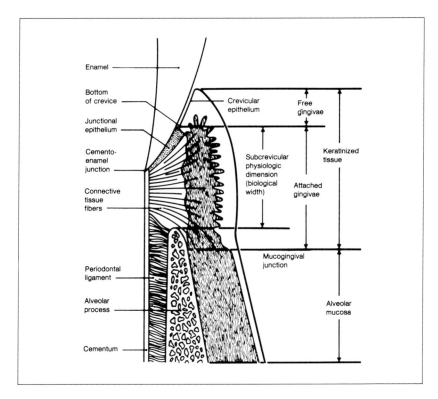

Fig 7-7 Diagram of the buccal portion of normal periodontium. Adapted from Wilson and Maynard.[8]

margin,[8] and it must be clinically perfect to avoid a rapid shift toward the bacterial populations associated with periodontal diseases.[9]

When a provisional restoration is placed, it should just cover the margins of the preparation and mimic the contours of the final restoration. Great care should be taken to fabricate a smooth, cleansable, well-fitting temporary restoration (Figs 7-6a and b).

Biologic width

In cases where a subgingival margin is necessary, extreme care must be taken to avoid impinging on the subcrevicular physiologic dimension (biologic width) (Fig 7-7). The biologic width is made up of the junctional epithelium (epithelial attachment) and the supraalveolar connective tissue found apical to the junctional epithelium.[10,11] This soft tissue attachment is found around all teeth and is probably constant for that patient in that area. The coronal-apical width ranges from 2 to 3 mm, with approximately half composed of junctional epithelium and half of connective

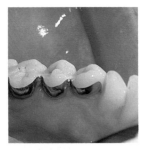

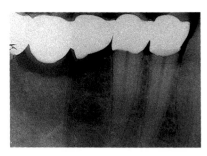

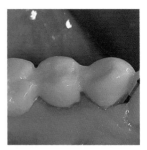

Figs 7-8a and b At her initial visit the patient was informed that she had no bone loss but the margins of the premolar crowns extended almost to the level of the alveolar bone. Crown lengthening was advised. The patient declined treatment. Despite excellent oral hygiene and dental prophylaxis every 3 months, bone loss and pocket formation ensued.

Fig 7-8c Provisional restorations were placed 4 years later and probing depths remained at 5 to 6 mm (the original probings were 3 mm).

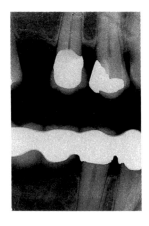

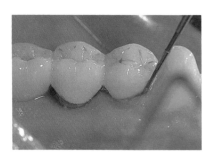

Figs 7-8d and e Crown lengthening was accomplished with osseous surgery, resulting in shallow probing depths and healthy tissue. (Final restorative dentistry courtesy of Dr Harry S. Wilbur.)

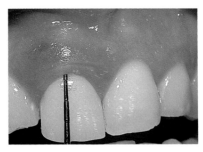

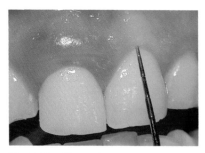

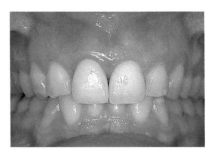

Fig 7-9a This patient presented with a chief complaint of gingival tenderness present since placement of a full crown on the maxillary right central incisor. When the facial surface of the tooth was explored, it was found that the tooth had been prepared several millimeters apical to the junctional epithelium (thus violating the biologic width), and bone loss was found, accompanied by 5 mm of probing depth.

Fig 7-9b The adjacent natural tooth had no inflammation or tissue hyperplasia.

Fig 7-9c After several rounds of closed scaling and root planing, the tissues healed and a provisional restoration was placed. (Final restorative dentistry courtesy of Dr Frank L. Higginbottom.)

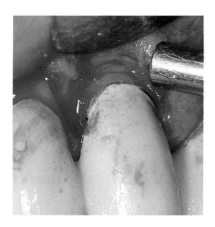

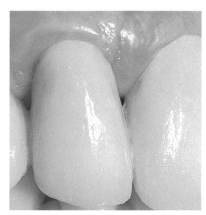

Fig 7-10a *(left)* This patient complained of tenderness that persisted after placement of a full crown, despite good oral hygiene efforts. When a flap was raised, only 1 mm of tooth structure was available for attachment of the soft tissues (biologic width).

Fig 7-10b *(right)* The tooth remains healthy and asymptomatic several years after 2 mm of facial bone was removed.

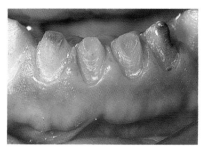

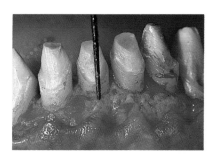

Fig 7-11a Shortened clinical crowns did not provide enough support for retention of full crown restorations.

Figs 7-11b and c Instead of impinging on the biologic width by carrying the margins into the soft tissue attachment, crown lengthening was performed.

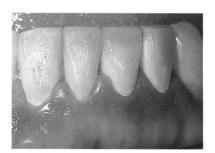

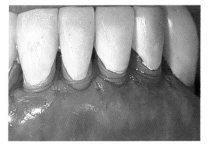

Figs 7-11d and e This produced increased clinical crown height compared to the preoperative view (Fig 7-11d) and the crown margins could now be placed in a position that would allow gingival health to be more easily maintained.

tissue fibers. This dimension tends to maintain itself even in the presence of disease or trauma. If this soft tissue is violated during restorative procedures, it may reform at a more apical level. In the medium or thick periodontium the crest of the free gingiva will usually remain in its original position, thus creating a periodontal pocket (Figs 7-8a to e and 7-9a to c).

This concept was clearly demonstrated by Tarnow and his group.[12] In their study, shoulder preparations were made at the gingival margins on the facial surfaces of teeth with chronic periodontitis but with probing depths of 4 mm or less in the test areas. A bevel was then intentionally prepared one half the distance between the apical extent of the clinical pocket and the coronal extent of the alveolar bone. Well-fabricated and fitted provisional restorations were then placed and the teeth and soft tissues removed in block sections from 1 to 8 weeks after placement of the temporary crowns. Histologic sections showed an apical progression of loss of soft tissue and bone resulting in a loss of attachment. In the thin periodontium this will result in gingival recession, and in a thicker periodontium pocket formation will occur. The biologic width that is violated only during the retraction phase will usually reattach if left undisturbed, but if a provisional restoration is placed on the area of the tooth previously occupied by the soft tissue, irreparable damage can occur within a few days (see Figs 7-6a and b). This means that neither preparation nor provisional restoration should invade the soft tissue. Similar problems can occur if the final restorations violate the biologic width. Where additional clinical crown length is needed, these problems can be avoided by apically positioning the soft and hard tissues before final crown preparation is performed. In cases where there is hyperplastic gingival tissue this can be accomplished by gingivoplasty. This hyperplastic tissue is rarely found in areas of esthetic concern and flap surgery with bone re-

moval is usually indicated (Figs 7-10a and b and 7-11a to e).

Marginal fit

The crown with inadequate marginal fit below the gingiva creates problems for the periodontium. It can result in radiographic bone loss,[13] loss of attachment,[14] and gingival inflammation.[15] This may be due to violation of the biologic width or more likely from increased retention of bacteria and their products.

At a glance

Margin placement, fit, and biologic width

- Gingival tissues require 2 to 3 mm of healthy tooth structure coronal to the alveolar crest to which to attach. This dimension is called the biologic width.
- All subgingival crown margins are a compromise and should not be used unless absolutely necessary.
- If you must place margins subgingivally, start with a healthy periodontium and place the margin 1 mm or less subgingivally.
- Subgingival margins that fit incorrectly lead to:
  - Change of microbial flora from healthy to disease-producing
  - Increased gingival inflammation
  - Apical migration of the junctional epithelium
  - Bone loss

Should you use removable or fixed restorations?

If the fabrication, placement, and maintenance of either of these classes of restoration are ideal, it will not matter to the periodontium which is used. However, in my practice removable devices seem to be more detrimental than fixed (Figs 7-12a and b and 7-13a and b). This may be because maintenance of removable devices is often not performed. In addition, removable devices usually cannot provide the type of rigid fixation desired in cases of advanced periodontal disease. In their defense, removable devices are easy to clean and more economical than fixed devices.

Trauma from occlusion as an etiologic factor in periodontal diseases

The idea that occlusion plays a part in the etiology of

periodontal diseases has been in the dental literature since the beginning of this century.[16] This concept was given a blow by the work of Orban and Weinmann[17] on human autopsy material when they concluded that there was no relation between occlusal trauma and pocket formation; however, later work suggested that this conclusion might be in error.[18]

Glickman and co-workers used histology to show what they believed to be signs in humans and animals that trauma from the occlusion caused the pathway of inflammation to change from midcrest of the alveolus to the periodontal ligament, thus creating angular defects.[19-23] These studies concentrated on the damage done to the alveolar bone. These works set the stage for a flurry of animal studies that looked at both alveolar bone and connective tissue reactions to trauma. For the most part, three animal groups were used: monkeys, beagle dogs, and humans.

Monkeys

Polson and co-workers[24,25] used the squirrel monkey

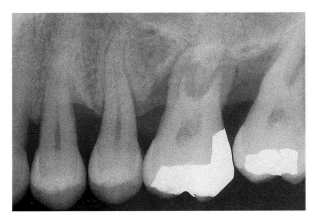

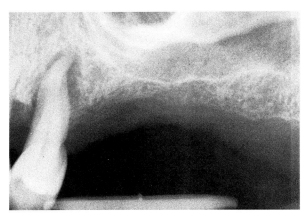

Fig 7-12a The radiograph was taken just before the removal of the molars and fabrication of a removable partial denture.

Fig 7-12b This view was taken 1 year after placement of the partial denture, showing radiographic evidence of trauma. The tooth was endodontically vital.

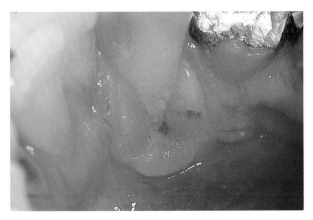

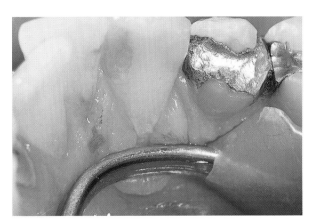

Figs 7-13a and b Soft tissue damage made by an ill-fitting, improperly designed removable partial denture.

for an experimental model in a series of studies. At first a single traumatic lesion was produced in the periodontal ligament using a heat probe. It was introduced 6 months after periodontitis was induced using silk ligatures. No difference was found between test and control animals as to connective tissue loss (pocket formation).

To study the effects of "jiggling" trauma, experimental periodontitis was produced and then large elastic ligatures were placed in the mesial or distal embrasure spaces. These ligatures were alternated on a regular basis, creating intermittent severe trauma. Periodontitis alone was compared to periodontitis plus trauma. In three of the four monkeys, trauma combined with periodontitis produced more radiographic and histologic evidence of bone loss, but there was no difference in the level of attachment.[26]

Later studies showed that when the periodontium was healthy but reduced, trauma had no effect on the level of the pocket.[27] Their conclusions were that one

should concentrate on reducing inflammation, not adjusting the occlusion.

Exceptions in monkey studies

There were exceptions to the rule that trauma played no part in pocket formation in monkeys. In Meitner's study[26] using four monkeys with induced periodontitis and superimposed jiggling forces, no significant differences were found in connective tissue loss in three of the four test areas when compared to controls. However, in one area (the distal area of the mandibular second premolar), significantly more loss of connective tissue was found compared to nontraumatized controls. In a second study performed years earlier, Waerhaug and Hansen[28] studied five monkeys on which they placed "high" gold crowns on teeth with surrounding gingivitis. Connective tissue loss was similar in the test area and in nonloaded controls except in one monkey. This monkey became ill during the study, so oral hygiene was discontinued. After the monkey recovered, the crown was removed 61 days after placement but oral hygiene was not restarted. After sacrifice it was found that the lingual surface of the control tooth on this monkey had a very deep pocket. These studies show that the data on monkeys indicate that trauma in these animals may be a co-destructive force in some cases.

Beagle dogs

Lindhe and Svanberg[29] did a series of studies on a colony of beagle dogs. One of the first studies included six dogs that had induced periodontitis from a soft diet. Later a cap splint that "jiggled" the test teeth was placed. Horizontal bone loss was found in both the test and control teeth. In the test teeth angular bony defects and apical migration of the junctional epithelium (pocket formation) were found. A later study showed that in reduced but healthy periodontia, occlusal trauma made no difference.[30] Their conclusions were that if the periodontium is kept healthy, then trauma from occlusion does not cause increased pocket formation. However, when both trauma and inflammation are present, they act as cofactors to "enhance the rate of progression of the disease."[31]

Humans

Clinical studies on humans are few where occlusal trauma is concerned. One study by Rosling et al[32] showed that when "hypermobile" teeth with surrounding severe periodontitis were treated with surgery followed by professional cleanings every 2 weeks for 2 years, complete healing of the surrounding bony defects occurred. This resulted in a gain of attachment level. The control group that received oral hygiene instruction initially and a professional cleaning every year lost attachment.

Another group studied 82 patients, 43 of whom were still in the study after 8 years. The patients were taken through initial therapy, which included oral hygiene, closed scaling and root planing, and occlusal adjustment. The patients then had open scaling and root planing, during Widman surgery or "pocket elimination" surgery. The following mobility criteria were used: M0—physiologic mobility, firm tooth; M1—slightly increased mobility; M2—definite to considerable increases in mobility but no impairment of function; M3—extreme mobility, a "loose" tooth that would be uncomfortable in function. Patients with M2 gained no new attachment after surgery, and those with M3 actually lost attachment. The authors attributed the

difference between their study and Rosling's study to the more effective plaque control seen in the Rosling group.[33]

In another paper, Pihlstrom and co-workers[34] evaluated 300 patients for the signs of trauma from occlusion and periodontitis. They found that teeth with mobility or fremitus had deeper pockets (more attachment loss) and more radiographic bone loss than teeth without these findings.

While there is still debate, the literature available on humans supports the association between periodontitis and trauma from occlusion. In addition, trauma may make a secondary contribution to gingival recession in patients who have a thin periodontium by causing dehiscences in thin buccal or lingual bone.[35]

In our practice we check and record clinical mobility and fremitus at the initial examination. We have found that many patients who have little clinical mobility exhibit fremitus. Once these problems have been identified, then we eliminate or ameliorate them. At present we try to treat all teeth with fremitus and clinical mobility of I+ and above. (For a discussion of the mobility scale, see chapter 2.)

In many of these patients elimination of mobility begins with a habit appliance. The device of choice is usually a maxillary hard acrylic resin guard that allows all of the mandibular teeth to touch in centric occlusion and has canine protection in lateral and protrusive movements. The patient is asked to wear this device when sleeping and to return 30 days later. If the patient reports that the guard is comfortable and if mobility of I or greater is still present or if the patient reports premature contacts immediately after removing the guard, then the occlusion is adjusted. Any remaining fremitus is removed at this time if possible. The adjustment begins by removing premature contacts in centric occlusion and then in lateral excursions. Occasionally maxillary and mandibular guards are needed in the same patient, when a single guard doesn't control mobility in the opposing arch.

When fremitus or mobility of Class II or greater cannot be eliminated in this manner, splinting is often needed in patients with uncontrolled disease or less than perfect compliance. This decision should not be made lightly because of the increased difficulty in cleaning and economic factors. The decision is easier when interproximal gingival recession is present, allowing use of an interproximal brush. Splinting can consist of either individual crowns joined together or an A-splint. This step usually coincides with reduction of gingival inflammation. Since better oral hygiene and subgingival scaling and root planing often reduce clinical mobility, the decision concerning the occlusion is often postponed until after the inflammation is reduced.

Trauma from occlusion as an etiologic factor in periodontal diseases

- A review of the current literature finds that in humans who do not clean optimally there is a good chance that trauma from occlusion superimposed on periodontitis exacerbates pocket formation when compared with patients whose teeth are not traumatized.
- In patients with generalized I+ tooth mobility or fremitus found after scaling and root planing who also have periodontitis, a maxillary hard acrylic resin bite guard is often helpful.
- If fremitus or mobility of I or greater is found after a bite guard has been used for 30 to 90 days, then occlusal adjustment is indicated in most of these cases.
- Splinting of teeth in humans with a II or greater mobility can be justified in patients who do not respond perfectly to active or maintenance therapy outlined in the first three steps. The advantage gained by splinting must be weighed against the increased difficulty in oral hygiene procedures.
- The decision to perform occlusal therapy is often postponed until after initial control of the inflammatory lesion.
- These steps are generalizations only—they must be individualized for each patient.

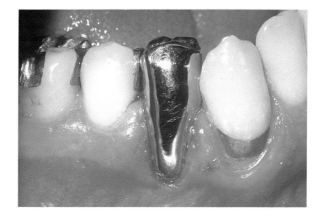

Fig 7-14 This crown had been redone several times because at that time regulations in the department where the work was performed required that full crown margins be carried below the soft tissue. Because there was no attached gingiva, the gingiva receded after each preparation and the work was redone. The free gingival margin was originally level with the adjacent tissue. (Photograph courtesy of Dr David Kaiser and the Graduate Periodontal Class of 1974 at the University of Washington.)

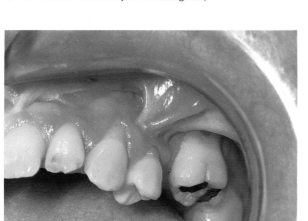

Fig 7-15a This patient had received a blow that resulted in intraoral tear. The results of the initial repair are seen.

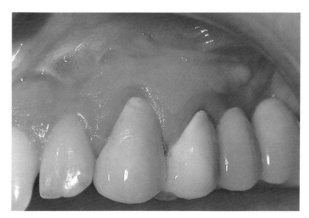

Fig 7-15b Before orthodontics and restorative dentistry were attempted, a free gingival graft was placed. (Restorative dentistry courtesy of Dr Harry S. Wilbur.)

Mucogingival considerations

Failure to recognize mucogingival problems can lead to less than optimal results in terms of health and esthetics (Fig 7-14), but intervention before restorative procedures can ameliorate or eliminate most of these problems (Figs 7-15a and b).

Whether a patient needs attached gingiva to sustain health has been the topic of much discussion. In people who clean well, minimal keratinized gingiva is needed.[36] The patients reported in these studies who did not have dental restorations at or below the gingival margin, were not undergoing orthodontic therapy, and who had inadequate home care and dropped from therapy showed continued recession.[36] In areas where restorative margins will enter the gingival crevice, the patient should have 5 mm of keratinized gingiva (2 mm of free gingiva and 3 mm of attached gingiva) (see Fig 7-7).[37] This suggestion seems to be supported by a study of restorations with subgingival

margins done in dogs[38] and by a recent study by Stetler and Bissada.[39] The latter study found more gingival recession in areas of inadequate attached gingiva.

At this time it seems prudent to have an adequate zone of keratinized and attached gingiva before restorative therapy is started in areas where recession should be retarded. This is especially true for those patients who have a thin periodontium or less than adequate oral hygiene or are less than perfect compliers to maintenance schedules (Fig 7-16). In clinical terms, those restorative patients whose gingiva is thin enough to allow the therapist to see a probe through the tissue are candidates for grafts before restorative margins are placed into the gingival sulcus (Fig 7-17).

Patients who are not having restorative dentistry or orthodontics (see chapter 8) come under different guidelines for maintaining the attached gingiva. Where no recession occurs from baseline, grafts

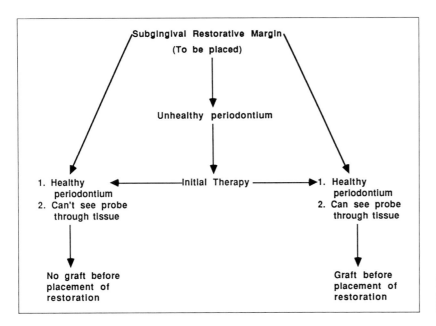

Fig 7-16 A decision tree for gingival grafting in restorative dentistry patients.

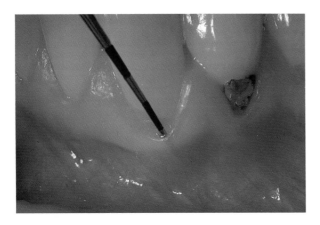

Fig 7-17 A thin periodontal probe can be seen through the soft tissue in an area where a subgingival margin will be placed. A soft tissue graft should be placed before restorative dentistry is begun.

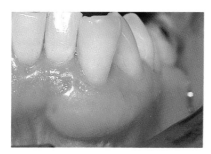

Fig 7-18a The gingival tissue had stripped away, leaving the root sensitive and the area at the depth of the vestibule tender and difficult to clean.

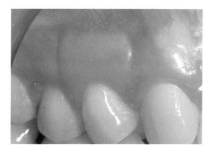

Fig 7-18b Because the tooth was not in trauma, was endodontically vital, and had no caries, a free gingival graft was placed. The grafted area is seen approximately 11 years after placement.

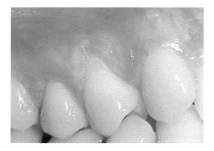

Fig 7-19a The facial surface of this premolar continued to strip away, causing a deformity that concerned the patient.

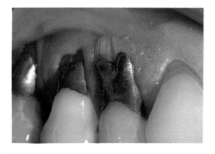

Fig 7-19b The area was repaired with a free gingival graft.

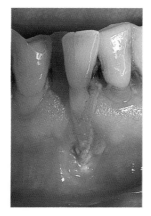

Fig 7-20a This area continued to strip away, and the longevity of the tooth has been shortened as a result. (Courtesy of Dr Curtis Becker.)

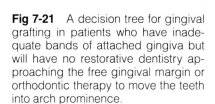

Fig 7-20b A second similar area is seen.

Fig 7-21 A decision tree for gingival grafting in patients who have inadequate bands of attached gingiva but will have no restorative dentistry approaching the free gingival margin or orthodontic therapy to move the teeth into arch prominence.

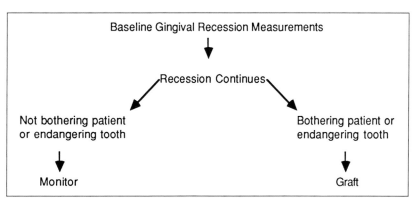

Baseline Gingival Recession Measurements

↓

Recession Continues

Not bothering patient or endangering tooth

Bothering patient or endangering tooth

↓

Monitor

↓

Graft

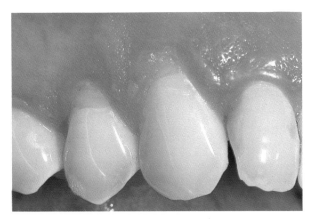

Fig 7-22a Esthetic concerns led this patient to have a free gingival graft placed to attempt coverage.

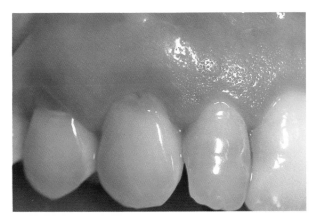

Fig 7-22b The patient dropped out of maintenance and reappeared 11 years later with a complaint of swelling in the area. (Suppuration can be seen at the orifice of the gingival crevice.)

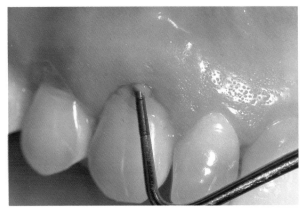

Fig 7-22c The graft, which originally had a probing depth of 3 mm, had become detached.

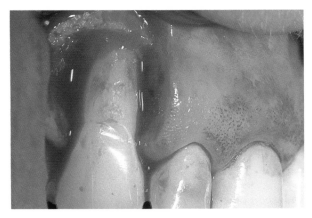

Fig 7-22d A replaced flap with root planing reattached the graft.

should not be placed regardless of the amount of attached gingiva present. The exception is the area that bothers the patient. When the area bothers the patient and recession is present, then grafts should be considered. Concerns of the patient could include thermal sensitivity (which could also be caused by occlusal trauma or caries), difficulty in cleaning (Figs 7-18a and b), esthetic deformities (Figs 7-19a and b), or recession that continues (Figs 7-20a and b). These can all warrant grafting (Fig 7-21).

With the finding that exposed roots could be routinely covered with free gingival grafts,[40,41] more of these procedures are being undertaken. Most are successful, but a small percentage will become detached (Figs 7-22a to d). You should be aware of this potential and check these grafts periodically.

- Procedures to gain attached and keratinized tissue should be considered in the following situations.
  - When gingival recession continues from a baseline measurement taken in health and the tooth may be lost
  - When the recession bothers the patient thermally or esthetically or creates a plaque trap
  - When a restorative margin will go below the gingiva and a periodontal probe placed in the sulcus can be seen through the tissue

II. Maintenance for the Removable Prosthesis

Eugene W. Dahl

The care provided by the patient and the dentist can directly affect the effectiveness of a prosthesis, which in turn affects the periodontium. The following section will deal with the maintenance of these devices. For completeness and because it applies to the overdenture, complete dentures are discussed.

Management of the removable prosthesis

The adaptation of a patient to a new dental prosthesis should be a controlled process. This portion of the treatment should be considered during treatment planning. The correct diagnosis and therapy are essential in managing the edentulous or partially dentate patient who is to receive a removable prosthesis.[42] There are some patients who have unrealistic expectations or emotional problems and cannot accept an artificial substitute for their natural dentition. These patients represent only a small portion of the total group of patients who are treated with removable prosthodontics.

The problems that occur after the delivery of a removable prosthesis should be considered as a part of the overall therapy, not the result of an incorrectly constructed prosthesis. If you have not compromised the basic prosthodontic principles of fabrication, which include (1) an accurate impression, (2) correct centric jaw relations, (3) correct vertical dimension of occlusion, (4) proper tooth selection and position, and (5) harmonious esthetics, then you can assume that comfort and function of the prosthesis can be attained by proper management of delivery and post-delivery problems.[43] If the basic principles have been followed, we will know we are not dealing with a defective prosthesis, but that it is a matter of patient adaptation to the prosthesis along with professional encouragement and care.

Instruction to the patient

At the time of denture delivery it is necessary to inform the patient that being able to speak, eat, and chew with the new prosthesis is a learned act. Inform the patient that there are millions of individuals wearing complete dentures who enjoy adequate comfort and efficiency with a removable prosthesis.[44] Written instructions should also be presented to patients at their dismissal to make them aware of all the potential obstacles they may encounter in mastering their new prosthesis. Figures 7-23 and 7-24 are examples of different sets of written instructions for patients with complete dentures, partial dentures, and immediate dentures.

INSTRUCTIONS FOR DENTURE PATIENTS

COMPLETE DENTURES: If all of your teeth in the upper jaw, lower jaw or both are missing, these teeth will be replaced by complete dentures. *Always bear in mind that no artificial replacement can possibly be as good as a sound set of natural teeth.* Complete dentures have many limitations, especially the lowers, and you must learn from experience what you can do and what you cannot do with your artificial teeth.

When you receive your new dentures, whether or not you have worn artificial teeth before, do not try to eat any foods that require hard chewing until after the necessary adjustments have been made and you have learned to use your dentures. It is advisable to read out loud to yourself to hasten your speech correction with new dentures.

Always remember that a complete lower denture is *much less* satisfactory than the upper, and for this reason we avoid as long as possible extraction of lower teeth that may serve to hold a partial denture.

Important: Regardless of what you may have been told in the past, *complete dentures should be left out of the mouth while you are sleeping.* They interfere with the normal circulation of blood in the underlying bone when left in the mouth all the time. Your mouth will tolerate dentures more comfortably for a much longer period of time if you will remove them when you sleep.

IMMEDIATE DENTURES: When all of your remaining teeth in either jaw are extracted and the teeth are replaced at the same appointment, the replacement is known as an immediate denture.

In the case of an immediate replacement, it is essential that you *do not attempt to remove it from your mouth.* You will be given an appointment for the following day at which time the dental practitioner will remove the denture and give you further instructions.

In *certain selected cases* an immediate denture has advantages over the conventional method of waiting for several weeks after extractions to construct the replacements. However, you must not try to eat any foods except those that require little or no chewing until after the soreness is gone from your mouth and the necessary adjustments have been made.

As healing progresses, your denture may become loose. This should be corrected by relining; otherwise, the tissues under the denture may become loose and flabby and the denture less stable.

CARE OF COMPLETE DENTURES

1. Before cleaning your dentures fill the washbasin with water. If you should drop them, water will break the fall, minimizing the danger of breakage. Clean your dentures at least twice a day with a soft toothbrush and facial soap.
2. Do not use scouring powder or abrasive hand soaps.
3. Do not place your dentures in hot water. Temperatures over 150° may warp them.
4. Dentures should be sterilized at least once a week. This can be done by placing them in a solution of household chlorine bleach.
5. Use one teaspoon of bleach to one cup of water; soak for 15 minutes.
6. To remove stains and calcium deposits (tartar), soak the dentures in full strength white vinegar for 15 minutes. If this is done regularly, stains are easily removed. If not, it may be necessary to leave dentures in vinegar for a longer period.
7. The vinegar can be used many times if it is stored in an airtight glass or plastic container.
8. If dentures are left out of the mouth more than 30 minutes, they should be stored in water.

PARTIAL DENTURES: When some but not all of your natural teeth are in good condition and in favorable locations, it is desirable to construct a partial denture. This has the advantage over a complete denture in that the remaining natural teeth will help to support and stabilize the teeth being replaced. This is especially important in the lower jaw as a complete lower denture is to be avoided as long as possible.

CARE OF PARTIAL DENTURES: Since a partial denture rests against natural teeth and has clasps that touch certain areas of the teeth, *the tendency toward decay of the teeth will be greater.* It is essential that you remove your partial denture after each meal, thoroughly clean it and your natural teeth. Be especially careful to clean the metal that touches the teeth. Do not use chlorine bleach to clean partial dentures since it will affect the metal. As with complete dentures, fill the washbasin with water to minimize the danger of breakage or warpage.

Fig 7-23

INSTRUCTIONS TO THE DENTURE PATIENT

Introduction
Nothing has been found to equal sound, natural teeth, but dental science has made great advancement in replacing them with artificial ones. A great deal of time and care is spent in the construction of these artificial substitutes to be certain they fit comfortably and harmonize with your facial contours. You must realize that you will have to expend even more time and effort to master the use of them. The successful use of your new dentures is dependent upon you and the effort you put forth to master them. You will undergo a period of "getting used" to them as you gradually overcome the usual feeling of awkwardness and self-consciousness. It will take determination and perseverance on your part to learn to master them, and the effort is well worthwhile. Remember that thousands of people wear dentures and you need not feel self-conscious about yours. Doubtless many of your friends have them without your being aware of it. Even your closest friends and family who know about your dentures will quickly forget if you do not remind them.

First Impressions
The first impression when the new dentures are placed in your mouth will be of fullness and looseness. This sensation will gradually disappear as the dentures settle into place, and your oral tissues become accustomed to them, and you will probably have difficulty in swallowing. The sensation of gagging also will be present. If you wear the dentures constantly except when sleeping, these difficulties will gradually disappear of their own accord. The sense of fullness will leave, the flow of saliva will decrease to normal, and the gagging sensation will cease and the feeling of looseness will disappear. You might notice a lack of taste at first.

Speech
You will probably notice a thickness in your speech, and you may perhaps lisp somewhat, perhaps even whistle your "s's" when you first attempt to speak with the new dentures. These difficulties usually correct themselves in a short time, merely through use. If you practice reading aloud in front of a mirror, the time will be considerably shortened. This will teach the tongue the new landmarks that must be touched in forming the various speech sounds, and will train the lips to relax, thus relieving the stiffness and muscular tightness so often felt at first. As a suggestion, try reading this information aloud in front of a mirror.

Appearance
At first you may think that your new teeth appear to be too prominent and too long. Remember that allowances must be made for the natural settling of the dentures and that the appearance will improve as they settle into place. For the same reason, the lips may appear too full and tend to change your facial expressions. However, as the dentures settle into place and the facial muscles relax, a more natural expression will result. If your former teeth did not have a pleasing appearance, you may have formed the habit of not opening your mouth very wide when talking or laughing. If this is so, try now to talk and laugh in a natural way before your mirror. You will be surprised how quickly it will restore your natural facial expression. In looking at yourself as other people see you, stand back about three feet from a wall mirror. Do not use a hand mirror.

Tenderness
You must expect some soreness and tenderness from your new artificial teeth. Sometimes pressure spots may be noticed immediately and these may be relieved by your dentist. Other tender spots may develop later, and will necessitate a return trip to your dentist for relief. Under no conditions cut or file the dentures yourself in order to relieve a sore spot. Take the dentures out of your mouth until you can arrange an appointment with your dentist, but be sure to replace them in your mouth at least two hours before keeping your appointment. You may bite your tongue or cheek at first. This usually corrects itself; however, if it persists, consult your dentist.

Eating
Patience, practice, and a fixed determination to succeed will be required to learn to eat with your new teeth. The patient who refuses to become discouraged is the one who best learns to use them. In chewing, your first attempts will be awkward. Start with soft foods which require very little chewing, and take small portions. Avoid sticky foods. Bread is difficult to chew. Crisp crackers or toast are less difficult. As the mouth tissues grow accustomed to their new task, more solid foods may be attempted. In biting through a morsel of food, do not bite with your front teeth and tear off the food, as you did with your natural teeth. You will dislodge your denture at the back. Instead, do a lot more chewing with your knife and fork on your plate.

Fig 7-24 Continues on p 114.

These points will help you.

1. Put your teeth together firmly and swallow frequently. This seats the dentures into place.

2. Take smaller morsels of food, so that the mouth is not opened too wide.

3. After chewing and swallowing, swallow again to seat the denture and to prepare it for the next morsel of food.

4. Do not attempt to bite off food such as apples, corn-on-the-cob, or celery by clenching the food with the teeth and pulling with your hand. Rather, cut or break the food into small pieces and place in the mouth.

5. Chew slowly and thoroughly.

6. At first, it may help you to balance the lower denture and to keep it seated in position if you learn to chew on both sides at once. As you become more adept, you will find it possible to chew on either side you wish.

7. Remember that the muscles and tissues of your jaws, lips, cheeks, and tongue must become accustomed to your new teeth before you can expect to become efficient in using them to chew hard foods.

8. Don't overdo the act of biting. Don't bring too much pressure on your gums by eating extremely tough, hard foods.

9. Too vigorous chewing may injure the tissues and cause conditions that result in gum shrinkage. This may result in your denture resting unevenly in your mouth and interfering with chewing efficiency.

10. Avoid nervous habits with your dentures such as "chewing" or "tripping" them. These habits are extremely hard to break when once established.

Fig 7-24 Continued from p 113.

Postinsertion appointments

Adjustments on the new dentures are anticipated and appointments should be scheduled at the delivery appointment. The appointments should be scheduled at 24 hours and the 3rd, 6th, and 9th postinsertion days.[45] When the patient presents for the first postinsertion appointment, you should have scheduled sufficient time to:

1. Correct any areas of mucosal irritation using pressure-indicating paste and disclosing wax
2. Perfect the occlusal relationship in centric relation, protrusive, and lateral relations
3. Give further encouragement

At the adjustment appointment, a differential diagnosis should be made as to the cause of the irritation. The most common complaints and the corrections required are shown in Table 7-1.

Oral health care

The patient must be made aware that the denture and also the soft tissue must be maintained for a healthy oral cavity.[46] Plaque and associated microorganisms on the tissue surface of the dentures are significant factors in the pathogenesis of denture stomatitis.[47–49] A routine denture cleaning regimen should be designed to remove and prevent reaccumulation of microbial plaque and to remove mucin, food debris, calculus, and exogenous discoloration.[50] There are many different methods to clean dentures:

1. Mechanical denture cleansing with a brush
2. Pastes and powder
3. Ultrasonic agitation
4. Chemical denture cleansing with alkaline peroxide or alkaline hypochlorite[51]

A brush, soap, and tap water is an effective mechanical cleansing method in maintaining denture hygiene. Acrylic resin is wear resistant, provided that a proper brush is used.[52,53] There is no experimental evidence that brushing with a toothpaste or polishing paste is more efficient than using soap.[47] A paste with an abrasive such as polymethyl methacrylate or sodium bicarbonate and a soft brush is recommended for removing plaque from the denture. The patient should be instructed to brush the denture thoroughly because plaque is difficult to remove.

Many commercial chemical denture cleansers are available. One study by Ghalichebaf et al[54] found that Mersene® (Richardson-Vicks, Inc) was the most effective agent in removing plaque from the denture

Table 7-1 Most common complaints about dentures and their corrective measures (continued on p 116)

Complaint	Causes	Treatments
Clicking	1. Tight lower lip (this may raise the dentures; try thinning lower labial flange) 2. Patient may not have had posterior teeth for some time (and may have been accustomed to carrying the mandible close to the maxilla) 3. Vertical dimension too great 4. Lack of retention and stability 5. Protrusive occlusion associated with the centric relationship	1. Check anterior mandibular denture flange for length and thickness 2. Carefully check vertical dimension; check for interocclusal distance; correct by grinding or resetting posterior teeth, or remake one denture 3. Replace mandibular second molar with acrylic resin teeth; place them out of occlusion in centric relation; space second molars equal to horizontal overbite 4. Correct centric occlusion 5. Patient remount of occlusion with new centric relation and protrusive records
Loose denture (drops when mouth is opened)	1. Premature contact in the second molar region; this may drive the maxillary denture forward 2. Case may have been closed during fabrication or grinding; this will cause premature contact of the teeth in centric and will drive the maxillary denture forward 3. Centric occlusion associated with a protrusive relationship 4. Weak post-dam 5. Overcompression of tissues of rugae and anterior to posterior palatine foramina 6. Overextension of flanges 7. Too long posteriorly	1. Reset mandibular second molars 2. Recheck centric, remount, and regrind occlusion 3. Patient remount of occlusion with new centric relation and protrusive records 4. Repost dam 5. Relieve area of overcompression 6. Carefully trim flanges 7. Shorten denture posteriorly
Loose denture (drops when chewing on one side)	1. Patient equation (patient has not learned to manipulate the tongue, cheeks, and lips) 2. Posterior teeth may be set too far buccally 3. Incorrect angulation of the posterior teeth (these teeth may be set with a lingual inclination) 4. Maxillary denture riding on median raphae 5. Lack of adaptation on side opposite to one being used 6. Lack of balance on side opposite to one being used 7. Faulty occlusion	1. Instruct patient as to his or her capabilities 2. Reset posterior teeth; may try reducing buccal cusps 3. Reduce buccal cusps 4. Reduce pressure in median raphae 5. Readapt flange area by adding material 6. Regrind occlusion 7. Regrind occlusion
Saliva gets under denture	1. Interference in lateral occlusion (causes a temporary shifting of the denture and saliva gets in) 2. Peripheral borders of denture too thick and square	1. Regrind occlusion 2. Trim and round over flanges

tissue surface in a 15-minute period. The second most effective cleansing solution was Calgon® (Beechman Products) with Clorox® (Clorox Co), but there was no statistically significant difference between Mersene and Calgon. The danger with the Calgon and Clorox solution is that hypochlorite cleaners may bleach the acrylic resin and may damage a cobalt-chromium alloy.[55]

Table 7-1 Continued

Complaint	Causes	Treatments
Denture is tight, then drops	1. If sudden, the trouble is mechanical 2. If slow, it may be saliva (thick, ropey saliva) 3. Overcompression of rugae and blood supply 4. Overextension posteriorly	1. Recheck and grind in occlusion 2. Rinse mouth with weak vinegar or lemon solution; physical checkup by physician 3. Relieve overcompression 4. Shorten posteriorly
Whistling	1. Labial frenum may be impinged 2. Uneven contour and thickness just lingual to anterior teeth 3. Lack of contour lingual to maxillary molars	1. Trim labial frenum area 2. Trim or add material lingual to maxillary anterior teeth 3. Add contour lingual to maxillary molars
Looseness of mandibular denture	1. Unbalanced occlusion 2. Shape and thickness of flanges incorrect 3. Overextended flanges from premolar to premolar on labial surface 4. Overextension of lingual flange distal to premolar area 5. Overextension of posterior border (interference with pterygomandibular raphae area) 6. Lack of sublingual extension	1. Regrind occlusion 2. Reshape flanges 3. Shorten flanges where indicated 4. Shorten flanges where indicated 5. Shorten flanges where indicated 6. Correct adaptation on lingual flange
Soreness of mandibular denture	1. Lack of extension and general overall retention 2. May result from areas of infection and root tips remaining in the denture-bearing area (if ulcer is perforated, it indicates a root tip in position) 3. Unbalanced occlusion (especially during lateral excursion of the mandible) 4. Vertical dimension too great 5. Teeth too large 6. Posterior teeth carried too far distally 7. Flabby or fibrous ridge tissue 8. Closure of bite due to settling (this causes an unbalanced occlusion) 9. Premature contact of second molars (causes soreness in lingual anterior region) 10. Locked occlusion (buccal cusps may be dragging in lateral excursion) 11. Case closed during grinding (will cause teeth to strike heavily on mesial inclines of mandibular teeth, causing soreness on inside of labial flanges)	1. Readapt to tissues (make new impression) 2. Remove root tips and areas of infection 3. Regrind occlusion 4. Decrease vertical dimension (by grinding, resetting teeth, or redoing) 5. Reset with smaller teeth or remove second molars 6. Remove mandibular second molars 7. Check impression technique 8. Recheck and regrind occlusion 9. Remove mandibular second molars 10. Shorten buccal cusps of maxillary denture 11. Recheck and regrind occlusion
Biting cheeks	1. Posterior teeth edge to edge 2. Posterior teeth carried too far buccally 3. Too much interocclusal distance 4. Loose denture bases	1. Round over buccal cusps of mandibular posterior teeth 2. Reset posterior teeth 3. Decrease interocclusal distance (reset posterior teeth or remake mandibular denture) 4. Correct adaptation of denture bases

- When treatment of the edentulous or partially dentate patient commences, discuss with the patient the problems he or she may encounter in accommodating to a removable prosthesis.
- A cooperative and informed patient is the key to success in adjusting to and maintaining a healthy oral cavity.
- Regular visits after delivery of the dentures allow inspection of the oral tissues, evaluation of the occlusion, monitoring of TMJ function, and changes in bony contours that may result in soft tissue impingements.
- Maintenance of a removable prosthesis is a dynamic process requiring participation of both patient and dentist.

III. Maintenance for Fixed Prosthodontics

Frank L. Higginbottom

Much of traditional dental practice is directed toward reconstructing lost tooth structure. In the past, little attention has been given to maintaining and extending the useful life of restorations. Because we have materials that are capable of extended wear, and because patients are demanding greater longevity for their restorations, it behooves us to reverse this trend. To help in this direction when formulating our treatment plan, we must consider the patient's ability to maintain the restorations we recommend. At the time a diagnosis and treatment plan are presented, you should begin to educate the patient about maintenance and its importance. This section will focus on problems that are encountered during the maintenance of dental restorations and present possible solutions. To facilitate this process, each prosthesis should be examined clinically at every maintenance visit and radiographically once a year.

The functional life of a restoration

The functional life of any dental restoration has two definitions: yours and the patient's. We have all seen patients who choose to extend the life of a dental restoration past the time that the professional considers prudent. Your task is to decide where pathology exists and whether this necessitates replacement

or repair, and then to inform the patient of the situation. These recommendations should take into account the longevity of both the patient and the dentition. In these situations we must understand our limitations and inform the patient of the difference between repair and replacement. We should ask ourselves whether repairs can adequately satisfy the same parameters as a new restoration. Can a repair provide:

1. Proper occlusion?
2. Cleansable contours?
3. Protection of existing teeth and tooth structure?
4. Proper esthetics?
5. Reduced maintenance in the future?

Composite resin restoration

Over the years much progress has been made in the field of tooth-colored filling materials. These restorations have a variable life expectancy that depends on proper diagnosis, the material, the placement technique, and maintenance.

Microleakage

All restorations have different rates of expansion and

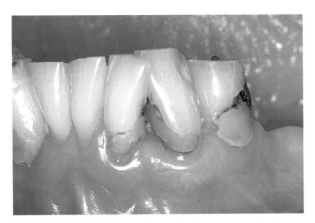

Fig 7-25 Microleakage in early to advanced stages leading to caries undermining of the composite resin restoration.

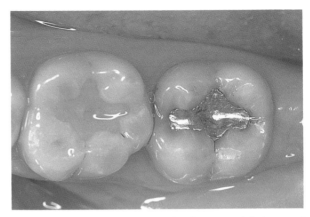

Fig 7-26 Loss of surface integrity due to particle loss and occlusal contacts of posterior restorations. Newer materials have fewer problems but still need to be maintained closely.

contraction relative to natural tooth structure. Thermal changes and functional stresses lead to marginal leakage. This problem can be reduced with proper bonding techniques and correct placement of the composite resin material. Also, protective liners need to be placed under all composite resins. However, even then, the possibility of failure exists. The first sign of this failure is staining of the cavosurface margin. As microleakage proceeds, discoloration undermines the restoration. This may first appear in areas where there is a "flash" of restorative material over unetched tooth structure. To reduce this problem, these areas should be smoothed to proper contour and polished at the time of placement or when discovered at a maintenance visit. When these areas of stain extend below the cavosurface, you must determine the extent of the microleakage and whether the restoration should be replaced, repaired, or observed at future visits (Fig 7-25). Most Class III restorations can be as easily replaced as repaired. Therefore, when these restorations appear to discolor because of undermining, they should be replaced with a newer hybrid material or a microfil composite resin. Posterior composite resins should be approached more aggressively when leakage is apparent. Leakage around these restorations will progress more rapidly because of increased occlusal stresses. There is therefore a greater possibility of leakage in Class II restorations, leading to undermining, eventual fracture, and possible pulpal involvement.

Loss of surface integrity

Loss of surface particles, which results in a rough surface and loss of occlusal contact, is seen particu-

larly in composite resins with larger filler particles used in posterior restorations. Large posterior composite resin restorations in stress-bearing regions are discouraged because friction, occlusal stress, and hydrolysis increase the breakdown rate (Fig 7-26). Newer materials such as hybrid composite resins limit these problems but should still be closely monitored.

Esthetics

Most composite resins eventually discolor. Fillers are lost, resulting in a roughened surface that attracts pellicle, plaque, and stain. This is a particular problem in older composite resin materials and shortens their useful life. This problem has been largely solved by microfil and hybrid composite resin materials, which have little surface loss. These new restorations produce a smoother surface, which may extend their life. When the patient with an existing restoration says that esthetics is a concern, replacement is the best choice. In Class V applications, surface roughness of these restorations is irritating to the gingiva, so margins should always be kept at least 1 mm coronal to the soft tissue. Replacement with microfil or hybrid composite resins is preferred in these areas (Fig 7-27).

Fracture

Fracture of an existing composite resin restoration may result from structural problems related to material strength or preparation design. The surrounding tooth structure should be evaluated for fracture or potential fracture before a replacement restoration is chosen (Fig 7-28). Despite claims of the composite

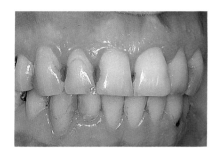

Fig 7-27 Surface roughness due to particle loss and leading to staining in anterior restorations. Replacing these restorations is usually better than repair.

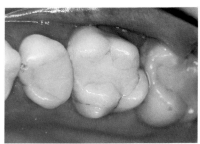

Fig 7-28 Failure of large posterior composite resin restorations that were inadequate at time of placement. For occlusal support and protection of surrounding tooth structure, these restorations are inadequate.

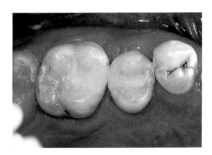

Fig 7-29 Conservative Class I and II posterior composite resin restorations are preferred because these materials do not support the occlusion or tooth structure well.

resin restoration's strengths, we must rely on sound restorative principles and cavity design for proper support and protection of remaining tooth structure. We sometimes fall victim to the patient's esthetic demands when selecting a restorative material and overestimate the material's durability. Guidelines for use of composite resin restorations to reduce problems include:

1. *Class I and II* restorations: use a hybrid or a large-particle composite resin; replace with a similar composite resin when the size of the restoration justifies replacement
2. *Class III* restorations: use microfil or hybrid composite restorative material for initial use and replacements
3. *Class IV* restorations: for initial and replacement uses, select a hybrid composite resin or a hybrid base veneered with microfil for esthetics; many Class IV restorations require a crown to protect the tooth adequately; composite resin should not be used in these situations
4. *Class V* restorations: microfil or hybrid composite resin is the proper choice for initial and replacement uses
5. *Direct composite resin veneers:* repair chipped or worn areas with microfil or hybrid composite resin and smooth any rough areas with disks; polish with Sof-Lex® disks (3M Dental Products Div)—*don't use prophy paste*

Composite resin placement

1. Prepare the tooth adequately for proposed restoration
2. Place pulpal protection with CaOH in deep areas
3. Place glass ionomer lining cement after conditioning dentin with polyacrylic acid

4. Acid etch all enamel
5. Apply dentin and enamel bonding agent
6. Place composite resin incrementally, allowing time for adequate curing of each addition
7. Finish

When placing posterior composite resin restorations, whether Class I or Class II, keep them small (Fig 7-29). They are not designed to support occlusion or protect unsupported tooth structure. If there is doubt, consider another restorative material, or place a crown.

Maintenance of the composite resin restoration

At each maintenance visit, evaluate the composite resin restoration for surface smoothness, marginal adaptation, and appearance. Where deficiencies exist, either polish, patch, or replace the restoration. Certain prophylactic procedures can create problems for composite resin restorations. Polishing with pumice will dull the surface and should be avoided. If polishing is necessary, it should be done with diamond polish, Sof-Lex disks, or commercially available composite polishing pastes. Commonly used prophylactic devices, such as air-powder abrasive machines and ultrasonic scalers, can be deleterious to these restorations.

Amalgam restoration

Amalgam has traditionally been the material of choice for posterior, tooth-confined Class I, II, and V restorations. Even with all its problems, this material has saved more teeth than any other. Properly placed and handled, it is most predictable and its shortcomings

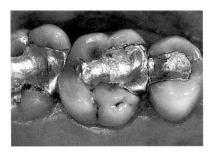

Fig 7-30 Cavosurface microleakage and ditching associated with breaking down of amalgam. These areas should be smoothed and polished to extend the life of the restoration.

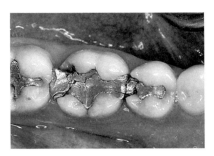

Fig 7-31 Fracture of restorations and surrounding tooth structure caused by large amalgam restorations with inadequate cuspal support.

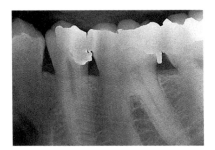

Fig 7-32a Large amalgam restorations with inadequate proximal contours.

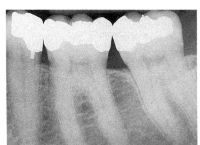

Fig 7-32b Correction with new properly contoured amalgam restorations.

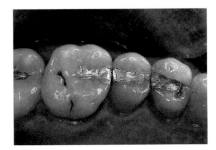

Fig 7-33 Properly prepared and placed amalgam restorations 7 years after placement.

are few. Its most serious physical property problems have been eliminated by the use of high copper–content alloys. Flow, creep, tarnish, and corrosion have been all but eliminated by reduction and elimination of the gamma 2 phase in the new alloys. However, the question of mercury contamination is still unresolved. You should evaluate this problem and reduce exposure where possible. The problems of thermal conductivity and appearance still exist, and the search for a suitable replacement continues.

Microleakage

Early breakdown is seen with ditching at the cavosurface (Fig 7-30). Many times microleakage is blamed, when in fact the problem is the breaking off of overextended areas, creating a rough margin. Roughness of these areas can be smoothed and repolished to extend the restoration's life. Softening or discoloration at the junction between the restoration and tooth structure caused by microleakage is an indication of caries. Radiographic evidence of leakage at the pulpal and gingival floor is an additional sign of failure. When radiographic evidence of failure exists, the restoration must be replaced.

Fracture

Fracture of the amalgam or surrounding tooth structure indicates failure of the restoration. When planning for replacement, you must consider the cause of the failure. When there is a fracture across the isthmus of a Class I or II restoration, suspect improper preparation design. Also, when any restoration extends more than one third the width from cusp tip to cusp tip, the tooth is significantly weakened. Therefore, when deciding between replacing or maintaining an existing amalgam restoration, consider its size and how much tooth structure will remain after removing the existing amalgam, unsupported tooth structure, and caries. Cracks or fractures in the surrounding tooth structure suggest that an amalgam restoration would not be an adequate replacement. An onlay or crown is indicated to protect the tooth adequately from future fracture (Fig 7-31).

Creep and flow relative to contour

Much has been said about creep and flow and their relation to amalgam failure. Interproximal overhangs and overcontouring resulting from these problems greatly shorten the restoration's life expectancy. They

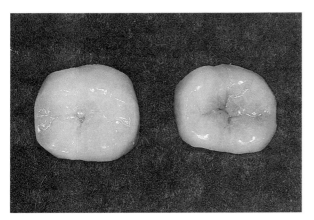

Fig 7-34a Conservative etched porcelain restorations with adequate cuspal support.

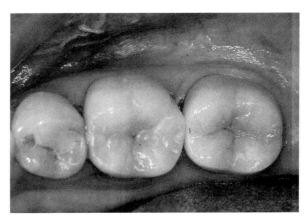

Fig 7-34b Immediately after placement.

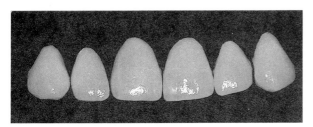

Fig 7-35a *(above)* Etched porcelain, composite resin–bonded restorations.

Fig 7-35b *(right)* The restorations a few months after placement, showing the positive response of the gingival tissues.

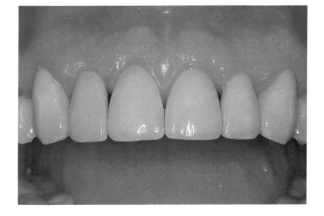

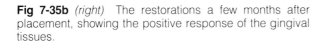

also create periodontal problems. When these problems occur, the patient does not have adequate access for removing plaque, which leads to periodontal breakdown, marginal tarnish, corrosion, and caries. Even though these areas could be maintained, they are doomed. You can attempt to remove or recontour these areas; however, this is rarely adequate or possible. The best time to create adequate proximal contours is at placement. Therefore, most amalgams with deficient contours need to be replaced (Figs 7-32a and b).

Maintenance of amalgam restorations

At maintenance visits, inspect amalgam restorations for signs of failure, areas of roughness, overhangs, and ditching. Polish the amalgam with pumice and Amalgloss (L.D. Caulk Co) to create a smoother, less plaque-retentive surface. If for some reason overhangs cannot be replaced they can be minimized by ultrasonic instrumentation, rotary or reciprocating handpieces, and abrasive strips. These measures will do much to extend the restoration's life (Fig 7-33).

Etched porcelain, composite resin–bonded restoration

Recently a great deal of information has surfaced regarding the use of porcelain inlay and onlay restorations and their anterior counterparts, porcelain laminates. These restorations are etched and then bonded to etched tooth structure using composite resin. Advocates claim conservative preparation of tooth structure and added protection from fracture resulting from bonding of the composite resin to the tooth and the restoration. The chances are good that this form of treatment will initially be overused and extended beyond its designed application. More traditional application of preparation design may be necessary to avoid tooth and restoration fracture and to protect the cusps. Maintenance includes smoothing any roughened marginal areas. Care should be taken in using ultrasonic instrumentation around these restorations. Clinical and radiographic examination of marginal areas for microleakage should also be performed (Figs 7-34a and b and 7-35a and b).

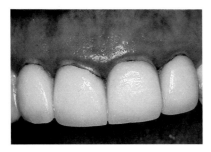

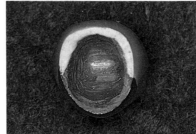

Fig 7-36 Marginal failure seen around fixed restorations; repair should be considered only if adequate marginal integrity and contour can be ensured.

Figs 7-37a and b Porcelain shoulder in conjunction with porcelain-fused-to-gold restorations. These margins can be fractured by ultrasonic cleaners or rough handling with curettes.

Full crown restoration

The full or partial veneer crown itself usually poses few maintenance problems. Besides crown displacement or occlusal adjustment, you should consider the following.

Recurrent caries in marginal areas

Where areas of decay occur at crown margins that are accessible, repairs may be possible. When the crown is otherwise satisfactory and there is access for caries removal and restoration placement, a gold foil, composite resin, or amalgam-reinforced glass ionomer may be placed to render the crown functional for an additional period. Amalgam is not satisfactory because of its increased tendency for tarnish and corrosion caused by dissimilar metals. Gold foil, while an ideal replacement, is not as practical because of access and difficulty in placement. Therefore, the best choice for repair is one of the newer composite resin materials or glass ionomer cement. Repair should be considered only if the placement can ensure adequate marginal integrity and contour (Fig 7-36).

Care for marginal integrity

Scaling and root planing around metal crown margins should be done where possible with a circumferential stroke to avoid disturbing the margin. Ultrasonic scalers should not be used. You should be very gentle (yet thorough) when root planing around porcelain labial margins and around porcelain jacket crowns. Avoid using ultrasonic scalers (Figs 7-37a and b).

Porcelain fracture

Today, with our increased concern for esthetics, a greater number of porcelain and metal ceramic restorations are being placed. When porcelain fracture occurs, it does not always render the restoration nonfunctional or unesthetic. These problems should be evaluated individually to determine whether the restoration can be smoothed, or whether repair or replacement is necessary. Many areas can be repaired with composite resin or porcelain repair kits. These repairs should not be considered to be as good as the original restoration. If a fracture occurs that is attributable to framework failure, any repair will have questionable longevity, and it might be better to replace the restoration and correct any underlying discrepancy in preparation and framework design. Also, if occlusal forces were judged to be the cause for failure, those factors should be altered or corrected (Fig 7-38).

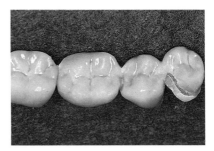

Fig 7-38 Fractured porcelain-fused-to-metal restorations (on the first premolar) associated with improper framework design.

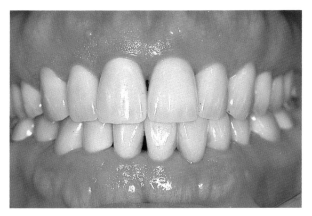

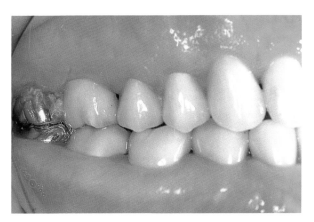

Figs 7-39a to c Multiple single fixed restorations with good contour to allow the patient to clean and maintain periodontal health.

Fig 7-39b

Multiple restorations

Special considerations apply to the maintenance of multiple restorations. Closer supervision than that used for patients with individual crowns is needed. Patients should be instructed to report any changes in their mouth. These changes would include gingival or tooth soreness, bleeding when cleaning, and sensitivity to thermal changes. Additionally, if the patient detects a bad taste emanating from a restoration, he or she should be encouraged to inform you prior to the regular maintenance visit. Patients with multiple restorations should have special attention paid to their occlusion at maintenance and in some instances may need to wear habit appliances to minimize occlusal trauma. This serves to protect restorations and a compromised periodontium (Figs 7-39a to c).

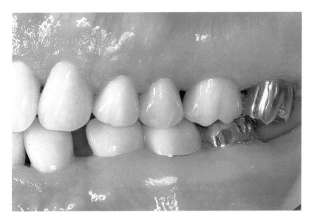

Fig 7-39c

Full-mouth fixed restorations

Maintenance of full-mouth fixed restorations should be minimal if the patient adheres to suggested oral hygiene and maintenance intervals. Evaluate wear and occlusion at each maintenance visit and make adjustments where appropriate. Full-mouth radiographs should be taken at regular intervals (at least every 2 years) to assess interproximal and periapical areas for problems. The patient should understand before therapy begins that repair or replacement of part or all of the restorations may be necessary in their lifetime. The frequency of repairs depends on the difficulty of the restoration, the patient's age, the number of missing teeth, the amount of supporting bone, the patient's bruxing and clenching habits, and adherence to suggested personal oral hygiene and maintenance schedules (Figs 7-40a to c).

Long-span fixed partial dentures

Special attention should be given to long fixed partial dentures, particularly to the possibility that one abutment may become displaced, or that connectors in the pontic areas may fail. Checks in the porcelain indicating framework failure should be noted and the patient informed. The patient's admission of problems or symptoms can be an insight to possible problems. In any case, it is most advantageous to detect problems early (Figs 7-41a and b and 7-42).

Periodontal prostheses

The patient who has been restored in conjunction with periodontal therapy has more challenging maintenance problems than the patient with a healthy periodontium. The first group has less supporting bone around the remaining teeth and often has multiple

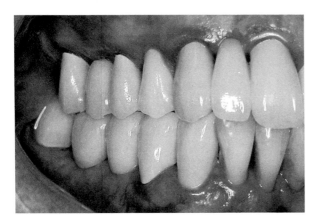

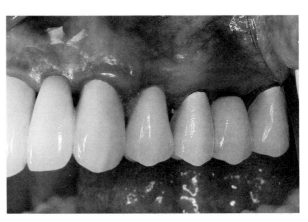

Figs 7-40a to c Multiple restorations involving fixed partial dentures and splinted units. This type of prosthesis requires close patient supervision.

Fig 7-40b

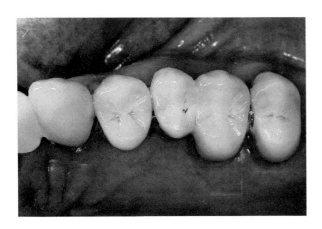

Fig 7-40c

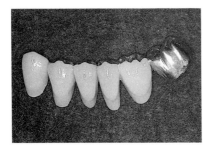

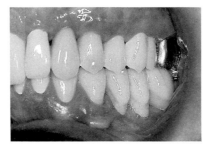

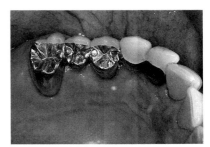

Figs 7-41a and b Long-span fixed restorations require close maintenance intervals because flexure may cause joint fracture or loss of retention of abutments.

Fig 7-42 Pier fixed partial denture used to avoid problems encountered when the fixed partial denture has no interlock. There is less chance of failure of abutments caused by individual movement.

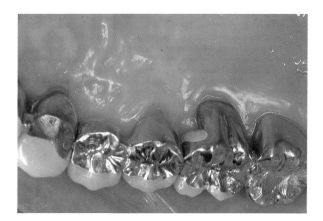

Fig 7-43 Periodontal-prosthetic patients present difficult maintenance problems. Weakened periodontal support and multiple splinted units need to be followed more carefully and at closer intervals than their nonperiodontally involved counterparts.

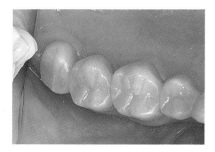 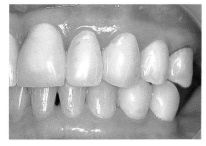 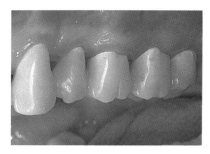

Figs 7-44a to c Properly designed provisional restorations seen in three different patients. Adequate access for periodontal health and maintenance is allowed during this stage of therapy to continue soft-tissue healing.

missing teeth. They generally have multiple abutted, longer-span fixed partial dentures and splinting to control mobility. Also, occlusal patterns are somewhat complicated. These patients cannot afford additional bone or tooth loss and need to understand that careful home care and frequent maintenance intervals are mandatory. Whether the superstructure is cemented directly to the teeth or placed on copings, it is necessary to supervise abutments closely and to tap out and recement these fixed partial dentures before caries or other breakdown occurs. Regardless of the means of cementation, with underlying individually mobile abutments there is great potential for cement washout and loss of fixation. The maintenance interval should be designed to intercept these problems at an early stage (Fig 7-43). These compromised patients also have greater difficulty in home care because of tortuous root morphology and furcation involvements. You should advise patients of potential areas of breakdown, because patients must bear a large share of the responsibility for maintaining their dentitions. Points of consideration for these patients include:

1. Proper maintenance intervals for reevaluation and adjustment (at least every 3 months)

2. Aggressive and frequent home care and instruction
3. Tap-out and recementation where applicable
4. Timely replacement or repair
5. Periodic occlusion adjustment and habit appliance therapy

Provisional restorations

Maintenance of provisional restorations is usually not of concern because as a rule, these are employed for a short time to protect and stabilize the teeth and edentulous spaces while the final prosthesis is being constructed. Usually this does not present maintenance problems. However, if the provisional restoration is placed before the patient is referred for periodontal care, or if the final restoration cannot be seated for some time, additional problems arise. A patient who is to be in provisional restorations for a protracted period of time (beyond 2 months) should be placed on a maintenance schedule to check for washout of cement, wear, fracture, and other problems. The original provisional restoration can usually be recemented, repaired, or relined. However, because of the nature of the material most often used

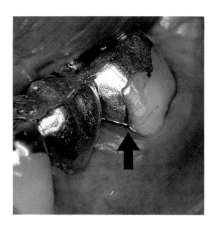

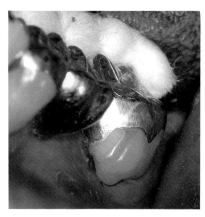

Fig 7-45a *(left)* Repair of marginal caries found on the mesial surface of this molar.

Fig 7-45b *(right)* If access is adequate and the defect can be cleaned, it may be repaired with composite resin or glass ionomer cement.

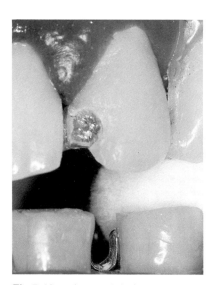

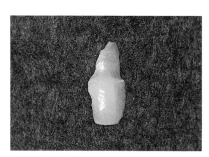

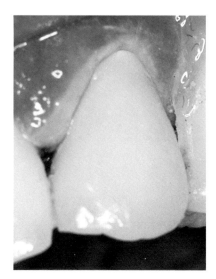

Fig 7-46a A porcelain fracture.

Fig 7-46b The fracture was repaired using a fractured piece of porcelain.

Fig 7-46c It was then rebonded to the fixed partial denture using porcelain repair kits containing porcelain etch, silane, and composite resin luting agent. (Courtesy of Dr Rick Roblee.)

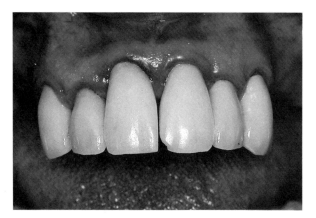

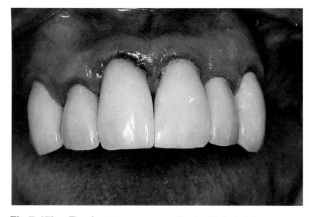

Fig 7-47a An incisal edge fracture.

Fig 7-47b The fracture was repaired with hybrid composite resin and porcelain repair kit, and the patient scheduled for periodontal care to regain health of the tissues.

(autopolymerizing acrylic resin), there is a point at which we must proceed with final restorations or replace the provisional restorations. This is essential in maintaining the patient's dental and periodontal health. It cannot be emphasized too strongly how important it is not to "lose" patients who are in provisional restorations. One needs only to have a patient surface after long absence with a "temporary" restoration that has washed out and an abutment that has silently decayed to the level of the gingiva to emphasize the need for maintenance care (Figs 7-44a to c). Inform patients of the importance of regular maintenance for their provisional restorations. Maintenance would include:

1. Regular prophylaxis recall
2. Recementation and repair every 2 to 3 months
3. Repair or replacement when necessary
4. Placement of final restorations as soon as possible

Repair of existing dental restorations

There are many considerations when problems arise with a dental restoration. Each situation must be evaluated individually as to advisability of repair versus replacement. Repair of existing restorations to extend their functional life might include the following measures.

Marginal caries repair

Marginal caries around existing restorations presents a special problem. Access for repair is not always possible, especially in interproximal areas and deep facial or lingual areas. When the existing restoration is otherwise satisfactory, marginal areas exhibit recurrent decay, and access seems adequate, repair is usually possible. As previously mentioned, where metal crown margins are involved, dissimilar metals hasten tarnish and corrosion breakdown, and composite restorative material or glass ionomer cement is advised. Repairs do not render the restoration as functional as it was when it was new, but they do extend its life. It is also sometimes possible to remove the cast restorations to gain better access for caries removal, and then reseat the restoration (Figs 7-45a and b).

Fractured porcelain

With the widespread use of porcelain restorations today, fractures of this material are seen with increasing frequency. With proper design and placement and patient compliance, these problems will be minimal. However, problems do occur and repairs are sometimes necessary. Any time a metal ceramic restoration fractures, you must decide whether or not the restoration is functionally or esthetically compromised. As mentioned previously, many times the restoration can be smoothed to enable continued function. Unfortunately porcelain fracture is not always so easily remedied. When porcelain needs repair, it can often be done in situ with composite resin or similar repair kits. When this is not satisfactory and the unit can be removed, it can be repaired in the laboratory by reveneering with porcelain and then be reinserted. Removal of porcelain units is not always easy, and additional damage may occur, particularly if the restoration needs to be cut off to avoid damage or fracture to the underlying tooth. Before removing these restorations, inform the patient of problems that may be encountered, including the possible need for replacement (Figs 7-46a to c and 7-47a and b).

Fracture of solder joints or connectors

Fixed partial dentures, whether cast in one piece or assembled in units and soldered, are subject to failure at the connectors. These areas are thinner and are often the first to show stress failure. This is especially a problem in larger units where stress in edentulous areas can produce fracture at the connectors. This can be due to inadequate strength in these areas or to improper soldering during construction of the fixed partial denture. It is sometimes possible to remove the units without damage to the remaining teeth or bridgework. Sometimes it may be necessary to cut the remaining units off to avoid removing large splints completely. Whenever the damage caused by removing the unit is judged to be excessive, repair is not possible. Assuming the units can be removed intact, a new model may also be necessary for reconstruction of the fixed partial denture. A soldering index should also be taken in the mouth or the fixed partial denture luted together in place. This should be done with DuraLay® (Reliance Dental Mfg Co) or similar materials. After the fixed partial denture is prepared for investing, it should be placed in a high-heat investment and prepared for soldering. If porcelain units are involved, oven soldering is recommended. After soldering and removal of investment material, the unit can be checked on the working model and margins smoothed on the dies. If the unit was cut or sectioned, additional repairs can be made in the laboratory. When repairs have been satisfactorily accomplished,

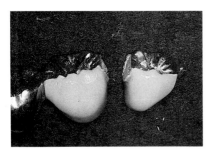

Fig 7-48a A fractured joint between premolars.

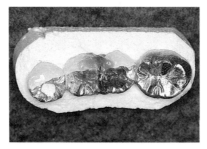

Fig 7-48b The fixed partial denture is recovered and luted together, invested, and soldered.

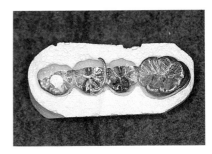

Fig 7-48c The fixed partial denture is recovered from investment and returned to service.

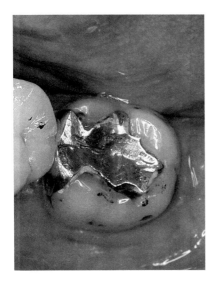

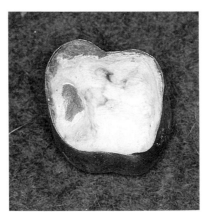

Fig 7-49 *(left)* A single mesioocclusal inlay that became displaced several times, showing cement margins and lack of cuspal protection. It should be replaced with a full-coverage restoration.

Fig 7-50 *(right)* A single restoration that became displaced, showing minimal loss of luting agent and that the restoration is still satisfactory. The restoration was replaced with a proper luting agent.

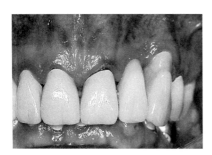

Fig 7-51a This restoration worked loose from both abutments.

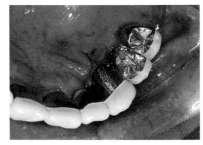

Fig 7-51b The fixed partial denture was retrieved by cutting both canine and premolar units.

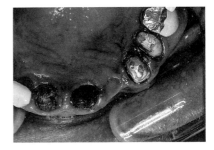

Fig 7-51c Examination revealed decay requiring endodontics on both central incisors.

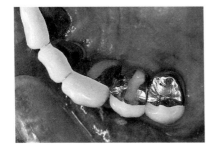

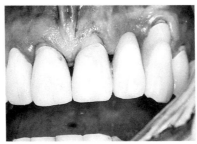

Figs 7-51d and e In this case the existing fixed partial denture was relined with acrylic resin to serve as a provisional restoration while the new restoration is fabricated.

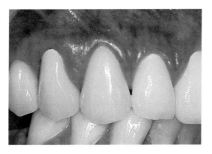
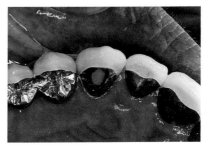
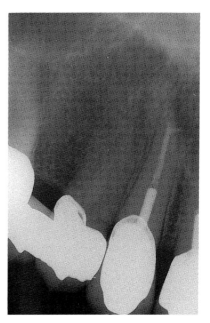

Fig 7-52a The anterior crown on this recently endodontically treated canine is still functional.

Figs 7-52b and c A stainless steel post was placed through endodontic access and closed with composite resin to salvage the crown.

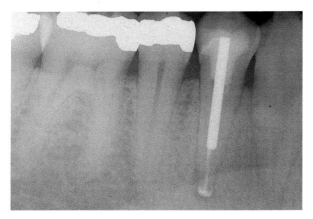
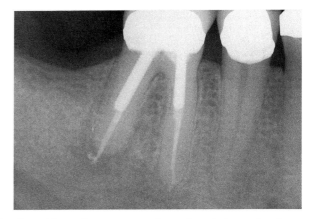

Figs 7-53a and b Periapical radiographs of intracoronal posts placed through access openings of posterior restorations.

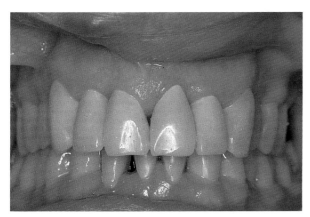
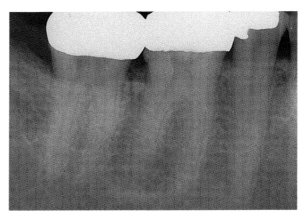

Fig 7-54 Long-term periodontal healing can be achieved with properly placed and supervised provisional restorations. These restorations were in place 8 months.

Fig 7-55 Improper crown contours such as those seen on this radiograph interfere with proper access for removal of bacteria and their products.

the fixed partial denture is replaced. The patient must understand before removal that continued function and longevity cannot be predicted. Also at times the difficulty and time involved with a repair may not justify the economics of this treatment (Figs 7-48a to c).

Displaced single restorations

Displaced single restorations should be evaluated for their possible continued usefulness and the reason(s) they became displaced. If the restoration and its retention are judged adequate, it may be recemented with a permanent luting agent. Care during recementation may produce superior results. Also, changing to a more retentive cement such as a glass ionomer may prove to be more successful. However, if retention is inadequate, the restoration will again fail. Under these circumstances the restoration can be temporarily recemented and the patient advised that it is compromised and replacement is planned (Figs 7-49 and 7-50).

Displaced fixed partial dentures

When one abutment on a fixed partial denture fails, it is best to discover it quickly. The fixed partial denture should be removed, preferably by tapping it out. If tap-out is not possible, the fixed partial denture should be cut off the secure abutment, avoiding irreparable damage to the margins or porcelain if possible. Next the teeth are examined for decay or fracture. The denture is evaluated for possible repair. When repairs to the denture are necessary, they can be performed in the laboratory. Problems with the underlying abutment can be varied. If there is decay, it can be removed and if enough of the abutment remains, the fixed partial denture can be replaced. The decayed areas can be blocked out, or the cementing agent can be allowed to fill these areas. If the abutment is decayed badly, then endodontics, along with a post and core buildup using the fixed partial denture as a matrix, will be necessary. It should always be determined why the abutment failed and whether the problem can be eliminated. Retention of the loosened abutment may be inadequate relative to the other abutment. There may be mobility of one of the abutments that would require a stress breaker between the units or additional teeth may need to be included. Also, long spans, particularly in the mandible, undergo flexing that will tend to dislodge the weaker abutment. As always, close supervision follows replacement.

Failure of intermediate abutments

As with any fixed partial denture, the failed unit must be removed and evaluated for replacement. Multiple-unit restorations present more problems because they are not as easy to remove. Sometimes the condition may have progressed to the point that the abutment must be sectioned out from under the fixed partial denture while it is in place; usually, however, the fixed partial denture is removed and evaluated. Failure may result from inadequate retention or from movement that is not tolerated by that unit. Usually it is learned too late that stress breakers were necessary in the original construction to allow for movement of larger units, but in some cases the provisional restoration would have been a problem as well, giving us a clue before the final fixed partial denture is placed (Figs 7-51a to e).

Repair of restorations after endodontics

After teeth have been treated endodontically, the access opening through the crown should be repaired. It is usually appropriate to place stainless steel posts into the root canal to reinforce the crown before covering the access opening. After the posts have been cemented, the core or pulp chamber area can be filled with cement or glass ionomer. The access opening can then be filled with alloy, composite resin, glass ionomer with alloy, or gold foil (see chapter 9). In some cases the chamber and access can be completely filled with composite resin or glass ionomer, greatly increasing the overall strength of the tooth (Figs 7-52a to c and 7-53a and b).

Maintaining the patients with periodontal diseases

Maintaining clinical health is not without problems for the patient with deepened probing depths (see chapter 6). However, many times the patient can be stabilized with the hope that more definitive measures can be performed later. The following factors contribute to maintenance problems for the patient with periodontal diseases (Fig 7-54).

1. *Dental plaque* is the primary extrinsic etiologic factor of inflammatory periodontal diseases. During initial therapy, instruct the patient in plaque removal techniques and perform scaling and root planing to remove tooth-borne bacteria that the patient cannot clean off alone.

2. *Restorations* can have major causal significance in periodontal lesions. Poor restorations exhibiting excessive contours and overhanging margins do not allow adequate plaque removal. Replace these during initial therapy. This is most easily accomplished with provisional restorations (Fig 7-55).

3. *Occlusal trauma* affects teeth adversely when compared to nontraumatized neighboring teeth. While the correctness of this view is still debated, this seems especially true for those teeth that have periodontitis and trauma from occlusion. As part of our therapy, we splint many teeth that exhibit what we consider excessive mobility after initial attempts to reduce inflammation (using oral hygiene and scaling and root planing) and trauma (with occlusal adjustment or habit appliances). We think this adds to patient comfort and to tooth longevity (Fig 7-56) (see pp 104–107 for a more in-depth discussion).

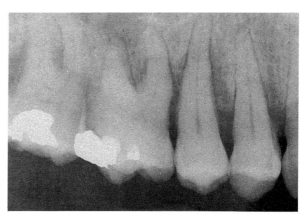

Fig 7-56 Trauma from occlusion is a factor in the progression of periodontitis when it accompanies inflammation. Evidence of traumatic occlusion often appears in radiographs as widened periodontal ligament spaces (seen here around a second premolar).

At a glance

Maintenance for fixed prosthodontics

- Consider the maintainability of each restoration during the original treatment planning stage.
- Composite resin materials have a place in posterior restorations but must be used selectively.
- Amalgam is still the restorative material of choice for many tooth-confined posterior restorations; composite resins show good promise for the future.
- Etched porcelain, composite resin–bonded restorations are part of a new generation of materials and still need to withstand the test of time.
- Full crown restorations should be in harmony with the occlusion and the periodontium and should allow easy access for oral hygiene.
- Multiple crowns that include splinting to control tooth mobility present special problems. These restorations need more frequent care than cases where the teeth are not splinted.
- Maintain provisional restorations that are to remain for more than 2 months on a regular basis.
- Many restorations fail or the periodontium fails because of improper restorative contours.
- Repair of existing restorations is often possible, thus extending their useful life.
- Design replacement or repairs so as to protect remaining tooth structure and periodontium and reduce future maintenance. Repairs should never be considered equivalent to new restorations (Figs 7-57a to c).

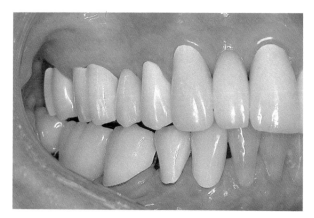

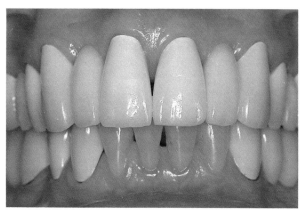

Figs 7-57a to c Finished fixed restorations exhibiting good contour, occlusion, esthetics, and function.

Fig 7-57b

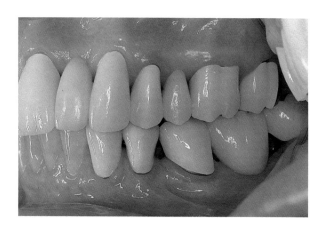

Fig 7-57c

References

1. Lang NP, Kiel RA, Anderhalden K: Clinical and microbiological effects of subgingival restorations with overhanging or clinically perfect margins. *J Clin Periodontol* 1983;10:563.
2. Löe H: Reactions of marginal periodontal tissues to restorative procedures. *Int Dent J* 1968;18:759.
3. Carranza FA, Romanelli JH: The effects of fillings and prosthetic appliances on the marginal gingiva. *Int Dent J* 1973; 23:64.
4. Müller HP: The effect of artificial crown margins at the gingival margin on the periodontal conditions in a group of periodontally supervised patients treated with fixed bridges. *J Clin Periodontol* 1986;13:97.
5. Silness J: Periodontal conditions in patients treated with dental bridges. II. The influence of full and partial crowns on plaque accumulation, development of gingivitis and pocket formation. *J Periodont Res* 1970;5:219.
6. Koth DL: Full crown restorations and gingival inflammation in a controlled population. *J Prosthet Dent* 1982;48:681.
7. Newcomb GM: The relationship between the location of subgingival crown margins and gingival inflammation. *J Periodontol* 1974;45:151.
8. Wilson RD, Maynard G: Intracrevicular restorative dentistry. *Int J Periodont Rest Dent* 1981;1(4):35.
9. Rodriguez-Ferrer HJ, Strahan JD, Newman HN: Effect on gingival health of removing overhanging margins of interproximal subgingival amalgam restorations. *J Clin Periodontol* 1980;7:457.
10. Gargiulo AW, Wentz FM, Orban B: Dimensions and relations of the dentogingival junction in humans. *J Periodontol* 1961;32:261.
11. Ingber JS, Rose LF, Coslet JG: The "biologic width"—A concept in periodontics and restorative dentistry. *Alpha Omegan* 1977;70:62.
12. Tarnow D, Stahl SS, Magner A, Zamzok J: Human gingival attachment responses to subgingival crown placement. Marginal remodeling. *J Clin Periodontol* 1986;13:563.
13. Bjorn AL, Bjorn H, Grkovic B: Marginal fit of restorations and its relation to periodontal bone level. Part II. Crowns. *Odontol Rev* 1970;21:337.
14. Than A, Duguid R, McKendrick AJW: Relationship between restorations and the level of the periodontal attachment. *J Clin Periodontol* 1982;9:193.
15. Richter WA, Veno H: Relationship of crown margin placement to gingival inflammation. *J Prosthet Dent* 1973;30:156.
16. Karolyi M, cited by Comar MD, Kollar JA, Gargiulo AW: Local irritation and occlusal trauma as co-factors in the periodontal disease process. *J Periodontol* 1969;40:193.
17. Orban B, Weinmann J: Signs of traumatic occlusion in average human jaws. *J Dent Res* 1933;13:216 (Abstr No 63).
18. Macapanpan IC, Weinmann J: Influence of injury to the periodontal membrane on the spread of gingival inflammation. *J Dent Res* 1954;33:263.
19. Glickman I, Weiss LA: Role of trauma from occlusion in initiation of periodontal pocket formation in experimental

animals. *J Periodontol* 1955;26:14.

20. Glickman I, Smulow JB: Alterations in the pathway of gingival inflammation into the underlying tissues induced by excessive occlusal forces. *J Periodontol* 1962;33:7.
21. Glickman I: Clinical significance of trauma from occlusion. *J Am Dent Assoc* 1965;70:607.
22. Glickman I, Smulow JB: Effect of excessive occlusal forces upon the pathway of gingival inflammation in humans. *J Periodontol* 1965;36:141.
23. Glickman I, Smulow JB: Further observations on the effect of trauma from occlusion in humans. *J Periodontol* 1967;38:280.
24. Polson AM: Trauma and progression of marginal periodontitis in squirrel monkeys. II. Co-destruction factors of periodontitis and mechanically-produced injury. *J Periodont Res* 1974;9:108.
25. Polson AM, Kennedy JE, Zander HA: Trauma and progression of marginal periodontitis in squirrel monkeys. I. Co-destructive factors of periodontitis and thermally-produced injury. *J Periodont Res* 1974;9:100.
26. Meitner SW: Co-destructive factors of marginal periodontitis and repetitive mechanical injury. *J Dent Res* 1975;54:C78.
27. Perrier M, Polson AM: The effect of progressive and increasing tooth hypermobility on reduced but healthy supporting tissues. *J Periodontol* 1982;53:152.
28. Waerhaug J, Hansen ER: Periodontal changes incident to prolonged occlusal overload in monkeys. *Acta Odontol Scand* 1966;24:91.
29. Lindhe J, Svanberg G: Influence of trauma from occlusion on progression of experimental periodontitis in the beagle dog. *J Clin Periodontol* 1974;1:3.
30. Lindhe J, Ericsson I: The influence of trauma from occlusion on reduced but healthy periodontal tissues in dogs. *J Clin Periodontol* 1976;3:110.
31. Lindhe J, Nyman S, Ericsson I: in Lindhe J (ed): *Textbook of Clinical Periodontology.* Copenhagen, Munksgaard, 1983, p 233.
32. Rosling B, Nyman S, Lindhe J: The effect of systematic plaque control on bone regeneration in infrabony pockets. *J Clin Periodontol* 1976;3:38.
33. Fleszar TJ, Knowles JW, Morrison EC, Burgett FG, Nissle RR, and Ramfjord SP: Tooth mobility and periodontal therapy. *J Clin Periodontol* 1980;7:495.
34. Pihlstrom BL, Anderson KA, Aeppli D, Schaffer EM: Association between signs of trauma from occlusion and periodontitis. *J Periodontol* 1986;57:1.
35. Gartrell JR, Mathews DP: Gingival recession: The condition, process, and treatment. *Dent Clin North Am* 1976;20(1):199–213.
36. Kennedy JE, Bird WC, Palcanis KG, Dorfman HS: A longitudinal evaluation of varying widths of attached gingiva. *J Clin Periodontol* 1985;12:667.
37. Maynard JG, Wilson RDK: Physiologic dimensions of the periodontium significant to the restorative dentist. *J Periodontol* 1979;50:170.
38. Ericsson I, Lindhe J: Recession in sites with inadequate width of the keratinized gingiva. An experimental study in the dog. *J Clin Periodontol* 1984;11:95.
39. Stetler K, Bissada NF: Significance of the width of keratinized gingiva on the periodontal status of teeth with submarginal restorations. *J Periodontol* 1987;58:696.
40. Miller, PD Jr: Root coverage using a free soft tissue autograft following citric acid application. I. Technique. *Int J Periodont Rest Dent* 1982;2(1):65.
41. Holbrook T, Ochsenbein C: Complete coverage of the denuded root surface with a one-stage gingival graft. *Int J Periodont Rest Dent* 1983;3(3):8.
42. Sharry JJ: *Complete Denture Prosthodontics,* 2nd ed. New York, McGraw-Hill, 1968, pp 270–284.
43. Sharry JJ: Symposium on Complete Denture Prosthesis. *Dent Clin North Am* November 1964;735–748.
44. Johnson DL, Stratton RJ: *Fundamentals of Removable Prosthodontics.* Chicago, Quintessence Publ Co, 1980, pp 253–267.
45. Heartwell CM: *Syllabus of Complete Dentures.* Philadelphia, Lea & Febiger, 1968, pp 335–345.
46. Langwell WH: Cleansing of artificial dentures. *Br Dent J* 1955;99:337.
47. Budtz-Jorgensen E: Clinical aspects of *Candida* infection in denture wearers. *J Am Dent Assoc* 1978;96:474.
48. Budtz-Jorgensen E: The significance of *Candida albicans* in denture stomatitis. *Scand J Dent Res* 1974;82:151.
49. Olsen I: Studies on oral yeast infections with emphasis on denture stomatitis. *Nor Tannlaegeforen Tid* 1976;86:497–501.
50. Neill DJ: A study of materials and methods employed in cleaning dentures. *Br Dent J* 1968;124:107.
51. Anthony DH, Gibbons P: The nature and behavior of denture cleansers. *J Prosthet Dent* 1958;8:796.
52. Pipko DJ, El-Sadeck M: An in vitro investigation of abrasion and staining of dental resins. *J Dent Res* 1972;51:689.
53. Sexson JC, Phillips RW: Studies on the effects of abrasives on acrylic resins. *J Prosthet Dent* 1951;1:454.
54. Ghalichebaf M, Graser GN, Zander HA: The efficacy of denture-cleansing agents. *J Prosthet Dent* 1982;48(5):515.
55. Rossiwald B: Can even acid-free cleansers cause corrosion of orthodontic expansion screws? *Quintessence Int* 1974;5:45–47.

Suggested readings

Amsterdam M, Vanarsdall RL: Periodontal prosthesis—Twenty-five years in retrospect. *Alpha Omegan* December, 1974.

Becker CM, Kaldahl WB: Current theories of crown contour, margin placement, and pontic design. *J Prosthet Dent* 1981;45:268.

Ingber JS, Rose LF, Coslet JG: The "biologic width"—A concept in periodontics and restorative dentistry. *Alpha Omegan* 1977;10:62.

Kraus BS, Jordan RE, Abrams L: *Dental Anatomy and Occlusion.* Baltimore, Williams & Wilkins, 1969.

Schluger S, Yuodelis RA, Page RC: *Periodontal Disease: Basic Phenomena, Clinical Management, and Occlusal Restorative Interrelationships.* Philadelphia, Lea & Febiger, 1977, chaps 17, 18, 26, 27, 28, 29.

Sorensen SE, Larsen IB, Jorgenson KD: Gingival and alveolar bone reaction to marginal fit of subgingival crown margins. *Scand J Dent Res* 1986; 94:109.

Chapter 8

Maintenance for Pediatric and Orthodontic Patients

I. Maintenance for Children from Birth Through Puberty

Francis L. Miranda

Philosophy of practice

This section deals with the diagnosis, maintenance, and prevention of dental diseases in children. The primary emphasis is in the area of pediatrics and pediatric orthodontics and its relation to periodontal care and will extend to the area of dental caries. This section also deals with orthodontic approaches other than full-arch fixed appliances, which will be covered in more detail on pp 142–149.

During the 22 years of my pediatric dental practice, I have attempted to provide my patients with the outlook and skills that will give them a reduced risk of dental diseases. Several events have significantly affected my approach to preventive maintenance. The first event occurred when I purchased an existing pediatric dental practice. This practice provided care that emphasized repair of problems as they occurred, not prevention. It emphasized expedient procedures for dealing with caries and early extraction of primary teeth without space maintenance. Attempting to change the attitude of the patients in this practice presented quite a challenge. They had not been introduced to a "wellness" approach to dental care, but had received therapy only for those problems at hand. This "poor child" approach promoted the idea that dental problems are inherited and therefore not controllable. These patients were not ready to accept techniques that emphasized early diagnosis and treatment of carious lesions; nor were they ready to accept responsibility for their own dental health. As a result of my desire to change my patients' and their parents' attitude, I began talking with colleagues. One of the people who affected me most was Dr Robert Barkley, an early advocate of prevention of dental diseases through improved oral hygiene. His mes-

sage was that people should take responsibility for their own oral health. After applying his principles for some time, I found that his ideas concerning practices of oral hygiene and their effect on preventing dental diseases were accurate, but few of my patients responded as I suggested. Within a short time I found that people in my practice would not change their behavior just because I could prove to them that there was bacteria in the mouth attacking soft and hard tissues. Slowly, the microscope and the disclosing wafers and the multiple visits went by the wayside. I thought I was losing the war with dental disease.

I then studied patient behavior to see how well patients responded to suggested recall visits. I found that only about 40% of my patients presented for recall. It was interesting to find that Wilson and his colleagues had similar percentages in their recall system (see p 14). Believing that we could do something, the staff changed the recall system to a 6-month preappointment scheduling. After a year passed, I evaluated the system and found the same compliance level.

Another way I evaluated the recall program showed similar compliance. Evaluation of 1,000 recall appointments disclosed that approximately 30% of these recall patients were seen within a month following the recall date previously set; another 30% were seen within the year following that date; and another 30% were seen more than 1 year later. This included only those seen on recall appointments. I then checked the number of recall cards that were not appointed during this period of time and were being carried forward. According to my calculations, only 20% of the patients were returning on the suggested schedule, another 20% were returning within a year of the recall date, and 20% drifted in whenever the feelings were right. About 40% of the total group were not influenced to return at all.

I contacted several pediatric dentists who had successful practices, and we brainstormed problems and solutions. We discovered that each of us were using different techniques for recall reminders, and that we were equally effective or ineffective (less than 50% within a year), however you wish to view this result.

These facts disturbed me, but they also awakened me to the realization that my attitude toward dental health does *not* carry over to my patients. I concluded that my attitude does not modify their behavior patterns. I now truly believe that only a new attitude on their part will accomplish this change.

The next and most significant event that influenced my philosophy occurred when my first second-generation patient came to the office, the child of a patient whom I had treated for many years. The mother had had many carious lesions and orthodontic therapy and was now bringing her child to me for the initial examination. The child had multiple lesions and generalized gingivitis. I was heartbroken. I had assumed that some modicum of oral health information would be transferred to the second generation. Here I found myself confronted by the same issues that had concerned me 20 years earlier. Here I was, two decades in practice and forced to question one of my basic beliefs: that my persistence and ethical practices could be meaningful if I improved the oral health of my patients. I must have expected that my professional life would be validated when my second-generation family was in better oral health.

From these experiences, I find that my philosophy of prevention involves two goals. The first goal is that my staff and I go to great lengths to inform the patients of their present oral health and show them how to improve on their present status. Second, we have found that having a specific goal for each patient is necessary. Currently we use the goal: no bleeding gingiva when the patient presents for his or her maintenance visit. We check and record this information at each recall visit and inform the patient of his or her progress. We also provide more information, assistance, and guidance where needed. We have found that both the parent and the patient must be aware of current status and progress for the system to be as successful as possible. There are no automatic procedures or videotapes for our patients. These come into the program as they are needed, and only after one-on-one training.

The dental profession has traditionally used a negative selling process to alert people to their dental needs. As a group we have threatened the patient with potential pain, pleaded that the teeth will be lost,

and cajoled that we can save their teeth, when in fact we were not always able to prove any of these claims. We have preached fire and brimstone dental prevention for years, yet we can get only 20% of the people to listen.

I believe two possibilities present themselves: one is to take the 20% of the population and give them the care they need and forget about the remaining 80%. The other possibility is to change our own attitude about prevention and provide information in a helpful manner, not condescendingly or negatively based. Then we can establish an environment at home and at the dental office in which it is easy for the patient and the parent to succeed and feel good about themselves, or fail and we can still feel good about ourselves. The remainder of this chapter will deal with specific procedures that can help patients achieve the goal of maintaining dental health.

Early prevention and maintenance

The first step in providing effective maintenance for the pediatric dental patient is to begin a preventive program in infancy. There is sufficient evidence to suggest that the child should be introduced to dental care around age 1. In my office, this introduction is classified as a "toddler visit." At this visit, the parents are informed of the importance of a wellness approach to dental care. This wellness approach stresses preventive oral hygiene techniques and early diagnosis. The treatment of carious lesions, gingival inflammation, and malocclusions will be discussed if and when they are discovered.

The parents are advised to develop a preventive program suited to their particular needs. The major emphasis is placed on the role of dental plaque in inflammation and caries formation. The parents are instructed to swab the teeth and gums with a soft washcloth moistened with lukewarm water. A small soft-bristled toothbrush may be substituted as the child becomes accustomed to the routine. Toothpaste is not necessary initially. The parents and the child may find the foaming action of the toothpaste disagreeable. A thorough daily cleaning at bedtime or after the infant's last feeding is stressed. The goal that is set for the parents to achieve is: *No bleeding.* Nursing and feeding habits are discussed at this initial visit. Many parents learn for the first time that the sugar present in formula or breast milk must not be allowed to remain in contact with the infant's teeth. As most children have progressed to some form of solid food by age 1, some diet counseling is necessary at the initial visit. Their first visit can be time consuming if not organized. Dental practices are busy, and with the help of a competent staff member, the visit goes quickly. The toddler visit will encourage the return of the family to your practice.

Preschool and elementary school–age children

Preschool-age children are the next group of children requiring special consideration. The medical history is reviewed with the parent at each recall. Included in each recall visit for every patient is an assessment of oral hygiene (see chapter 2). The child's progress is charted. Also included in each recall visit is an assessment of the occlusal status. The parents are given a copy at each recall, which serves as an update of the status of their child.

Preschool and elementary school–age children rarely possess the coordination or attention span necessary to clean the teeth and gingiva properly. Both parent and child must be given oral hygiene instruction. Several techniques for performing brushing and flossing are demonstrated to the parents. The child's head may be rested against a wall or in the parent's lap for support during oral hygiene practices (Fig 8-1). Gentle restraint may be necessary for the active child. The circular brushing technique is demonstrated for the parents. Toothpaste is *not* used during demonstrations. Flossing instructions are also demonstrated. It is useful to introduce the use of floss holders to the parents, as many parents are not accustomed to using floss on a regular basis, and we have found that the floss holder is helpful when working in someone else's mouth.

We like to have the parent take responsibility for maintaining the oral health of the child. Children must also develop good hygiene practices on their own. After the parent has performed a thorough cleaning of the teeth, we suggest that a small amount of fluoridated toothpaste is placed on a toothbrush. The child is encouraged to brush his or her own teeth to develop coordination and good habits.

As long as the child has a balanced diet, supplements are not necessary. The balanced diet will provide all of the essential vitamins and minerals. Because many children receive supplements containing iron, brown or yellowish orange stains may be present at recall and may be removed with pumice and a rubber cup. We show the parent this at the cleaning appointment; it helps them understand why we clean the teeth.

During the school-age years, the dental office becomes the most important source of oral hygiene information. When children go to school, parents seem to give the child a new level of responsibility that

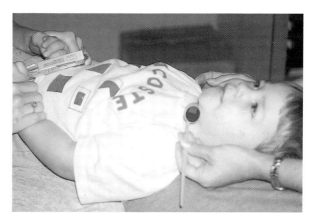

Fig 8-1 Positioning of a child in the laps of the mother and dental assistant. The parent is lightly restraining the child and can observe first hand the examination and the training for oral cleaning.

is above the level that the child is able to accept and master. Parents seem to stop providing routine oral hygiene care to children of this age. In dental practice in a fluoridated area, my office detects the highest incidence of gingival inflammation and caries during these elementary school years.

The office must develop routines that are effective at any age. For this reason, I teach my dental auxiliaries the need for a simple guideline for success: *no bleeding gingiva*, a measuring system that the layperson can learn to identify with.

The charting system that we use throughout these routine preventive visits is simple and straightforward:

Examination

We check for:

1. New decay and possible or recurrent decay
2. Areas where patient may not be cleaning well
3. Condition of gingiva and oral mucosa
4. Irregularities in restorations
5. Shift in occlusion
6. Rate of exfoliation and eruption

Hygiene charts

1. Age
2. Plaque index is calculated according to the amount of plaque found on six teeth: buccal maxillary right first molar, lingual mandibular right first molar, labial maxillary right central incisor, lingual mandibular right lateral incisor, buccal maxillary left first molar, and lingual mandibular left first molar. If first permanent molars are missing, grade according to the last tooth in each arch, and if the

central or lateral incisors are missing, grade the tooth closest to the midline.

  0—No plaque or debris present, no stain
  1—Plaque covering not more than one third of the tooth surface
  2—Plaque covering more than one third but not over two thirds
  3—Plaque covering more than two thirds of the tooth surface

Plaque index = sum of each plaque score of all six teeth

3. Gingival index pertains to the condition of the gingiva in the same areas used for the plaque index.

  0—No gingival inflammation or bleeding; gingiva is pink and has good contour
  1—Slight bleeding (one or two areas)
  2—Bleeding in a few areas (three or four)
  3—Bleeding in multiple areas (five or six) with generalized inflammation of the gingiva

4. Calculus index pertains only to the mandibular anterior teeth.

  0—No calculus present
  1—Mild amounts of calculus in various areas (eg, mesiodistal surfaces on several teeth)
  2—Moderate amounts of calculus
  3—Severe amounts of calculus making a continuous band on the tooth surface

5. Coordination and attitude is made up of two separate scores.

  Coordination
  1—Child still requires help to work with a toothbrush
  2—Child is able to brush own teeth but not effectively
  3—Child does well with the toothbrush but is not able to use floss well
  4—Child brushes and flosses fairly well but can do better job
  5—Child does very well with toothbrush and floss

  Attitude
  1—Attitude of the child is excellent
  2—Attitude is high
  3—Attitude is low
  4—Negative attitude

Teenagers

Teenagers seem to be the most perplexing age group we deal with. Teenagers have many activities that take precedence in their schedules and give little attention to maintaining health in general. Their diet is poor and their hygiene deteriorates. The prevalence of caries rises and their gingival health declines. In fact, repetition and fluoride seem to be the only successful measures available. Communication is often difficult with teenagers, so we must continuously look for ways to relate with this group and not turn them away. If sincere interest and concern are demonstrated by the auxiliaries and the dentist, the patient will usually respond well. A rapport should be established first, then an improved oral hygiene can be accomplished. Responsibility for maintenance of dental health is very difficult to establish in the teen. We must not be condescending but be concerned and consistent. The most important is true concern for the person. The next most important step is that the teaching be consistent.

Again, I have come to the conclusion that the most effective goal is to achieve no bleeding around the teeth. That goal is not difficult for the teen to understand. If he or she detects any bleeding then he or she must be told that it will take at least a week for this to heal, assuming that he or she cleans the teeth and gingival crevices thoroughly each day.

Handicapped patients

Handicapped patients must be considered according to the level of parental maintenance necessary for their wellness. Each type, and thereby various maintenance problems, must be evaluated individually. Then the responsibility for maintenance can be established. That person needs to demonstrate this understanding.

We use the same criteria as before to evaluate these patients.

Restorative maintenance

Maintenance of dental restorations in the primary, mixed, and young permanent teeth is similar to that described in other areas of this text (see chapter 7). There are some unique problems in the pediatric patient, and these will be discussed.

The stainless steel crown is a mainstay of many pediatric dental practices. Many graduate programs advocate placing and maintaining the margins of these crowns subgingivally. In practice, however, this presents problems and is unrealistic. The anatomic form and dimensions of the primary first molar make placement of the margin subgingivally extremely difficult without negatively affecting the gingival tissue along the buccal margin. The stainless steel crown

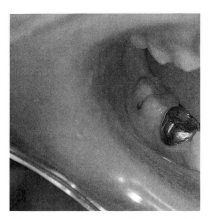

Fig 8-2 Gingival margins around a crown at 1 year post-treatment.

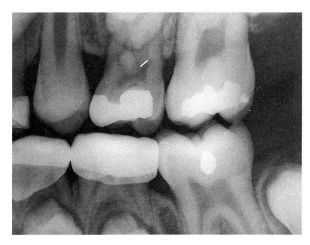

Fig 8-3 Radiograph of posttreatment restorations. Note the interdental alveolar bone and multiple restorations.

margin is usually placed outside the dimensions of the natural tooth. Hence, it is expected that some gingival irritation will occur at the margins of recently placed stainless steel crowns. To help reduce this problem, extreme care must be used to remove all dental cement from the crown margin, a source of chronic inflammation.

Margins of stainless steel crowns that have required trimming should be polished and adapted to the tooth as well as possible to minimize gingival irritation. The satisfactory steel crown restoration should be able to be flossed without causing the floss to fray or tear. A close-fitting crown presents the least likelihood of cement leakage and gingival irritation. They must be checked regularly (Figs 8-2 and 8-3).

Another problem in primary teeth is the amalgam restoration. It needs the same considerations as in the permanent dentition. The most common defect in the amalgam in the primary dentition is the isthmus fracture. If this restoration fractures, it must be replaced immediately. Usually this is followed by a pulpotomy and steel crown because of the rapid course of infection into the primary molar dentin and the proximity of the pulpal tissue.

The composite resin restoration presents a unique dilemma. The mercury controversy and the esthetics of the composite resin restoration make it easy to consider using the composite resin restoration routinely. But these restorations are prone to leakage, and the recurrent carious lesion is difficult to detect until considerable damage has occurred. To combat this problem, I suggest examining all composite resin restorations with a fiber optic light to check for any change in translucency and thoroughly inspecting all composite resin or sealant margins. The staff should

also alert the parents to the unique problems associated with composite resin restorations. To minimize problems, the finished composite resin restoration should also have good margins, have contours acceptable to the gingival tissues, and be easy to clean with dental floss. (The ultimate mechanical test is that floss does not fray or tear.)

Pulpotomies

Teeth treated by pulpotomy techniques must be monitored with radiographs annually because they are prone to root resorption. The bite-wing radiograph is not always sufficient for detecting root resorption in the mixed dentition. More radiographs are suggested for those patients who have extensive dental treatment (Figs 8-4 and 8-5a to f).

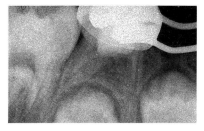

Fig 8-4 Abnormal root resorption on primary molar being used for space maintainer abutment. The molar had pulp therapy.

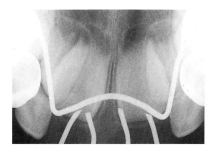
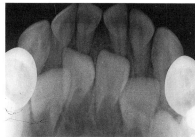

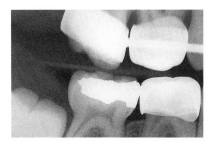
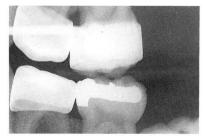

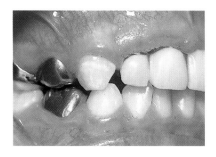
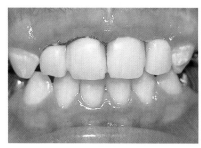

Figs 8-5a to d Posttherapy radiographs of restorations and space maintainer cemented to second primary molars replacing primary incisors.

Fig 8-5c *(left)*

Fig 8-5d *(right)*

Figs 8-5e and f Clinical views of the patient.

Tooth position maintenance

Eruption problems

It is usually necessary to have a band of attached gingival tissue around each tooth (for a discussion, see chapter 7). The position of the permanent tooth when it emerges into the oral cavity determines how much gingival tissue, if any, will be present around the tooth.[1] Teeth that might erupt into alveolar mucosa if left alone may need to be surgically exposed in order to create the desired band of gingiva.[2] Erupting teeth should be evaluated to make sure there is an adequate band of gingiva. Any tooth having less than 1.5 mm of attached gingiva should be evaluated critically, the parent advised, and the child referred for corroboration (see pp 150–158).

The same problem can arise in areas that have more than 1.5 mm of attached gingiva but are not healthy and cannot be maintained by the patient. The parent should be advised and the problem explained

(Figs 8-6a and b). In our practice, these problems are seen most commonly in the mandibular incisors and maxillary canines.

Space maintenance problems

Space maintenance has two aspects: *(1)* the spaces to be maintained, and *(2)* the appliances themselves. All teeth lost 6 months before eruption of the permanent replacements should have the space maintained in the ideal arch. If the arch is not ideal, the amount of crowding and the potential symmetry or asymmetry must be evaluated by the dentist.

Because the space you are usually maintaining could be in an arch that needs correction, an orthodontic evaluation is usually necessary. This evaluation should be a complete visual examination of potential orthodontic problems.

Replacement of primary anterior teeth is offered along with the usual space maintainer replacement

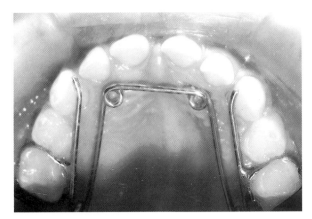

Fig 8-6a Intraoral appliance (quad-helix) for expansion of the maxillary arch. Multiple food traps must be shown to parent.

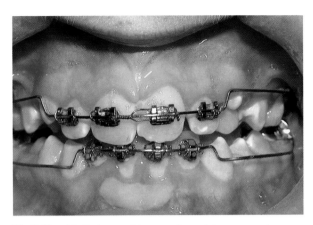

Fig 8-6b Multiple problems of maintenance demonstrated by eruption of permanent teeth, brackets, and arch wires.

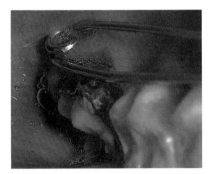

Fig 8-7 Appliance embedded in palatal tissue.

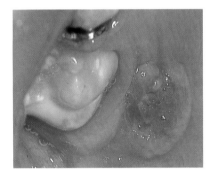

Fig 8-8 The tissue underneath the embedded appliance seen in Fig 8-7 will require follow-up evaluation.

(see Figs 8-5a to f). With the advent of composite resins and orthodontic resin cements for brackets, maintaining the primary molar space has become an easier task. There are many competent textbooks that demonstrate these techniques.

The anterior tooth space maintainer currently used in our practice is bonding the maxillary molars accompanied by acrylic resin teeth and a small acrylic resin pad. Single teeth without acrylic resin support result in gingival irritation when the occlusion embeds the teeth into the tissue. It is difficult to provide ideal occlusion with a prosthesis in the primary dentition. There are times when the anterior tooth replacement prosthesis will result in a bite opening appliance. This needs to be kept to a minimum but will not cause uncontrollable problems.

All space maintainers and orthodontic appliances need to be evaluated on a regular basis for gingival health and positional integrity. The appliances may become bent, broken, or dislodged without the child becoming aware of the problem. I believe a 3-month period is a reasonable time for periodic evaluations.

Fixed appliances

The fixed appliances in pediatric orthodontics usually comprise several bands and multiple wires. The major problem with the appliances is their becoming embedded in tissues (Figs 8-7 and 8-8) and collecting food. Parents must be instructed in the potential problems.

Occasionally the appliances must be removed for a short period of time for healing to take place before replacement of the appliance.

Removable appliances

Maintenance of gingival health while the patient is wearing a removable orthodontic appliance should center around the fit of the clasps and the positioning of the springs. When either of these wires is positioned incorrectly, the gingiva will react to the irritation. The reaction will usually be in the form of swelling and subsequent bleeding.

Management of this bleeding problem involves the

same preventive techniques described previously for gingival tissues.

Food debris must also be removed from the appliance itself. The same techniques can be used, but the patient or parent must be informed about the regularity of the procedure.

───────── *At a glance* ─────────

Maintenance for children from birth through puberty

- Stainless steel crowns should have closely fitting, well-polished margins to facilitate oral hygiene.
- Composite resin restorations require close inspection at maintenance visits because of frequent breakdown and marginal leakage.
- Pulpotomies must be closely checked at maintenance for abnormal root resorption.
- In my opinion, areas that have 1.5 mm or more of attached gingiva have fewer problems than those with less width.
- Any primary teeth lost in an ideal arch more than 6 months before eruption of the permanent replacement should have a space maintainer.
- Space maintainers and orthodontic appliances need supervision more often than the customary caries evaluation time.
- There should be no areas of bleeding gingiva or swollen and unmanageable tissue.

II. Maintenance for the Adult in Fixed Appliances

Robert E. (Gene) Lamberth

Retention and maintenance for the orthodontic patient is no different from retention and maintenance for the fixed-prosthetic patient, the removable-prosthetic patient, the oral surgery patient, or the periodontal patient. The dentist should maintain and retain the health of the stomatologic system. Every oral procedure we do for the patient and every procedure the patient does for himself or herself is performed with that goal in mind. The quality of our results in maintenance and retention is the measure of our success.

Early orthodontists emphasized the need for retention following active therapy. Dewey and Anderson[3] stated that the forces of retention are natural and mechanical. This statement is as true today as it was then. They stated further that natural forces are those that govern occlusion; they are cuspal relation, harmony in size and relation of the arches, muscular pressure, approximal contact, cell metabolism, and atmospheric pressures. Strang[4] said, "Following the corrective period of treatment, the teeth must be maintained in their new location by mechanical restraint to permit a remodeling of the structural form of the alveolar process. . . . The permanency of the results of active treatment is in direct proportion to the ability of the operator to establish a balance of force play upon these dental units by a strategical adjustment of the teeth during treatment combined with the elimination of structural deficiencies and abnormal actions of environment tissues." If the imbalances that caused the malocclusion originally are not diagnosed and eliminated during the course of orthodontic therapy, then those forces will still be active following debanding and postretention. Stability of the case will be questionable, to say the least, and extended retention will be necessary.

Strang goes on to say, "For this reason the preliminary analysis of every case must include a study of the deformed dentures from the viewpoint of malformed teeth in harmony with environmental forces." The preservation of this balance or the renewal of this

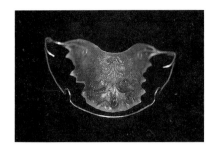 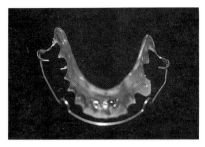

Figs 8-9a and b Maxillary Hawley retainers are the most commonly used retainers. They are easily adjustable.

condition as part of treatment is the key to success when mechanical restraint is removed.

Retention considerations

If orthodontic therapy is maintained within the principles and parameters of good orthomechanics, if physiologic balances have not been grossly violated, and if principles of good occlusion have been adhered to, then retention stability and maintenance of the orthodontic patient is greatly enhanced and will be successful.

Retention consideration begins at the time of diagnosis and treatment planning. Because bone remodels during orthodontic treatment, there is always some degree of tooth mobility following fixed appliance removal. Retainers help stabilize the teeth until new bone has been laid down and the integrity of the attachment apparatus has been reestablished. Retention for the patient with missing teeth, for the periodontally involved patient, and for the patient with muscle imbalance may be planned differently than in patients without these problems. For these types of considerations, it is important that a total treatment plan (including restorative therapy, prosthodontics, periodontal therapy, oral surgery, psychological, and myofunctional considerations) be formulated prior to therapy. Retention is planned in view of the complete treatment plan. However, final retention decisions are ultimately made just prior to debanding, and original retention plans may be modified as needed.

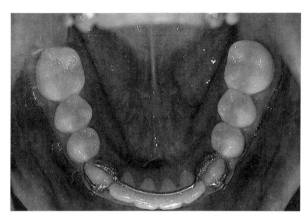

Figs 8-10a and b Cemented mandibular canine-to-canine retainers provide rigid retention for anterior teeth and are not easily adjusted. They allow for little physiologic settling.

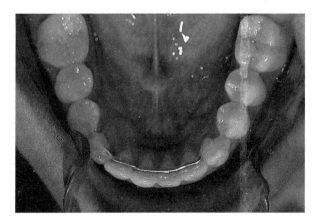

Fig 8-10b

Types of retention

Hawley retainer

Probably the most widely used retainer is the removable Hawley-type appliance (Figs 8-9a and b). This retainer can be fabricated with auxiliary springs, hooks, or an anterior bite ramp.

Removable-fixed retainer

Another widely used mode of retention is a combination of a removable retainer and a fixed mandibular retainer. This fixed retainer may be referred to as a three-to-three retainer or canine-to-canine retainer (Figs 8-10a and b). However, these fixed retainers can reach from premolar to premolar or molar to molar

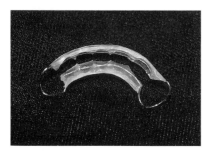
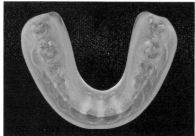
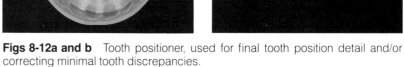

Fig 8-11 Mandibular spring-loaded retainer. This is an effective active appliance to realign maxillary and mandibular incisor crowding.

Figs 8-12a and b Tooth positioner, used for final tooth position detail and/or correcting minimal tooth discrepancies.

and can be used in the maxilla and mandible. Oral hygiene around this type of retainer is difficult and should be monitored closely.

Spring-loaded retainer

An effective appliance to regain and maintain incisor relapse is the spring-loaded retainer (Fig 8-11). This is fabricated from a model that has had the crowded teeth removed and then waxed back in proper relationship to each other and the opposing dentition. The appliance is then fabricated to the newly waxed position. It may be necessary to use judicious interproximal polishing concurrent with appliance wear. After the dentition has been moved, the appliance can then function as a retainer worn only at night.

Positioner

Another form of retainer is the "tooth positioner" appliance (Figs 8-12a and b). Fabricated from rubber or polyurethane, the positioner is active when placed and becomes passive as tooth movement occurs, whereas removable or fixed retainers (with the exception of a spring-loaded retainer) are for the most part passive. The positioner retainer is fabricated from an ideal wax setup on a semiadjustable articulator. When the patient closes into the appliance, it becomes active. After it has moved the teeth to coincide with the waxed position, it then becomes passive, retaining the teeth. This appliance is often misused in an attempt to achieve a correction that was not accomplished in active therapy, or is used in place of fixed-appliance therapy. I have found this approach for the most part to be unsuccessful. However, this appliance can be of help in making the final delicate adjustments needed for a well-treated case.

Removable splints, night guards, habit appliances

The splint retainer (Figs 8-13a and b) serves to retain and stabilize periodontally involved teeth while in place (see chapter 3). There is occlusal coverage, with lateral and protrusive functions built into the appliance.[5] It also serves as a habit device for the patient who clenches, and it helps stabilize the temporomandibular joints and musculature in the sensitive patient with temporomandibular problems. This type of retainer can be fabricated to support and stabilize mandibular repositioning, and it is often used prior to extensive restorative dentistry. After restorative dentistry it is often necessary to fabricate a new splint. Again, the need for treatment planning and sequencing with the restorative dentist and periodontist is paramount.

Kloehn

Still another form of retention is the Kloehn headgear (Fig 8-14) used either alone or in conjunction with removable or removable-fixed retention. This type of retention should be considered in a patient who is suspected of continued Class II growth tendencies or in whom Class II mechanics (elastics) have been used extensively. Headgear is worn at night and is an effective countermeasure to continued growth of the maxillae and/or physiologic rebound.

Functional appliance

Functional appliances (Figs 8-15a and b) can be used to reinforce and retain orthopedic correction following functional orthopedics. This would mean wearing the appliance only at night. The reintroduction of functional jaw orthopedics in the United States from Europe in the late 1960s opened a new era of

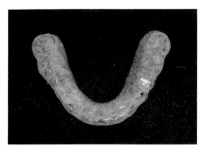

Fig 8-13a Maxillary splint retainer. This is an effective retainer that offers occlusal protection and stabilization of the periodontal and/or temporomandibular joint patient.

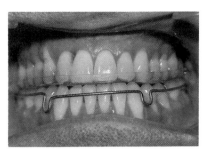

Fig 8-13b Maxillary splint retainer with mandibular Hawley retainer. The splint should be adjusted to the occlusion with the mandibular Hawley appliance in place at least 24 hours prior to adjustment.

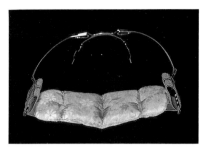

Fig 8-14 Kloehn headgear, used on patients with suspected continuation of growth or to counter physiologic rebound.

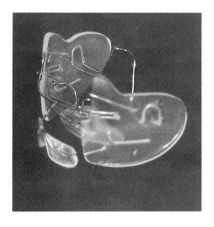

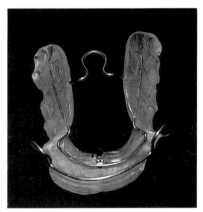

Fig 8-15a *(left)* Fränkel orthopedic corrector, used to help correct skeletal and dental discrepancies, and for maintenance of position after treatment.

Fig 8-15b *(right)* Bionator orthopedic corrector. It has a similar function to the Fränkel appliance.

treatment modalities. This has been especially true for the growing patient. No longer is it desirable to wait for the patient to exfoliate all the primary dentition before referring him or her to the orthodontist. Not only can abnormal growth problems be addressed early, but arch width and arch length can be increased for the patient with crowded teeth. Thus a patient who was destined for extraction now can be spared this necessity. Fixed-appliance wear is usually reduced by at least 12 months.

After skeletal discrepancies have been corrected, the functional appliance may be worn at night while awaiting eruption and development of the permanent dentition.

Occlusal equilibration

Occlusal equilibration can be an effective means of stabilization. A mutually protected occlusion may be defined as the occlusion and function of the masticatory apparatus that is physiologically acceptable to the patient. This balanced occlusion tends to be more stable than an unbalanced occlusion. Maximal occlu-

sal contacts in centric relation in harmony with lateral and protrusive excursion can best be achieved by minute adjustments of the occlusal surfaces of the dentition. Refinement of occlusal contacts cannot be perfected with orthomechanics alone. A thorough knowledge of occlusion and equilibration techniques is necessary to achieve the final balance and harmony needed for a physiologic occlusion (see chapter 3). It appears that a well-balanced occlusion in harmony with the temporomandibular system and muscles of mastication is an effective means of stabilizing and maintaining this portion of the stomatologic system.

A-splint

Still another effective means of retention for the periodontal patient is the A-splint (Fig 8-16). This is usually placed by the restorative dentist or periodontist and is considered a temporary means of stabilization. It can be used while awaiting further periodontal therapy or evaluations, but in cases when fixed stabilization is

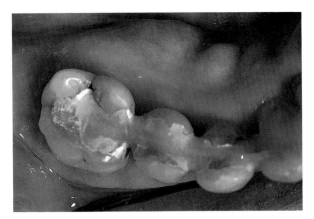

Fig 8-16 A wire and composite resin A-splint.

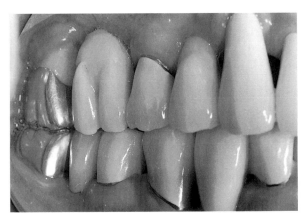

Fig 8-17 Postorthodontic retention provided by crowns that have been splinted together. (Courtesy of Dr Frank Higginbottom).

needed and cost is a concern, these splints may serve for a number of years.

Splinting with fixed partial dentures

In some cases, fixed splints that use full or partial crown restorations can be helpful (Fig 8-17). In such cases the periodontal support may be compromised or an edentulous area may have been planned into the case to minimize tooth movement or treatment time (see chapter 3).

Considerations prior to debanding

As the time for debanding approaches, decisions are made concerning treatment results, problems encountered during treatment, and the final disposition of the patient. As previously stated, patients with growth problems or muscle imbalances (tongue thrust or other aberrant habits) or who will need extensive restorative dentistry will be retained differently than patients without these situations. Communication with other dentists involved in the patient's treatment sequencing is extremely important at this time. The patient who will be having extensive restorative dentistry must be retained with consideration for space maintenance, abutment position, and occlusal plane integrity. The periodontal patient must be retained in conjunction with short-range and long-range periodontal considerations. For the benefit of the patient, the restorative dentist must sequence treatment with all other dental professionals involved in the patient's care. If the generalist has had the orthodontic patient on recall and has followed the progress of

the patient through communication with the orthodontist, he or she should be well apprised of the patient's status. Ideally, the generalist should see the patient prior to debanding and concur that treatment objectives have been reached and that functional, esthetic, and tooth-position requirements have been fulfilled. Communication between the different disciplines of dentistry always benefits the patient. If there is a problem with treatment, or treatment has been compromised, it is best to know this prior to debanding.

Considerations after debanding

For the orthodontic patient who has completed treatment without complications, retention considerations are minimal. These patients wear retainers full time for a period of 6 months. The retention used for the majority of patients in our office is a maxillary Hawley retainer and a mandibular fixed retainer. The maxillary Hawley retainer is worn full time for the first 6 months and then worn only at night for another 12 to 18 months. Subsequent wear is enough to keep the appliance fitting. (In most patients this means wearing the retainer two or three times per week at night.) The mandibular fixed retainer is worn until a decision is made concerning the mandibular third molars. If it appears that eruption of these teeth will be uneventful and they will have normal function, they are maintained. However, if these teeth are impacted and eruption is doubtful, then their removal is suggested along with the maxillary third molars. If on occasion the maxillary third molars have been retained and are in occlusion with the mandibular second molars, they are left. If second molars have been removed and third molars are being allowed to erupt, the mandibular retainer may be left until the third molars are in normal function. Continue to see these retention patients on your routine recall, monitoring with the orthodontist the continuity of retainer wear, oral hygiene, and the condition of the appliances. Continue to check for loose or broken retainers, leaking bands, and the stability of the dentition, including the occlusion and temporomandibular joint dysfunction. Also during this time, special attention is given to periodontal health, and particularly to gingival health and the overall integrity of the periodontal apparatus (see chapter 3). Be alert for teeth in traumatic occlusion causing excessive mobility, fremitus, or discomfort. Many patients who receive retainers no longer feel it is necessary to keep orthodontic appointments and fail to return for follow-up care. It is important that you and your dental hygienist encourage these patients to return to the orthodontist for follow-up. Unless you want responsibility for all aspects of orthodontic retention, it would be advisable not to remove retentive appliances for the patient.

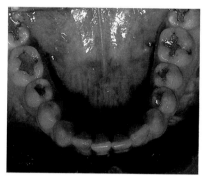

Fig 8-18   Recurrence of crowding. Incisal recrowding is a continual problem.

situations. The supracrestal fiberotomy also seems beneficial in preventing rotational relapses.

With the advent of bonding procedures, tooth size discrepancy problems resulting in diastemata can often be addressed in this manner. In many instances, tooth buildup interproximally or in extreme circumstances bonding the teeth together will correct the problem.

Problems that occur during retention

Relapse

Recurrence of crowding (Fig 8-18) is commonly seen, especially in the mandibular incisors. A different type of retention with minimal interproximal enamel polishing can usually remedy this problem (see p 144). Other manifestations of relapse may include reopening of anterior or posterior open bites and reclosing of anterior closed bites, resulting in spacing in the maxillary anterior teeth, fremitus, mobility, and crowding of mandibular anterior teeth. When these problems arise, it is prudent to consult the attending orthodontist. The generalist should be aware that extremely tight contacts as a result of placement of amalgam, crowns, or fixed partial dentures can cause sufficient tooth movement to begin crowding of the dentition. Clenching, bruxing, other parafunctional habits, misdiagnosis, unbalanced growth, and a too great of an interincisal angle contribute to incisal problems.

Recurrence of diastemata, especially in the maxillary anterior region, and opening of posterior contacts is a common problem. The very nature of anterior diastemata makes them difficult to manage. Tooth size discrepancies and thick labial frenulum are certainly possible causes. Occasionally, frenulum repositioning is necessary, and the incision of supracrestal fibers seems to be an adjunct in stabilizing these

Centric relation–centric occlusion discrepancy

Centric relation–centric occlusion problems result from an improper diagnosis, not completing treatment to centric relation–centric occlusion harmony, a continued Class II growth pattern, an aberrant swallowing pattern forcing a skeletal discrepancy, or overuse of Class II mechanics with resulting physiologic rebound (Figs 8-19a and b). Again, it is prudent to notify the attending orthodontist.

Skeletal problems (growth)

Abnormal growth patterns can still be active after debanding (Fig 8-20). This is especially true in young men because of their continued growth beyond age 20. Ideally this should have been recognized at the time of treatment, but growth prediction is an estimate for even the best diagnostician. Many of these patients will have to be rebanded in conjunction with an orthognathic surgical procedure to correct the skeletal discrepancy. This should be done when you are relatively sure that growth sites are no longer active.

Muscular problems

One of the most common causes of bites reopening or failure to close bites during treatment relates to a

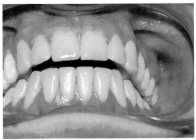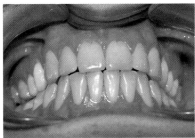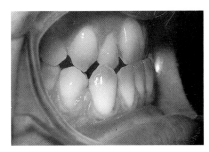

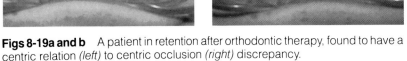

Figs 8-19a and b A patient in retention after orthodontic therapy, found to have a centric relation *(left)* to centric occlusion *(right)* discrepancy.

Fig 8-20 Continued skeletal growth after debanding.

myofunctional imbalance manifested by "tongue thrusting" or a "deviate swallowing" pattern. We normally swallow approximately 2,000 times per day with 2 to 7 pounds of pressure exerted with each swallow.[6] With this type of force on or between the dentition, there will be movement of the dentition until a physiologic balance is reached. The child with allergies offers another example of muscular imbalance. Because most children with allergies have occluded or partially occluded nasal air passages, nasal respiration is either labored or nonexistent. This patient is normally a mouth-breathing patient with a low tongue posture. It is not unusual to see skeletal development with a constricted maxilla, manifested often by a posterior crossbite and/or an anterior or posterior open bite. This patient presents a real challenge. Normal growth will not and cannot take place in the presence of abnormal muscle behavior. Unless nasal airways are established before debanding and aberrant swallowing patterns corrected, treatment will at best be compromised, and retention and stability will be difficult.

It is not uncommon after many years out of retention for the patient to become aware of spacing and movement in the anterior dentition. This may be related to a myofunctional problem that has been present for years and manifests itself with periodontal breakdown. Because of adequate periodontal structures and counterbalance of the lips and cheeks, until this time there has been no deleterious effect on the dentition. However, if periodontal health is diminished, accompanied by substantial bone loss and possibly pressure from clenching or bruxing, there can be a change in physiologic balance. Thus the force field that has countered the muscle imbalance has become altered, resulting in tooth movement.

Williamson[7] states that all tongue thrusting results from a discoordination between the temporomandibular joints and occlusion. In essence, he says that the tongue is placed between the teeth as a protective mechanism to cushion the forces of the malocclu-

sion. Once the joint is restored in harmony with the occlusion, the bite will close on its own.

Williamson[8] also states that the tongue acts as a protective mechanism between the teeth to alleviate discomfort in the presence of internal joint derangements or myofascial pain. The resting posture may result in an open bite. Because the mandible is held slightly open due to the discomfort, the tongue is reflexly protruded.

Habits

Any habit can have a deleterious effect on the dentition. This would include digital, lip, or cheek sucking, pipe smoking, "tooth doodling," clenching, bruxing, or any habit that would tend to influence tooth movement or wear. These habits should be brought to the patient's attention and reduced or ameliorated where possible.

Open contacts

Open contacts or opening of extraction sites is a common problem encountered during the retention period. Often forces of occlusion will tend to separate contact areas. Occlusal equilibration can help eliminate the conflicting force and will allow the contacts to close spontaneously or with adjustment to the retainer. The opening of extraction sites is often related to improper root paralleling during active treatment or to soft-tissue pile-ups or overextension of elastic fibers in the gingiva. Tipping the teeth to close extraction sites usually results in reopening of the sites. It will usually be necessary to replace the fixed appliances and complete therapy. In some cases this can be accompanied by a supracrestal fiberotomy, which can help to reduce relapse. Destruction of a buccal or lingual alveolar wall during extraction may result in diminished alveolar width; such a bone defect may not accommodate a root that is wider than the available alveolar width, thus resulting in open contact. Improper retainer design with occlusal wires crossing interproximally may force contacts to open. Redesigning the retainer will usually eliminate the problem.

Temporomandibular joint problems

Temporomandibular joint problems often occur during the retention phase or begin during active therapy and are not resolved. Grummons[9] has shown that contrary to popular thought, TMJ dysfunction may not be more prevalent in orthodontic extraction cases.

As previously mentioned, the harmony of the TMJs should be monitored during and after the course of active therapy with the orthodontist. At the first sign of internal derangement, abnormal joint noises, myofascial pain, myalgia, or pain in or around the joint, the attending orthodontist should be notified (see chapter 12). If this is a new problem, proper attention should be given immediately. If it is a recurrence of a long-standing problem, its management should have been decided upon at the time of diagnosis and treatment planning. Many of the myofascial pain-dysfunction problems are transitional and disappear within a short time. However, if the muscle pain lingers, a minimal amount of equilibration or initiation of splint therapy may be necessary to reestablish joint stability and occlusal harmony.

Periodontal maintenance of the patient during active orthodontic treatment

During active orthodontic therapy, it is to the patient's advantage to continue to see the generalist and/or periodontist for routine maintenance. This might vary from 2-week to 3-month intervals. The periodontally involved patient should be seen on a frequent basis for subgingival scaling and root planing, to monitor the occlusion, and to eliminate fremitus. The clinical signs of inflammation must be eliminated prior to orthodontic care and be kept under control during therapy (see chapter 3). If this cannot be done, continued orthodontics may lead to a deterioration of periodontal health. Shared maintenance not only benefits the patient by adding a different dental perspective, but it keeps the generalist or periodontist in touch with treatment progress and any developing problems. At these visits the dental therapist should be acutely observant of periodontal health, especially with regard to gingival tissue health (stripping, bleeding, hyperplasia, oral hygiene, probing depths), caries, and decalcification (see chapter 2). The dentist and hygienist should also be alert for loose or leaking bands, brackets, broken appliances, and overall patient attitude. The dentist also should observe centric relation–centric occlusion discrepancies, TMJ dysfunction, and related myofascial pain, headaches, or other symptoms related to internal derangement of the joint. The orthodontist should anticipate and will appreciate a call from the generalist or periodontist relative to any findings.

At a glance

Maintenance for the adult in fixed appliances

- Orthodontic retention should be planned and discussed with the patient before therapy begins.
- There are a number of ways to retain teeth once active treatment is complete. A knowledge of each approach is needed so the dentist can choose the appropriate retention modality.
- The introduction of functional appliances has opened a new arena for treatment. Patients who can benefit from this kind of therapy should be referred before loss of the primary dentition.
- Problems arising during maintenance may include crowding, relapse, centric relation–centric occlusion discrepancy, growth disharmony, muscular problems, habits, open contacts, and temporomandibular joint problems. Onset of any of these problems should trigger an orthodontic consultation.
- The generalist and/or the periodontist should participate in maintaining the dentition and periodontium during and after orthodontic care.

III. Periodontal Maintenance for the Orthodontic Patient

Thomas G. Wilson, Jr

Periodontal diseases

Childhood through puberty

The vast majority of patients from childhood through puberty who receive fixed orthodontic devices develop gingivitis. This gingivitis usually disappears clinically after removal of appliances.[10] However, during orthodontic therapy a small number develop periodontitis de novo or exacerbate a previously existing condition (Fig 8-21); consequently, every patient should be evaluated for periodontal problems before, during, and after orthodontic therapy.

Chronic gingivitis

This is the most common periodontal problem and is often encountered in children. The diagnosis is made when bleeding upon probing is seen in depths of 3 mm or less. Problems occur when this inflammatory lesion moves apically to involve the alveolar bone. Fortunately, in the vast majority of orthodontic cases this does not occur. Maintenance for these patients involves the same procedures as with adults—increased emphasis on oral hygiene and frequent recall for professional prophylaxes.

Prepubertal periodontitis

This form of periodontitis occurs at the time of eruption of the primary teeth. It has a generalized and a localized form. The former is characterized by severe gingival inflammation, rapid bone destruction, and marked changes in peripheral white blood cells. Otitis media and upper respiratory infection are often seen. The localized form features little or no gingival inflammation and is amenable to treatment by curettage and antibiotics.[11] These patients are not orthodontic candidates unless the bony destruction can be halted and held in check.

Localized juvenile periodontitis

This problem occurs around the onset of puberty and is therefore occasionally seen in orthodontic patients.[12] It is characterized by localized bone loss (usually vertical) seen around first molars and maxillary incisors. Two bacterial species have been found

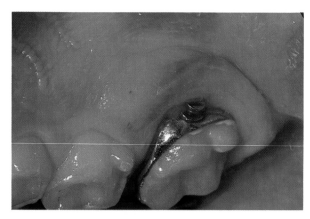

Fig 8-21 A periodontal abscess associated with the placement of an orthodontic band that violated the biologic width (see chapter 7). The lesion probed 7 mm, but it resolved when the band was removed and the area treated using closed subgingival scaling and root planing.

to be associated with these lesions (*Actinobacillus actinomycetemcomitans* and *Actinobacillus capnocytophagia*). Bone loss can occur rapidly, and therefore this problem should be treated aggressively (Fig 8-22). These problems are occasionally discovered during orthodontic care, and if treated and followed closely these patients can have orthodontic movement of the involved teeth.

Adults

Chronic periodontitis

This is the most common form of periodontitis and is often encountered in adult orthodontic patients. Its hallmark is slow, progressive bone loss. In patients with less than optimal oral hygiene or maintenance, the combination of orthodontic trauma and periodontitis can hasten pocket formation (Figs 8-23a to c).

Rapidly progressive adult periodontitis

This disease is characterized by rapid generalized bone destruction. These patients should have their disease process under control before orthodontics begins and should be monitored very closely during therapy.[13]

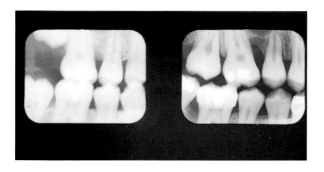

Fig 8-22 A radiograph exposed at age 12 revealed a radiolucent bony lesion on the mesial surface of the maxillary first molar *(left)* that was exacerbated by orthodontic therapy. At age 14, following orthodontic care without the benefit of periodontal care *(right)*, the probing depth was 9 mm.

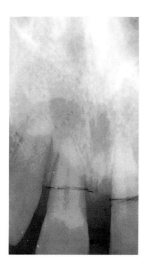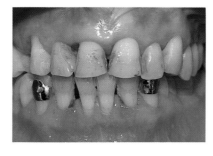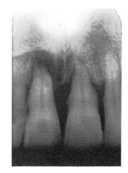

Fig 8-23a *(left)* The bone loss seen in this radiograph was demonstrated to the patient with a pencil line drawn on the film before orthodontic care was started.

Figs 8-23b and c *(middle and right)* Unfortunately, the inflammatory lesions were not treated during orthodontic care, resulting in clinical and radiographic bone loss. The central incisors are endodontically vital.

Refractory periodontitis

This group of patients has extensive, rapid bone loss following traditional periodontal therapy. In some cases the disease is quiescent for months or years only to appear in the form of rapid bone loss. At times this bone loss occurs during tooth movement. In those cases, tooth movement should be stopped, the periodontal problem treated, and the patient reevaluated to determine whether or not orthodontic therapy should be resumed.

——— *At a glance* ———

Periodontal diseases in orthodontic patients

■ Because periodontal diseases affect children and young adults, you must gather the same periodontal information on these patients as you gather for adults.
■ For patients with periodontal problems, frequent maintenance and optimal oral hygiene are important.

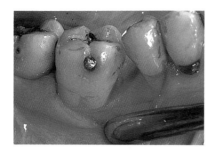

Fig 8-24a A full-thickness mucoperiosteal flap was raised before orthodontic procedures were initiated. Note the two-wall bony crater on the mesial surface of the second molar (the third molar was extracted at the time of this surgery).

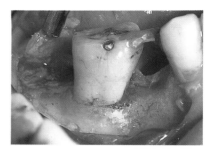

Fig 8-24b This is the bony picture found 6 months after orthodontic therapy was completed; the bony defect seen before orthodontics has resolved without bone removal.

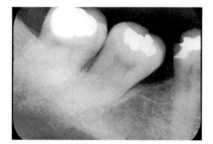

Fig 8-24c Pretreatment radiograph of the teeth seen in Fig 8-24a.

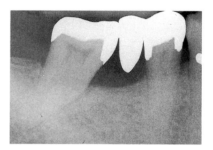

Fig 8-24d Radiograph taken 13 years after therapy.

Is orthodontics beneficial to the periodontium?

Although there is debate on either side, some saying there is benefit from orthodontic care[14–16] and some saying no,[17–20] in my opinion the efficacy of the patient's oral hygiene and the timeliness of maintenance visits dictate the longevity of the dentition to a greater degree than does orthodontic therapy. There are specific areas, however, where orthodontic therapy is definitely beneficial to the periodontium; they include the following:

1. If a patient has an overbite that impinges on periodontal tissues[20]
2. To reduce trauma from the teeth in cases of anterior open bite and other severe malocclusions
3. To change the topography of the periodontium around tipped teeth[21,22]

There are also negative aspects to orthodontic care.

1. Orthodontic therapy results in a small loss of attachment even in well-maintained cases.[23,24] This may occur because many orthodontists still place bands subgingivally in adults. While this may not cause immediately evident problems, it may set up

negative changes in the sulcus ecosystem similar to those seen in the placement of subgingival margins of improper fit.[25–27] The effects could be far reaching. To help with these problems we suggest that you use bonded brackets above the gingiva where possible, use removable devices whenever possible, take care to ensure that any flash around brackets is trimmed well short of gingival tissues, and place band margins coronal to the gingival margin.
2. Orthodontics may exacerbate a preexisting periodontal condition.[28]
3. Orthodontic therapy may create mucogingival problems.[29]

Preventing or ameliorating periodontal problems associated with orthodontic therapy

Before orthodontic therapy

Every potential candidate for orthodontic therapy should have a thorough periodontal screening before

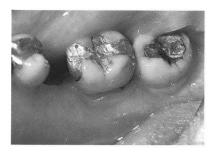

Fig 8-25a A more advanced bony lesion associated with a tipped mandibular molar. The original clinical picture.

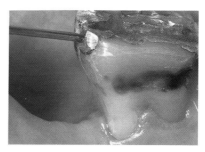

Fig 8-25b The clinical view 9 years after completion of therapy.

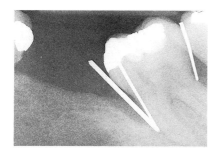

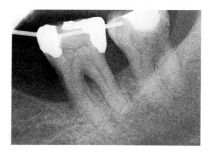

Figs 8-25c and d Radiographs from the same periods. The original bony defect is shown in Fig 8-25c and its resolution (without bone removal) and a second surgery 7 years after completion of orthodontic therapy is shown in Fig 8-25d. The tooth was cleaned thoroughly before orthodontic therapy (using a flap approach for improved access), then uprighted and extruded with fixed appliances.

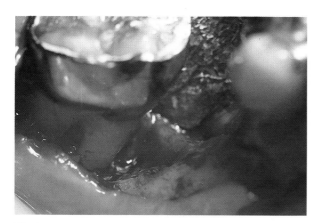

Fig 8-25e When flaps were lifted to facilitate root planing, small flecks of calculus could be seen despite previous closed scaling.

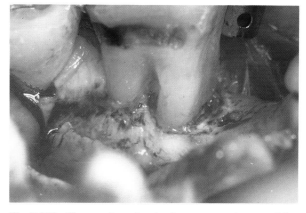

Fig 8-25f Six months after tooth movement ceased the area was reopened, revealing a positive remodeling of the alveolar housing when compared to Fig 8-25e. The probing depths were within normal limits.

tooth movement begins. This should include an evaluation of oral hygiene, a check for inflammatory periodontal diseases, an examination for the presence of trauma from occlusion, and an examination for potential mucogingival problems (see chapter 2).

Oral hygiene

It is important for the potential orthodontic candidate

to have optimal oral hygiene. Absence of proper cleaning can have extremely negative consequences for children and adults who have periodontitis before tooth movement starts. Each individual should be taught to use the most effective means possible for interproximal cleaning. Where space is available, floss or interproximal brushes are optimal; where they cannot or will not be used, then a mechanical toothbrush with individually rotating tufts is recom-

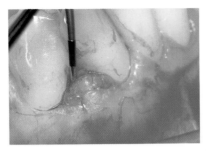

Fig 8-26a *(above)* A pathologically deepened sulcus (7 mm) was found on the mesial surface of this premolar before orthodontic therapy. The root was cleaned under local anesthetic with closed subgingival scaling and root planing.

Fig 8-26b *(right)* After frequent maintenance visits during orthodontic therapy, the area has a reduced probing depth (3 mm) but is still associated with slight bleeding upon probing. For this reason the maintenance intervals are kept short (usually every 6 weeks).

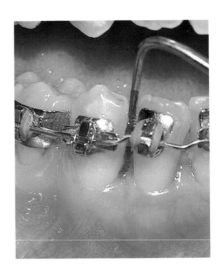

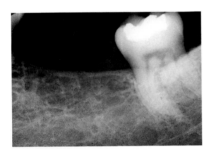

Fig 8-27a Radiograph taken before orthodontic care. Bleeding upon probing associated with 3-mm probing depths was seen. The therapist failed to adjust the occlusion or refer the patient for periodontal care.

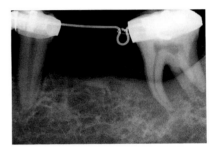

Fig 8-27b Radiograph 9 months after initiation of orthodontic therapy.

mended.[30] An oral irrigator is a poor third choice. Using well-trimmed, bonded brackets and keeping bands as far away from the base of the sulcus as possible leaves more room for effective cleaning.[31]

Inflammatory periodontal diseases

The patient should be screened for the presence of inflammatory periodontal diseases in the usual manner (see chapter 2). If any problems are found, they must be corrected before orthodontic therapy begins. Subgingival deposits should be removed by the most conservative, expeditious manner possible. This usually means closed subgingival scaling and root planing, but in deeper pockets a flap approach is often necessary. Bone should not be removed during surgical procedures performed at this stage (Figs 8-24a to d to 8-26a and b).

Trauma from occlusion

This is best evidenced by the presence of fremitus, which should be eliminated before tooth movement begins in patients who manifest inflammatory disease by bleeding upon probing around the tooth in question after initial therapy. Failure to perform this step can lead to dramatic problems (Figs 8-27a and b). For a discussion of the role of trauma from occlusion and its role in inflammatory periodontal diseases, see chapter 7.

Mucogingival problems

At present there is a question about when or indeed whether gaining additional attached gingiva is necessary before orthodontic therapy. It would seem that where oral hygiene is optimal and orthodontics is not

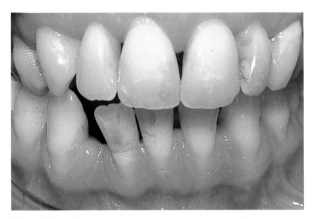

Fig 8-28a This patient was advised to have free gingival grafts before orthodontics that would retain the teeth anterior to their initial position.

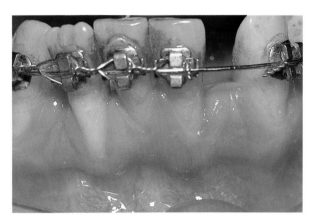

Fig 8-28b The patient refused the suggested treatment and despite optimal oral hygiene, stripping continued.

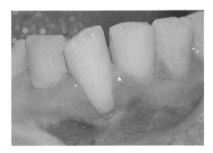

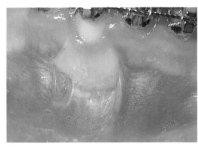

Fig 8-29a This patient was about to begin orthodontic care that would result in anterior positioning of the left central incisor.

Figs 8-29b and c A free gingival graft was placed, and the area fared well during orthodontic therapy.

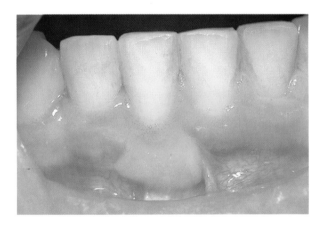

Fig 8-29d The graft 5 years posttherapy.

to be done, grafts are seldom needed.[32] However, because perfect oral cleanliness is rare, grafts may be needed before tooth movement begins,[33] because if the teeth are moved through the cortical plate, recession often occurs in a thin periodontium.[34] If oral hygiene is good and these same teeth are retracted, little residual damage ensues.[35] However, if oral hygiene is not optimal or if these teeth must be held in a prominent position, permanent and often progressive gingival recession can occur (Figs 8-28a and b and 8-29a to d). In my practice, grafts are placed before orthodontics begins on teeth that have all of the following conditions: 1 mm or less of attached gingiva, thin gingival tissues, less than optimal oral hygiene, and when this tooth is to be moved and held in a prominent position.

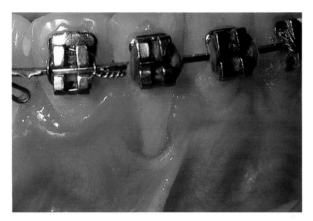

Fig 8-30a Stripping of the soft tissues occurred when this incisor was moved into facial prominence.

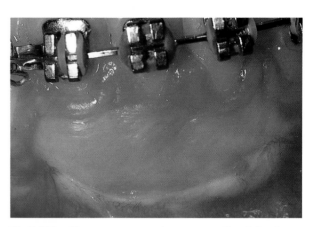

Fig 8-30b The area was no longer sensitive following a free gingival graft to repair the lesion.

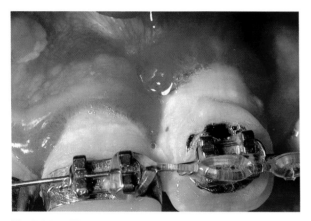

Fig 8-31a The central incisor erupted high in the alveolar mucosa and brought this tissue along as it was moved incisally.

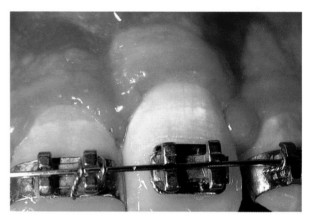

Fig 8-31b The area was bothering the patient both functionally and esthetically until it was repaired with a graft, here seen shortly postoperatively.

During orthodontic care

Oral hygiene

You should simply continue to monitor, record, and attempt to improve oral hygiene at each maintenance visit.

Inflammatory periodontal diseases

The patient with less than optimal oral hygiene or with preexisting (or developing) periodontitis should be seen for a periodontal prophylaxis at intervals similar to other patients with these problems. Maintenance intervals are set by bleeding upon probing and probing depth changes (see chapter 6).

Trauma from occlusion

Fremitus should be monitored and eliminated where present in patients who have clinical signs of inflammatory periodontal diseases (see chapter 7). In extreme situations the fabrication of a disarticulating device may be warranted.

Mucogingival problems

These are detected by referring to premovement baseline measurements of gingival recession and treated as previously described (Figs 8-30a and b and 8-31a and b). A special condition exists when impacted teeth must be uncovered (Figs 8-32a to d and 8-33a to d).

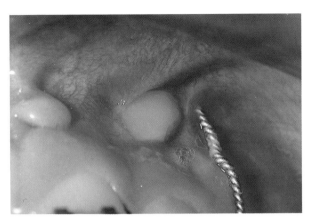 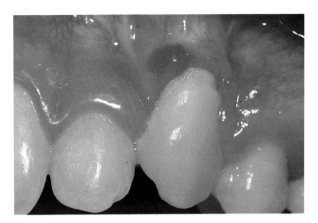

Figs 8-32a and b A canine uncovered with a window procedure brings the alveolar mucosa incisally as it erupts.

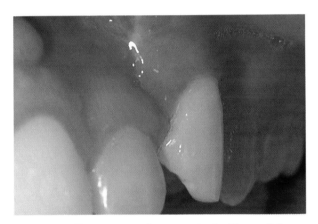 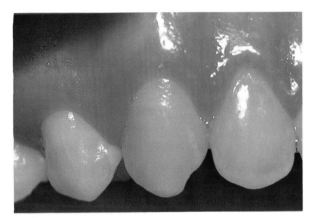

Fig 8-32c The area was later repaired with a soft tissue graft.

Fig 8-32d The opposite canine erupted into attached gingiva and erupted normally.

After orthodontic care

Oral hygiene

This parameter should be monitored as with any other patient.

Inflammatory periodontal disease

The patient should be kept on appropriate maintenance then reevaluated 6 months after tooth movement ends. At this time, any remaining deepened probing depths should be dealt with.

Trauma from occlusion

Monitoring of fremitus and tooth mobility should be continued and evaluated 6 months after cessation of active orthodontics. At that time a final treatment plan to control the occlusion should be developed. For bruxers, a maxillary hard acrylic resin habit appliance should be worn in place of the typical orthodontic retainer. For a discussion of this aspect of therapy, see chapter 7.

Mucogingival problems

It frequently takes time for gingival recession to occur after orthodontics has been completed. Therefore, this parameter must be closely monitored.

Figs 8-33a to d   A canine that was uncovered using an apically positioned flap to reposition the keratinized gingiva.

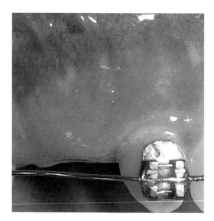

Fig 8-33a

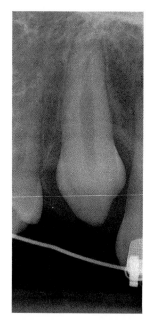

Fig 8-33b

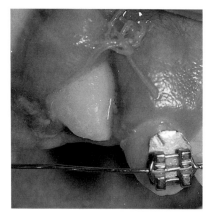

Fig 8-33c

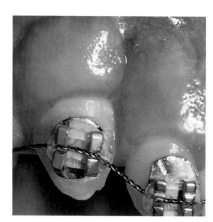

Fig 8-33d

At a glance

Preventing periodontal problems during orthodontic care

- Prevention depends on examination before, during, and after orthodontic care.
- Oral hygiene, especially in interproximal areas, is of optimal importance in these patients.
- Preexisting gingivitis and periodontitis should be controlled with scaling and root planing (open or closed) before orthodontics begins and kept under control by the same approach during and up to 6 months after treatment. Residual pockets should be dealt with at this time.
- In patients with periodontitis, fremitus should be eliminated at each orthodontic and maintenance visit.

References

1. Ochsenbein C, Maynard JG: The problem of attached gingiva in children. *J Dent Child* 1974;41:263.
2. Vanarsdall RL, Corn H: Soft-tissue management of labially positioned unerupted teeth. *Am J Orthod* 1977;72:53.
3. Dewey M, revised by Anderson GM: *Practical Orthodontia*, 5th ed. St Louis, CV Mosby Co, 1935, p 463.
4. Strang RHW: *Textbook of Orthodontics*. Philadelphia, Lea & Febiger, 1943, pp 598–599.
5. Becker CM, Kaiser DA, Lemm RB: A simplified technique for fabrication of night guards. *J Prosthet Dent* 1974;32:582.
6. Straub WJ: Malfunction of the tongue. II. The abnormal swallowing habit: its causes, effects, and results in relation to orthodontic treatment and speech therapy. *Am J Orthod* 1961;47:596.
7. Williamson EH: Lecture notes, November, 1985.
8. Williamson EH: Treatment of internal derangement and closure of posterior open bite in the adult. *Facial Orthop and Temporomandibular Arthrol* 1986;3:3.
9. Grummons D: Lecture notes, December, 1984.
10. Zachrisson S, Zachrisson BU: Gingival condition associated with orthodontic treatment. *Angle Orthod* 1972;42:26.
11. Page RC, Bowen T, Altman L, Vandesteen E, Ochs H, Mackenzie P, Osterberg S, Engel LD, Williams BL: Prepubertal periodontitis. I. Definition of a clinical disease entity. *J Periodontol* 1983;54:257.
12. Topoll HH, Lange DE: Juvenile periodontitis. Pathogenesis and treatment: A case documentation. *Int J Periodont Rest Dent* 1988;8:57.
13. Wilson TG, Higginbottom FL, Lamberth RE, Adcock JE, Schoen J: Rapidly progressive periodontitis in young adults: Two case studies with 10-year follow-up. The role of active and maintenance therapy. *Int J Periodont Rest Dent* 1989;9:107–121.
14. Alexander AG, Tipnis AK: The effect of irregularity of teeth and the degree of overbite and overjet on the gingival health. *Br Dent J* 1970;128:539.
15. Buckley LA: The relationship between malocclusion and periodontal disease. *J Periodontol* 1972;43:415.
16. Kessler M: Interrelationships between orthodontics and periodontics. *Am J Orthod* 1976;70:154.
17. Geiger AM, Wasserman BH, Turgeon LR: Relation of occlusion and periodontal disease. Part VIII. Relationship of crowding and spacing to periodontal destruction and gingival inflammation. *J Periodontol* 1974;45:43.
18. Ingervall B, Jacobsson U, Nyman S: A clinical study of the relationship between crowding of teeth, plaque and gingival condition. *J Clin Periodontol* 1977;4:214.
19. Prichard JF: The effect of bicuspid extraction orthodontics on the periodontium. Findings in 100 consecutive cases. *J Periodontol* 1975;46:534.
20. Gould MSE, Picton DCA: The relation between irregularities of the teeth and periodontal disease. A pilot study. *Br Dent J* 1966;121:20.
21. Brown IS: The effects of orthodontic therapy on certain kinds of periodontal defects. I. Clinical findings. *J Periodontol* 1973;44:742.
22. Cohen DW: Areas of common concern to orthodontics and periodontics, in McNamara JA, Ribbens KA (eds): *Malocclusion and the Periodontium*. Ann Arbor, Center for Human Growth and Development, University of Michigan, 1984, p 73.
23. Zachrisson BU, Alnaes L: Periodontal condition in orthodontically treated and untreated individuals. I. Loss of attachment, gingival pocket depth and clinical crown height. *Angle Orthod* 1973;43:402.
24. Alstad S, Zachrisson BU: Longitudinal study of periodontal condition associated with orthodontic treatment in adolescents. *Am J Orthod* 1979;76:277.
25. Bjorn AL, Bjorn H, Grkovic B: Marginal fit of restorations and its relation to periodontal bone level. Part II. Crowns. *Odontol Rev* 1970;21:337.
26. Than A, Duguid R, McKendrick AJW: Relationship between restorations and the level of the periodontal attachment. *J Clin Periodontol* 1982;9:193.
27. Richter WA, Ueno H: Relationship of crown margin placement to gingival inflammation. *J Prosthet Dent* 1973;30:156.
28. Ericson I, Thilander B, Lindhe J, Okamoto H: The effect of orthodontic tilting movements on the periodontal tissues of infected and noninfected dentitions in dogs. *J Clin Periodontol* 1977;4:278.
29. Klar LA: *An evaluation of occlusion in post-orthodontic patients*. Master's thesis, Cleveland: Case Western Reserve University, 1977.
30. Long DE, Killoy WJ: Evaluation of the effectiveness of the Interplak™ home plaque removal instrument on plaque removal and orthodontic patients. *Compend Cont Educ Dent* 1985;6:S156.
31. Zachrisson BU: Clinical implications of recent ortho-perio research findings, in Hösl E, Zachrisson BU, Baldauf A (eds): *Orthodontics and Periodontics*. Chicago, Quintessence Publ Co, 1985, p 109.
32. Kennedy JE, Bird WC, Palcanis KG, Dorfman HS: A longitudinal evaluation of varying widths of attached gingiva. *J Clin Periodontol* 1985;12:667.
33. Maynard JG, Ochsenbein C: Mucogingival problems, prevalence and therapy in children. *J Periodontol* 1975;46:543.
34. Engelking G, Zachrisson BU: Effects of incisor repositioning on monkey periodontium after expansion through the cortical plate. *Am J Orthod* 1982;82:23.
35. Steiner GG, Pearson JK, Ainamo J: Changes of the marginal periodontium as a result of labial tooth movement in monkeys. *J Periodontol* 1981;52:314.

Chapter 9

Periodontal-Endodontic Problems Encountered During Maintenance

Justin E. Aurbach / Thomas G. Wilson, Jr

Because their clinical presentations can be so similar, differentiating among periodontal and endodontic problems can be vexing. The practitioner must decide if the problem is a periodontal pocket, periodontal abscess, endodontic problem, or a combined periodontal-endodontic lesion. Diagnosis of periodontal pockets has been covered in detail in chapter 2. This chapter will deal with the pure endodontic lesion, the combined periodontal-endodontic lesion, and the periodontal abscess.

Diagnosis of the pure endodontic problem

Medical and dental history

Chief complaint

1. Pain, swelling, a loose tooth, or a dark tooth may indicate endodontic involvement.
2. Ask if the patient can positively identify the offending tooth. Ask additional leading but specific questions to help elaborate on the history, particularly with regard to all aspects of pain.

Duration of pain

1. Intermittent, continuous, or only when stimulated?
2. Does it last seconds, minutes, or hours?
3. Is pain spontaneous or only when stimulated?

Type of pain

1. Is tooth painful to hot or cold liquids?
2. Does cold relieve pain from heat?
3. Is tooth painful while chewing?
4. Does it throb?

5. Is it painful at gum line?
6. Is it painful during tooth brushing or flossing?

Pulps do not contain proprioceptive nerve fibers; the periodontal ligament does. In cases of vague pulpal pain, the offending tooth will eventually identify itself and the pain will localize once the inflammatory process involves the periodontal ligament. This is especially important in large reconstructive cases.

Visual examination

Conditions that may indicate endodontic lesions:

1. Facial asymmetry—extraoral swelling
2. Changes in color or contour in soft tissues surrounding teeth
3. Presence of caries
4. Extensive restorations
5. Fractures
6. Discolored teeth (nonvital teeth may appear darker)
7. Sinus tracts (these are rarely associated with periodontal lesions)

Conditions that can be occasionally associated with endodontic lesions:

1. Cervical erosion
2. Gingival recession
3. Developmental defects of teeth
4. Abrasions

Clinical examination

1. *Palpation—swelling, tenderness, lymphadenopathy.* Swelling seen with endodontic lesions is usually located in the apical regions of the tooth, whereas periodontal lesions usually swell around the gingival

margin. Lymphadenopathy is rarely associated with periodontal conditions.

2. *Percussion—pain from an acute apical periodontitis.* Sensitivity to percussion indicates that the inflammatory process has extended from pulp into the periodontal ligament space. The pressure buildup from edema (in the periodontal ligament) in this space can be tremendous and the pain excruciating when the tooth is percussed (tapped). According to Seltzer and Bender,[1] "Percussion is an important diagnostic test for detection of partial or total necrosis of pulp tissue."

3. *Probing.* A periodontal screening should be done and the results compared with the suspected tooth (see chapter 2). It is unusual to see a periodontal problem manifest as the only deep probing depth in the mouth. When an endodontic lesion drains through the periodontal ligament, it usually results in a single deep, narrow pocket. Periodontal diseases usually present with broad pockets in the coronal aspect that narrow apically.

4. *Tooth mobility.* The nonworking end of two single-ended instruments can be used to test for tooth mobility. Causes for mobility include:
   a. Pressure from an acute apical abscess
   b. Advanced periodontal disease
   c. Root fracture
   d. Chronic bruxism or clenching
   e. Trauma—fracture of labial plate

Clinical tests

Electric pulp tests

The electric pulp tester is an instrument that uses a gradient electric (DC) current to elicit a response from susceptible pulpal elements. The electric pulp test does not truly measure pulp vitality, which is determined by the presence (vitality) or absence (nonvitality) of a vascular supply. The results of electric pulp testing are always subject to the error of human interpretation and should be evaluated with results from other diagnostic aids before establishing a final diagnosis. It is fortunate that most nonvital teeth have lost all sensory innervation. Electric pulp testing does not give absolute values for particular conditions in specific teeth, and results must be interpreted on an individual basis. Thus, a standard threshold must be established for each individual. Results of testing from the tooth in question must be compared with values obtained from adjacent teeth and the contralateral tooth of same type. It has been shown that considerable loss of blood supply may occur before there is sufficient degeneration of nerve supply to

alter the electrical response, and so it is hoped that instruments to judge this parameter will be developed. The battery-operated tester manufactured by Analytic Technology is preferred. It has automatic progression in current, the rate of which can be controlled; low-battery indicators; a light on the handle that indicates a complete circuit; and mini-tips that can be placed on the enamel or cementum of many crowned teeth.

As with many tests, there are limitations of reliability. The accuracy of results can be influenced by numerous factors.

False-positive reactions. Circumstances leading to false-positive reactions to electric pulp tests are:

1. Mental and emotional state. Extremely apprehensive patients may have an abnormally low pain threshold response to clinical diagnostic tests. Children in particular may be apprehensive; they may not fully understand what the sensation is, or when and how to respond.
2. Pain threshold level. Each individual has a different pain threshold, which makes it imperative that the results of the tooth in question be compared with a normal contralateral tooth or adjacent tooth. For example, a patient losing sleep because of a toothache or the anxiety of anticipating dental treatment is apt to have a lower pain threshold and will respond more quickly to the stimulus. The same tooth may give different responses when tested a few minutes or days apart.
3. Saliva on the tooth or the prolonged drying of a tooth (with moisture loss from the enamel), causing increased electrical resistance.[2]
4. Electrode positioned too close to marginal gingiva. This may elicit a response from the gingival tissue rather than from the tooth.[2]
5. Transfer of electric current from a nonvital tooth to a vital tooth via large approximal metallic restorations. To avoid this, separate the proximal contacts with small strips of rubber dam.[2]

False-negative responses. Circumstances leading to false-negative responses are:

1. Diffuse calcification of the pulp tissue.[2]
2. Large amounts of reparative "irritational" dentin obliterating the pulp chamber and insulating the vital pulp from the electrical stimulus.[2] This often is the result of extensive restorations or pulp-capping procedures.
3. An immature tooth with an incompletely formed apex. Such a tooth will often give unreliable responses.[2]

4. Poor contact between the electrode and tooth surface.
5. Failure to turn pulp tester on or plug it in; dead batteries.
6. Teeth recently traumatized or having undergone recent orthodontic movement may respond irregularly or not at all to vitality tests.[3] Some traumatized teeth may regain their ability to respond to vitality testing. For this reason, several electric pulp tests should be performed on a tooth, and results should be averaged to form a baseline for future reference.[2]
7. Analgesics, alcohol, sedatives, and tranquilizers may mask the patient's true reaction to the stimulus by raising the pain threshold.[2]
8. Primary teeth do not provide reliable information to electric pulp tests. Permanent teeth with immature apices will give a misleading response to such tests. Frequently, there may be no response (or a very high response) when the pulp is completely vital. Elderly individuals with diffuse calcification and near obliteration of pulp canals will often show little or no response to pulp tests.
9. A multicanaled tooth with vital pulp tissue in only one canal. Such a tooth may respond with a high "normal."[2]

Directions to patients. In all vitality tests the patient should be told in advance why the test is being performed, what to expect, and how to respond so that he or she will be less apprehensive. The patient can respond by raising a hand when the stimulus is first felt. Test a normal tooth first to acquaint the patient with the sensation.

Pulp testing technique. Isolate the tooth or teeth to be tested with cotton rolls and air dry them.

All pulp testers require an electrolyte medium for conduction from the probe to hard tissue. I prefer electrocardiography gel. The probe is dipped into the gel and placed on the cervical portion of the crown of the tooth without contacting the gingiva, making sure the tip of the probe is on sound enamel, dentin, or cementum. Electric pulp testing on dentin or cementum will cause an almost immediate response compared with teeth covered with sound enamel. To prevent a false reading, the probe and conductor must not touch any restoration.

The finding of multiple nonreactive teeth should be disregarded, particularly when apparently normal teeth are involved, because individual patients may be stoic or have a high pain threshold. Conversely, some patients may be excitable and react quickly to minimal stimulation.

The electric pulp test can be a valuable aid in determining whether a problem is of pulpal or periodontal origin. Some of the clinical symptoms of an acute alveolar and acute periodontal abscess are similar. Pulp evaluation is a necessary adjunct in periodontal diagnosis to determine the correct course of treatment for lesions possibly requiring endodontic therapy in addition to periodontal therapy.

Thermal pulp tests

It is the opinion of many endodontic clinicians that thermal testing is the most reliable indicator of pulp health and vitality. Thermal testing is quite valuable in detecting pulpitis and as an adjunct in the differentiation of reversible and irreversible pulpal inflammation.

Cold tests. Cold tests are easily performed with ice or ethyl chloride. Ethyl chloride is sprayed onto a cotton pellet until ice crystals form then applied to the tooth for 5 seconds.[2] I prefer to freeze water in empty anesthetic carpules or in the covers from disposable needles.

Cold tests cannot be repeated immediately. Pulp tissue learns rapidly to accommodate to cold stimuli. A prolonged hypersensitive response (pain that lingers after removal of stimulus) is an abnormal response indicating irreversibly inflamed pulpal tissue.

Heat tests. To test a tooth with heat, use white baseplate gutta-percha wrapped around a plastic instrument that has been warmed in a flame. Heat until the material just begins to smoke and apply to the cervical area of the tooth. A temperature of over 150°F should be reached, which is sufficient to gain a response from an inflamed pulp. The material should be warmed out of the patient's line of vision to avoid undue anticipation and unreliable response. A prolonged hypersensitive response (pain that lingers after stimulus has been removed) usually signifies irreversible pulpitis. Generally, a normal pulp will show a moderate response to both heat and cold; when the stimulus is withdrawn, the mild discomfort dissipates almost immediately. The total absence of a response to thermal and electric pulp tests strongly suggests the presence of pulpal necrosis.

Test cavity

The test cavity examination, usually considered a last resort, is used to determine pulp vitality only if the results of other tests have proved inconclusive. Without the use of an anesthetic, a pulpal response will occur in a tooth with a vital pulp when a bur penetrates the dentinoenamel junction. After the patient understands why this test is being performed and

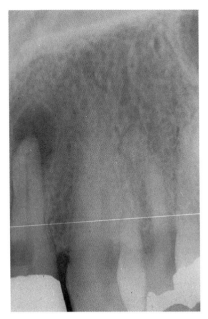

Fig 9-1a A preoperative radiograph showing external resorption on the mesial surface of a maxillary lateral incisor.

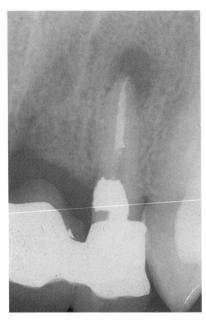

Fig 9-1b The external lesion was repaired with amalgam.

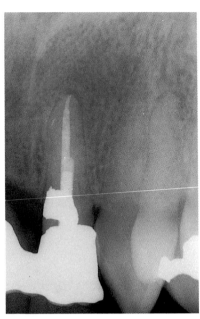

Fig 9-1c Radiograph 10 years later.

what to expect, a small half-round high-speed bur with a copious water spray is drilled through the dentinoenamel junction. The patient will feel a sharp painful sensation if the pulp is vital. Conversely, if the pulp chamber is reached with no response, the pulp is necrotic or partially necrotic.

Anesthetic tests

Anesthetic tests can separate pain between mandibular and maxillary arches to localize the arch in question. Selective infiltration in the maxilla can locate a specific tooth.

Transillumination

When a beam of light from a fiber optic light source is passed through a normal tooth, it will appear clear and pinkish. A necrotic tooth will usually appear opaque and darker than adjacent teeth. This is also helpful in locating fractures.

Radiographic examination

To make a diagnosis, you should obtain high-quality, parallel, long-cone radiographs. Bisecting-angle radiographs are not acceptable for endodontic diagnosis. At least two preoperative periapical radiographs

should be taken. To help gain a three-dimensional perspective, the second film is taken with the vertical angulation of the x-ray cone remaining unchanged, but the horizontal angulation is varied between 5° and 15°. With a properly oriented central beam, differences in radiographic shadows can be interpreted with greater accuracy.

The status of pulpal health, even necrosis, cannot be determined radiographically, although certain findings can arouse suspicion of degenerative change: deep carious lesions with possible pulp exposure and deep restorations; pulp cappings; pulpotomies; pulp stones; pathologic canal calcifications; internal or external root resorption (Figs 9-1a to c); radiolucent lesions (circumscribed or diffuse) at or near the root apex; root fractures; severe periodontal disease.

Bite-wing radiographs are an aid when there is no periapical involvement. In general, the deeper the caries (Figs 9-2a and b) and the more extensive the restoration, the greater the probability of pulpal involvement.

The use of a strong magnifying lens and good lighting are helpful when examining radiographs.

A radiolucent lesion need not be at the root apex to indicate pulpal degeneration or inflammation. Toxins resulting from tissue necrosis in lateral canals or accessory canals can result in osseous destruction anywhere along the root (Figs 9-3a to c) or floor of the

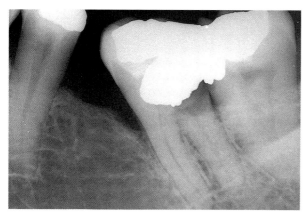

Fig 9-2a Extensive caries has invaded this mandibular molar.

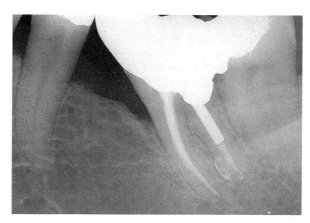

Fig 9-2b Radiograph taken 10 years after endodontic therapy and repair of the carious lesion.

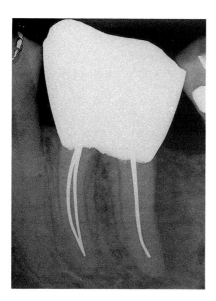

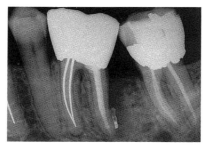

Figs 9-3a and b Re-treatment of a failing distal root on a mandibular molar.

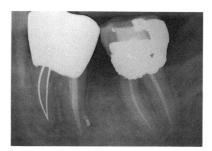

Fig 9-3c A 3-year followup showing return of bony tissues.

pulp chamber. Conversely, a lateral canal can be a portal of entry for potentially destructive toxins in teeth with severe periodontitis. If osseous loss extends far enough apically to expose the foramen of a lateral canal, toxins from periodontal pathogens can enter a healthy pulp and produce inflammation and necrosis in an otherwise healthy tooth. Periodontal disease that extends to the apical foramen can result in pathologic changes in the pulp. The incidence of calcifications in the pulp chamber or canal increases in the presence of periodontal disease or extensive restorations.

Other endodontic problems that can be seen radiographically include internal resorption. The pulp expands at the expense of the dentin and must be removed as soon as possible to prevent perforation of the root, which worsens the prognosis.

Root fractures can result in pulpal degeneration. They can be difficult to detect radiographically. The vertical root fracture can rarely be identified on radiographs, except in advanced root separation. It is easy to confuse horizontal fractures with osseous trabeculae; however, the lines of osseous trabeculae extend beyond the root border. Fractures will also frequently cause a widening of the periodontal ligament space.

The cracked or fractured tooth

A tooth with a long-standing crack or vertical fracture may exhibit vertical bone loss. Clinically these teeth exhibit the total spectrum of pulpal and periodontal diseases, depending on the age and severity of the fracture. Diagnosis of fractured teeth is normally straightforward; however, cracked teeth can exhibit bizarre symptoms and pose a diagnostic challenge. Radiographs can show cracks in the later stages but are usually not helpful in the early stages, especially if the crack runs mesiodistally. Having patients bite down on a rubber disk placed on one cusp at a time

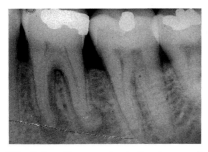

Fig 9-4a The cracked distal root of this mandibular molar was removed.

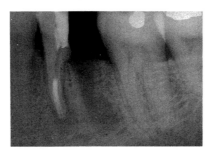

Fig 9-4b The mesial root was treated endodontically.

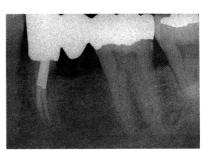

Fig 9-4c A 15-year followup.

can occasionally elicit the sharp pain characteristic of these cracks (Figs 9-4a to c).

Developmental grooves

Developmental grooves like those frequently found in maxillary central and lateral incisors are most certainly capable of causing localized periodontitis and osseous destruction along the root surface.[4–6] These grooves or invaginations usually traverse from the cingulum apically through enamel, cementum, and dentin. When plaque reaches the groove, it incites a self-sustaining periodontitis. The pattern of osseous deterioration is tubular and follows the path of the groove. Clinically these lesions may be asymptomatic or demonstrate acute or chronic periodontal symptoms. Pulps in these teeth can become secondarily involved. The prognosis varies with the apical limit of the groove.

Diagnosis of the combined periodontal-endodontic lesion

Periodontal-endodontic lesions are caused by both periodontal and endodontic problems existing simultaneously on the same tooth.[7] When both pulpal and periodontal diseases are present around a tooth, each disease may progress until the lesions unite. A necrotic pulp along with plaque, calculus, and periodontitis will be present in various degrees (Figs 9-5a to c).

Endodontic component

The formation of a sinus tract through the periodontal ligament has been shown to be a part of the natural history of pulp disease around some teeth.[8] This tract originates from the apex or a lateral canal and may eventually extend along the root surface and exit

through the gingival sulcus. This sinus tract cannot be considered a true periodontal pocket, but rather is a fistula that opens into the gingival sulcus. It can be differentiated from a periodontal pocket because the resulting tract is usually narrow and deep, whereas most periodontal lesions are broad at the coronal end and narrow apically. Radiographically, it appears as a lucency extending along the mesial or distal root surface or into the bifurcation area.

Clinically, exudate may be evident in the sulcus, and some swelling may be present (this is especially true in furcations), resembling a periodontal abscess. Often this presents as the only area or the most serious area of bone loss. These tracts can usually be traced with a silver point or gutta-percha cone passed toward the source of initiation—the apex or lateral canal. There usually is no pain or at most only minor discomfort. In most cases, complete resolution of apical lesions can be anticipated with routine endodontic treatment.

Periodontal component

The clinical and radiographic signs that accompany advancement of periodontal diseases to the point of tooth loss are well known. In the periodontally involved tooth, endodontic evaluation procedures usually elicit a clinically normal pulpal response. The bony lesion of periodontal diseases is usually more widespread than that of lesions of endodontic origin. Purely periodontal lesions respond to management using the principles of periodontal therapy outlined in chapter 3.

Endodontic lesions with secondary periodontal involvement

If a primary endodontic lesion is left untreated, it may become secondarily involved with a periodontal disease already existing around the tooth. If this should

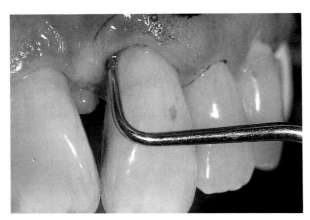

Fig 9-5a A combination periodontal/endodontic defect. Suppuration was seen on the mesial surface of this nonvital tooth, which continued after endodontic therapy.

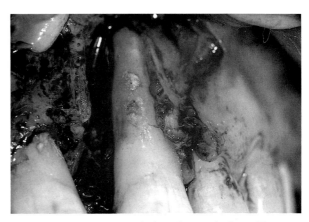

Fig 9-5b When repeated closed root planing with anesthesia also failed to make the patient comfortable, a flap was raised and the residual calculus removed.

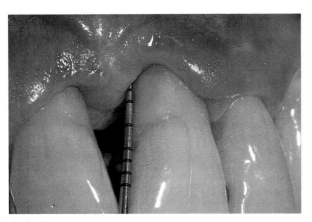

Fig 9-5c This combined therapy resulted in an asymptomatic tooth with greatly reduced probing depths.

occur, not only does the diagnosis become more difficult, but the prognosis and treatment may be altered.

From a diagnostic standpoint, these lesions have a necrotic root canal system and a periodontal lesion demonstrable by a probe or radiograph. When this situation occurs, endodontic and periodontic therapy are necessary to resolve the problem.[9,10] If the endodontic therapy is adequate, the prognosis depends on the severity of the periodontal involvement and the efficacy of periodontal therapy.

Periodontal lesions with secondary endodontic involvement

Periodontal diseases can affect the dental pulp via dentinal tubules, lateral canals, accessory canals, and other connecting structures. Lateral and accessory canals are a normal anatomic component of many teeth, especially in the apical third of the root and in the furcations. The presence of lateral canals and their distribution have been demonstrated by numerous methods. Saunders[11] used a microradiographic technique to visualize lateral canals in the pulp chamber floor of a vital human molar; numerous vessels were shown coursing between the pulp and the periodontal ligament.

The effect of periodontal disease on the pulp does not appear to be as clear cut or as prevalent as the effect of pulp disease on the periodontium.

Cahn[12] was the first to demonstrate that degenerative changes occur in the pulps of periodontally involved teeth. In the mid-1950s and through the 1960s, a controversy emerged as to whether or not periodontal diseases have any effect on the dental pulp.[13–17] Seventy-four periodontally involved teeth were studied histologically by Rubach and Mitchell.[18] They found periodontal disease affecting the dental pulp in 11 teeth. Stahl[19] found pulpal changes in rat molars where the overlying gingiva had been injured. Irregular dentin formation was seen in areas of the pulp opposite the site of gingival inflammation in 21 of 69 specimens. Stahl also reported noting similar irregular dentin formation in some human cadaver specimens at sites opposite periodontal lesions. Seltzer et al[20] found numerous atrophic pulps in periodontally involved teeth free of caries or restorations. Of these, 37% exhibited inflammatory pulpal changes and approximately 10% had totally necrotic pulps. Investigators then focused on the mechanism for this apparent interaction between periodontal disease and pulpal health. Seltzer et al[21] extracted periodontally involved teeth without caries or restorations and found that 37% had some degree of pulpal inflammation or necrosis or both. Others demonstrated direct inflammatory extension of periodontal inflammation through lateral canals. However, they did not demonstrate that total pulpal necrosis would result from inflamed lateral canals.[21,22] Lanjeland et al[22] believed that as long as the main canal is not seriously damaged, the pulp may not succumb. Lowman et al[23] showed that periodontal therapy may increase pulpal inflammation. By planing the roots of molars and then drawing a dye through the canals they were able to demonstrate the presence of patent canals in 59% of the molars. The incidence of patent canals in the coronal and middle third of maxillary molars was 55%; it was 63% in mandibular molars. The unplaned teeth had a significantly lower percentage of patent canals. Koenings et al[24] showed accessory canal openings with the scanning electron microscope and found more canals in maxillary molars than in mandibular molars. The intimate relationship between periodontal vascular plexus and pulpal blood vessels has been graphically demonstrated.[25–28] Besides vascular communications, connective tissue fibers run from the dental pulp to the periodontal ligament.

Repair of the periodontal component of the lesion

Osseous lesions of both endodontic and periodontal origin are easier to treat if detected early. Primary endodontic lesions will usually heal completely after endodontic therapy. In lesions having an endodontic and a periodontal component, the lesion of endodontic origin *may* heal. The periodontal lesion can then be treated separately (usually 3 to 6 months after endodontic therapy is completed). Regeneration of appreciable amounts of bone lost to periodontal disease is rare except in three-way bony lesions, after acute abscess therapy and with some advanced regenerative procedures.

Repair of the endodontic component of the lesion

Though much work on periodontal healing mechanisms has been done and is in progress, no studies have shown how endodontic lesions fistulating through the periodontal ligament heal. In primary endodontic lesions there is apparently no apical migration of the epithelial attachment.[7,29] Perhaps apical migration is retarded in the presence of this type of inflammation. If cemental fibers are removed from the

root surface, the epithelial attachment will migrate apically until new fiber support is found. If there is no long-term exposure to the oral environment (bacteria, toxins, and such), it is possible that when (or if) the endodontic lesion fistulates through the periodontal ligament space, the cementum and its fibers may not be irreversibly disturbed.

Researchers have proposed that the induction mechanism for healing may reside in the fibers, cementum, or dentin.[29–32] If the fibers are disturbed, the cementum may induce new cementum and fiber formation to effect healing. Or, if the fibers and cementum are affected, the dentin may induce new cementum and fiber formation. Though it has been suggested that the root does not contain a bone inductive principle, it may be a co-inducer with bone.[31] Clinically these lesions heal following endodontic treatment.

In lesions secondarily involved by periodontal disease, healing of the portion of the lesion not affected by periodontal disease can occur following endodontic treatment. Thus, the prognosis of lesions with secondary periodontal involvement also depends on the efficacy of the periodontal therapy. In general, the greater the periodontal involvement, the poorer the prognosis. Conversely, the more the lesion is the result of pulpal disease, the better the prognosis. Healing potential should dictate the course of treatment.

Differential diagnosis

Although the radiographic appearance of periodontal and endodontic lesions may be similar, you must resist the temptation to generalize and label all of them as combined lesions. Roentgenographically there are differences between endodontic and periodontal lesions. If the lesion is of periodontal origin, usually other teeth besides the one in question will have bone loss. A periapical lesion that does not communicate with the periodontal pocket is probably of endodontic origin. If a furcation lesion exists around only one tooth, endodontic procedures should be employed first, provided that this is consistent with clinical findings. In addition, testing will usually show that the pulps of endodontically involved teeth are nonvital.

For a summary of diagnostic information see Figs 9-6a to c.

USUAL DIFFERENTIAL DIAGNOSIS OF DENTAL PAIN (TOOTH)

	Pulpal	Periapical	Periodontal
Type of Pain	sharp, lancating	dull, continuous	dull or absent
Swelling	absent	generalized	localized
Color of Tooth	normal	darkened	normal
Percussion	normal	sensitive	usually normal*
Lateral Coronal Pressure	normal	slightly sensitive	more sensitive
Extrusion of Tooth	absent	extruded	absent*
Lymphatic Involvement	absent	enlarged	absent
Pulp Vitality Tests	responsive	no response	normal
Palpation	absent	muco-buccal fold	attached gingiva
Coronal Radiographic Examination	caries, recent fillings, trauma, morphologic changes	deep caries, fillings, trauma, etc. morphologic changes	pocket, calculus
Radicular Radiographic Examination	morphologic changes -more irregular -internal resorption -calcific metamorphosis -thickened pdl -condensing osteitis	morphologic changes -more irregular -internal resorption -calcific metamorphosis -loss of lamina dura -condensing osteitis -periradicular osteoporosis -pocket widen apically	normal canal morphology pocket wider

*Except in cases of traumatic occlusion.

Fig 9-6a

PERIRADICULAR (PERIAPICAL) PATHOSIS OF PULPAL ORIGIN

Diagnosis	Pain	Radiographic	Percussion	Palpation	Fistula/Swelling	Mobility	Minimum Emergency Treatment
Acute *Apical Periodontitis	Spontaneous pain may be present or absent	Range from none to large peri-radicular lesions	ALWAYS Responsive	Sometimes Responsive	None	Sometimes	1) Pulpectomy 2) Relief of occlusion
Chronic *Apical Periodontitis (sometimes called chronic radiolucency)	NONE	ALWAYS Range from expansion of pdl to large peri-radicular lesions	NO Response	NO Response	NONE	Rarely	Not an emergency condition
Acute *Apical Abscess A) Primary B) Secondary** (Recrudescent)	Constant dull ache--often severe; may exhibit fever or lymph-adenopathy	A) Primary--none B) Secondary** (Recrudescent) Periradicular radiolucent lesion (sometimes called chronic granuloma)	Always Responsive	Usually Responsive	SWELLING and/or PURULENT DRAINAGE from Root Canal System	Usually	1) Drainage through incision--if fluctuant and/or RCS*** 2) Debridement of RCS*** 3) Antibiotics if: A) Drainage not obtained B) Systemic mani-festations C) Specific medical indications
Chronic *Apical Abscess (suppurative apical perio-dontitis)	None--possible occasional mild soreness	Periradicular radiolucent lesion	No Response	Area of fistula may be sore	FISTULA	Rarely	Not an emergency condition

*"Apical" is a term of common usage. "Periradicular" is a better term, as the pathosis may occur at any point surrounding the root.
**Sometimes called "Phoenix".
***If cellulitis (hard, unyielding swelling) prepare canal(s) and palliative treatment.

MUSOD/
William Kelly, D.D.S.
Harold Gerstein, D.D.S.

Fig 9-6b

PULPAL PATHOSIS

Diagnosis	Symptoms			Signs			Minimum Emergency Care
	Pain	Stimulus	Duration	Mastication Percussion	Radiographic	E.P.T.*	
Dentinal Sensitivity	Sharp, Localized	1) Sweets 2) Thermal 3) Physical Abrasion	Only while stimulus present--Seconds	No Response	No Changes	Responds Normally	1) Cover exposed dentin 2) Desensitizing procedures
Reversible Pulpitis **Hyperemia	Sharp, Localized	1) Sweets 2) Thermal, mostly cold Not spontaneous	Several seconds after stimulus is removed	No Response	No Changes	Responds Normally	1) Eliminate cause 2) Sedative temporary 3) Time
Irreversible Pulpitis A) mild B) moderate C) severe	A) Mild B) Moderate C) Severe Often spontaneous, diffuse and referred	Thermal, often spontaneous	Minutes to hours after stimulus removed--often continuous	Often in moderate and severe cases	1) None 2) Thickened pdl and/or break in lamina dura	1) Responds normally 2) hypo and hyper responses common 3) rarely no response	1) Pulpotomy if no response to percussion 2) Pulpectomy
Irreversible Pulpitis Subtype Internal Resorption	None	None	None	No Response	Balloon expansion of pulp canal	Responds Normally	Not an emergency in pure form
Irreversible Pulpitis Subtype Hyperplastic Pulpitis	Usually absent unless mechanically stimulated	Mechanical	While stimulus present	No response unless impinging on pulp polyp	1) Usually none 2) Possible thickening of pdl	Visual diagnosis renders this test unnecessary	Pulpotomy
Non-vital Pulp (pulpal necrosis)	Pain and radiographic changes may be associated with periradicular pathosis that may result from pulpal necrosis					No Response	Not emergency unless associated with symptomatic periradicular pathosis

*Electric Pulp Test
**Historical Terminology

MUSOD/
William Kelly, D.D.S.
Harold Gerstein, D.D.S.

Fig 9-6c

- Periodontal and pulpal lesions can occur as separate entities, or one disease process can affect the other, causing a combined pulpal-periodontal lesion.
- A periodontal lesion may produce atrophic changes in the pulp when products from the periodontal lesion enter the pulp through accessory canals or possibly across untreated tooth surface.
- Pulpal lesions may secondarily involve (and mimic) preexisting periodontal lesions.
- When pulpal and periodontal lesions coexist on the same tooth, the pulpal lesion usually should be treated first and allowed to heal before definitive periodontal therapy.

Endodontic techniques

Numerous techniques have been used that satisfy the previously presented objectives. All techniques can be expected to produce a certain degree of success. Euchopercha, chloropercha, and chlororosen techniques duplicate internal anatomy well; however, apical movement of these materials is hard to control, and shrinkage and inflammation from the solvents can occur.[2]

Lateral condensation of gutta-percha in conjunction with a nonsolvent cement has been used. Pressing gutta-percha cones laterally against one another and against the dentinal walls of the pulp canal produces the appearance of a dense, well-adapted filling. Unfortunately, the gutta-percha cones never merge into a homogeneous mass, as occurs with gutta-percha solvent techniques.[33] Recent evidence indicates that an apical seal with "lateral condensation" is enhanced when the spreader is used very close to the apex. In these instances the spreader acts essentially as a vertical compactor. In reality, most molar root canals presumably filled by lateral condensation have actually been filled by the method of a single gutta-percha cone generously engulfed in sealer.

Silver cones (points) in conjunction with sealer previously enjoyed great popularity as obturation materials. Silver cones have the advantage of being able to negotiate narrow and severely curved canals (Figs 9-7a to c). When handled well, they are able to seal the apices of many root canals. Unfortunately, because silver cones are preformed, they are not able to adapt to the convolutions seen in the majority of root canal systems. When apical foramina are ovoid, it is impossible to seal canals without relying heavily on cement. A large number of failures have occurred when cement has resorbed, resulting in seepage not only apically but along the entire body of the silver cone (Figs 9-8a and b).

Paste root canal fillings have been used for more than a century. Their appeal is twofold: *(1)* they can serve as vehicles for pharmacologic agents or may be pharmacologic agents in and of themselves, and *(2)* they can be extruded into canals that have been inadequately cleaned and shaped.

Some successes can be seen with paste fillings, but no amount of chemical disinfection will neutralize grossly contaminated root canal systems. A thoroughly debrided canal requires little pharmacologic assistance. Pharmacologic pastes are an anachronism whose appeal of simplicity ensures their retention in the dental armamentarium despite the unpredictability of their results.

Vertical compaction of warm gutta-percha

It is fortunate that gutta-percha can be softened by heat and chemical action. The technique of vertical compaction of warm gutta-percha depends on this plus the ability to place vertical compactors into the root canals. The change in the shape of the prepared canals makes this possible.[2,34] These changes are as much a product of the need for total cleaning and organic substrate removal as of the requirements of vertical compaction. Well-prepared canals are cleaner; cleaner canals contain fewer microorganisms and less toxic substrate. Better shaping has led to better cleaning, which allows for the ease of placement of instruments to compact the softened gutta-percha directly into the deepest part of root canal preparations. Through the use of this technique, accessory canals are routinely obturated in the cervical and middle thirds of the root as well as apical bifidities, trifidities, and delta formations. Occasionally, auxiliary canals leading to the base of infrabony pockets and into previously resistant bifurcation and trifurcation lesions are also filled.

The technique requires prefitting the appropriate compactors (Schilder compactors or the like) into the

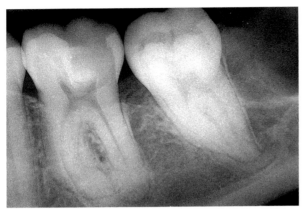 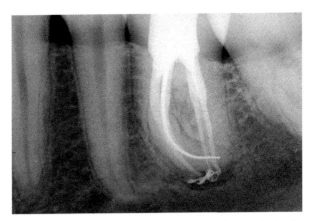

Figs 9-7a and b Silver cones were used in severely curved canals after a large carious exposure caused an endodontic lesion.

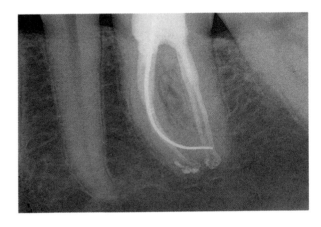

Fig 9-7c Fourteen years later the tooth is asymptomatic.

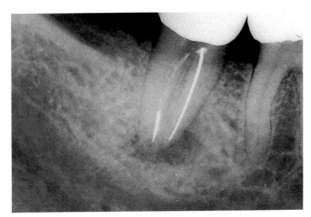 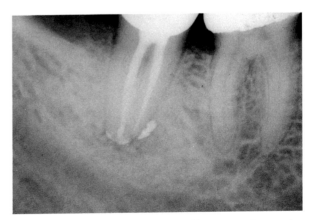

Fig 9-8a Failing endodontic therapy.

Fig 9-8b Successful retreatment with warm gutta-percha technique (1 year later).

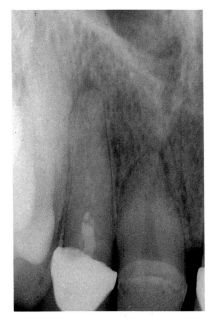
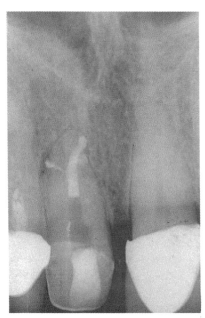
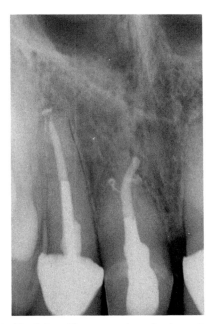

Fig 9-9a A necrotic central incisor next to a failing paste-treated canal in a maxillary lateral incisor.

Fig 9-9b Both teeth were treated.

Fig 9-9c Five years later both teeth were asymptomatic.

prepared canal, selecting and preparing a master gutta-percha cone, placing the master cone into the canal with a small amount of sealer, softening the gutta-percha in a controlled manner with a heat transfer instrument (spreader, Schilder heat transfer instrument, Analytic Technology Touch 'n Heat), and then gradually vertically compacting the softened gutta-percha mass into the cleaned and shaped root canal system. A microfilm of root canal cement (Richert sealer or Roth 811) should surround the final gutta-percha filling. Vertical compaction produces a dense, homogeneous, gutta-percha filling with minimal cement content.

This technique is predicated on trapping the maximum cushion of softened gutta-percha with appropriate compactors and moving the material toward the apex. Any thermoplastic technique that does not incorporate vertical compaction will result in a gradual volume reduction of the root canal filling[35] (Figs 9-9a to c).

Endodontic surgery

As early as the fourth century AD, incision and drainage were used to treat the acute apical abscess.[36] Although the need for endodontic surgery has been greatly reduced in the last 15 years, a need still exists for surgical procedures to manage problems that cannot be eliminated by conventional techniques.

Surgery can be useful in the following situations:

1. To establish drainage
2. To relieve pain—by triphination when routine procedures fail to give pain relief
3. To overcome anatomic complications:
   a. Calcified canals
   b. A pulp stone that cannot be bypassed with conventional techniques
   c. Nonnegotiable root curvatures
   d. Incomplete apical development
   e. Root resorptions—external root resorption can occur on any surface of the root including the apex. Conventional procedures are often inadequate for sealing perforations when the root resorption occurs on the lateral aspect of the root. In such cases it may be necessary to gain access surgically and seal the defect directly. Prognosis may be especially poor in cases occurring near the cervical area because they are inaccessible, lack osteogenic potential, and are usually complicated by a secondary periodontal pocket.
   f. Bony fenestration. A lack of bone covering the root apex is not uncommon, and because the neurovascular bundle is protected by overlying mucosa, the tooth remains functionally

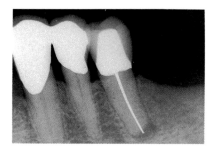 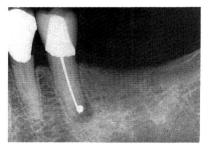 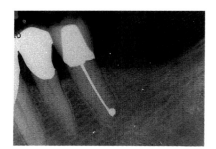

Figs 9-10a and b A failing silver cone on a 75-year-old patient required a retrofill with amalgam to obtain the successful result. **Fig 9-10c** Two years posttreatment.

healthy. However, when the pulp necroses, the apical pathosis often creates inflammation that will not respond in spite of a radiographically successful root canal filling. Apical surgery can reduce the root length and place the remainder of the root into bone.

g. Iatrogenic problems:
   i. Nonsoluble material associated with a failing root canal. Many pastes are insoluble and drilling out the material invites perforation. In such cases surgery with concomitant reverse fill is indicated. Also, when silver cone or gutta-percha cannot be removed, a surgical approach is the only alternative. Surgical exposure and reverse fill may be required when the canal is blocked by debris, dowel or post, an irretrievable broken instrument, or file fragment.
   ii. Impassable ledges
   iii. Perforations occur when an endodontic instrument that is not precurved is forced through the wall of the canal. Perforations can also occur during dowel preparation. This happens most often when an engine-driven bur or reamer is used in postpreparation. Some perforations require surgical access to the site, and the prognosis depends upon the size, location, and accessibility.
4. Overinstrumentation
5. Gross overfills
6. Persistent preobturation pain
7. Persistent postobturation pain
8. Failure to heal
9. Trauma
10. Root fractures with pulpal necrosis. Not all root fractures result in pulp death, but when necrosis does occur, the coronal segment frequently separates from the apical segment. When this happens, treatment is predicated on the type and location of the fracture.

a. If the displaced segment is small and the remaining root satisfies an acceptable crown-root ratio, root canal therapy is performed to the fracture and the apical segment is removed.
b. If the crown-root ratio is inadequate, you might consider using a vitalium stabilizer. Such a choice may or may not preclude removing the apical root segment.
c. When the root fracture is parallel with the long axis of the root, the prognosis is poor and usually the tooth is lost.
11. Failure of previously endodontically treated teeth
12. Inability to control exudate
13. Recurrent exacerbations
14. Need for biopsy

Radicular cyst

Many pathologists believe that it is necessary to eradicate the apical lesion when it is a radicular cyst. Pathologists disagree with the rationale of limiting endodontic surgery to the improvement of the apical seal without total excision of pathologic periapical tissue. Contradictions to such objections follow.

1. The definitive diagnosis of a cystic area cannot be made by radiograph solely (though the larger the lesion, the greater the chance that it is cystic).[37]
2. A statistical analysis of large lesions removed for biopsy shows a high percentage of cysts.[38]
3. A statistical analysis of the healing of teeth with similarly large lesions, subsequent to conventional endodontic treatment without surgery, shows a high degree of success.[39]

It becomes obvious that some of the periapical lesions that heal must be cysts. Therefore it is not always mandatory to remove all pathologic tissue to obtain complete periapical repair.

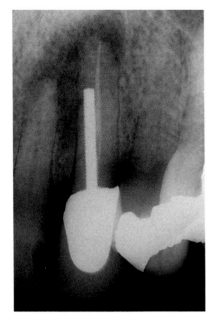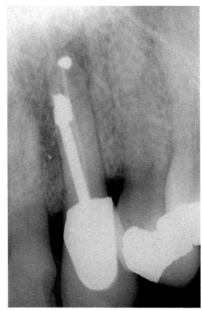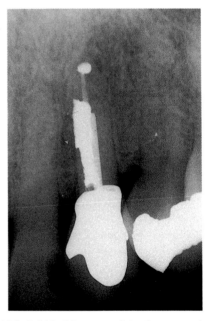

Figs 9-11a and b The perforation of a post into the periodontal ligament space of a maxillary lateral incisor necessitated an apicoectomy with retrofill amalgam and repair of the perforation with amalgam.

Fig 9-11c These procedures seemed successful initially.

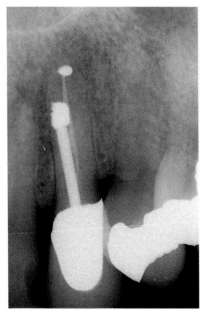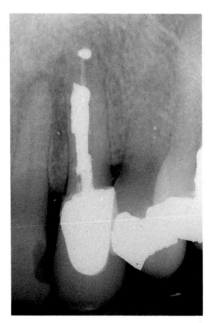

Fig 9-11d The area around the perforation later started to break down, however.

Fig 9-11e Removal of the post was necessary, as was obturating the space with amalgam.

Fig 9-11f Nine years later the second repair is holding.

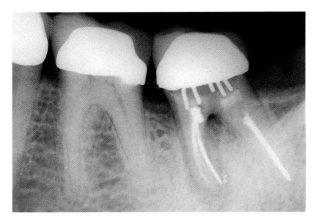
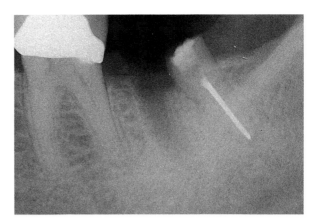

Figs 9-12a and b The mesial root of the second molar cracked subsequent to a pin buildup in the area and was removed.

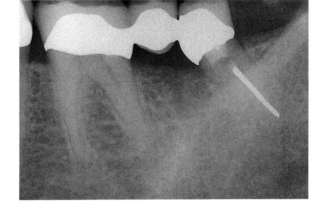

Fig 9-12c Two years later the lesion has healed well radiographically.

Endodontic surgery classification

Endodontic surgery may be classified as follows:

1. Periapical surgery (Figs 9-10a to c and 9-11a to f)
   a. Curettage
   b. Apicoectomy
   c. Retrograde filling at the apical foramen
2. Intentional replantation
3. Root amputation
4. Hemisection (Figs 9-12a to c)

Replantation and intentional replantation

The complete displacement of a tooth from its socket most frequently occurs between ages 7 and 10 years. Avulsions occur most commonly in this age range because of the unsettled condition of the periodontal ligament caused by the continuous eruption of the teeth.[40] These avulsions are usually the result of fights or falls. In adults the most common cause is automobile accidents.[41] The teeth most frequently affected are the maxillary central incisors.[40]

The most important fact in the history is the elapsed time between the accident (injury) and the time of replantation. Radiographs should be taken to determine any alveolar fractures or root tips.

The treatment is to replace the tooth in the socket to obtain ligament reattachment. The second objective is to restore the appearance no matter how guarded the prognosis.[41]

To obtain the best prognosis, you should examine the avulsed tooth to see that no gross fractures of crown or root are present. The alveolar socket should be evaluated for fracture, as such injuries result in excessive amounts of resorption. The prognosis decreases markedly in the presence of periodontal disease.

There has been much investigation into the optimal time a tooth can be removed from its alveolar environment and replanted successfully. Success in such cases is the absence of resorption, mobility, swelling, and pain.[42] The shorter the extraoral period, the more promising the prognosis.[43,44] Therefore, time is a most important factor. The major effect of a prolonged extraoral period is the degree of damage to the periodontal ligament fibers by drying (dessication), contamination,[45] manipulation,[44] or chemicals. The viability of the periodontal ligament fibers has a direct bearing on the ultimate prognosis of the tooth in question.[46–48] The chance of survival for a replanted tooth is directly proportional to the quantity of viable periodontal ligament fibers present.[49]

Time is the main factor in expressing success percentages, because this is easier to express than units of periodontal ligament fibers. Of teeth replanted within 30 minutes after injury, 90% achieve primary healing with no subsequent resorption.[42] The percentage of success diminishes as the extraoral time increases to 60 minutes.[42] Beyond 90 minutes, there is a dramatic drop in success rate. Resorption is seen in 95% of teeth replanted after 90 minutes.[14]

Procedure

1. Place tooth in warm saline solution to prevent drying of periodontal fibers.[56] Failure to do so produces extensive resorption.[44,46,51–53] If there is obvious contamination, irrigate the surface thoroughly with sterile saline.
2. Do not attempt to sterilize or disinfect the root surface.[46,49,50,54] These procedures and chemicals damage viable periodontal fibers and cementum. Maintenance of the viability of these fibers is critical to the prognosis.[44,52,53] If the fibers' viability can be maintained for 1 hour,[46] extensive replacement resorption can be prevented.[14,48,51,53] The presence of some viable fibers slows replacement resorption and prolongs the life of the tooth.[14]
3. To remove the clot from the socket, irrigate but do not curette.
4. Replant the tooth immediately.[44,55]
5. Stabilization for 7 to 10 days is adequate only in the case of an alveolar fracture. To maintain stabilization for a prolonged period, use of monofilament fishing line and direct bonding is preferred.
6. Endodontic therapy should be initiated 5 to 7 days after replantation and the canal obturated with calcium hydroxide. The calcium hydroxide is replaced in 14 days, then again in 3 months. The procedure seems to reduce the inflammatory re-

sorption. The canal can be obturated with guttapercha after 9 to 12 months. These replanted teeth should be checked at 3-month intervals for 2 to 5 years. Evaluation should include radiographs to check for root integrity.

Primary healing occurs in nearly all cases. The majority of replanted teeth succumb to resorption.[41,42] Consequently, the prognosis for long-term retention is poor.[41,44,55]

Treatment of a periodontal abscess

The periodontal abscess is often encountered in clinical practice. Other areas of this chapter have covered the differential diagnosis of the lesion. This section will deal with treatment.

Periodontal abscesses often occur because of closure of the orifice of an existing periodontal pocket.[56,57] In order to treat these problems successfully, drainage must be established. This can be accomplished in two ways—through the pocket or by incision and drainage remote to the sulcular area. In many cases the former occurs spontaneously and is often not reported by the patient. In patients who are still swollen, the area is anesthetized with local anesthetic (preferably at a site distant from the abscess). If time permits and deep probing depths are encountered in firm tissue, a full-thickness mucoperiosteal flap is raised, the area thoroughly curetted, and the tissue replaced. In most cases, this is not feasible and the area should be drained through the pocket if possible. In abscesses that are fluctuant and distant from the mouth of the pocket, I prefer a horizontal incision. Placement of a drain is rarely necessary. The patient is then given a prescription for doxycycline hyclate 100 mg twice a day to be used for 7 days. Hourly warm saline rinses are suggested for use in the first 24 hours after drainage.

The patient is then reappointed at least 7 days later for reevaluation. At that time, a diagnosis of any chronic periodontal problem is made and appropriate treatment is recommended. This final step is often overlooked by the treating dentist and patient and will result in further problems where underlying periodontal disease exists.

References

1. Seltzer S, Bender IB: *The Dental Pulp: Biologic Considerations in Dental Procedures.* Philadelphia, JB Lippincott Co, 1965, p 337.
2. Cohen S, Burns RC: *Pathways of the Pulp.* St Louis, CV Mosby Co, 1976, pp 12–15.
3. Bhaskar SN, Rappaport HM: Dental vitality tests and pulp status. *J Am Dent Assoc* 1973;86:409.
4. Everett FG, Kramer GM: The disto-lingual groove in the maxillary lateral incisor: A periodontal hazard. *J Periodontol* 1972;43:352.
5. Lee KW, Lee EC, Poor KY: Palato-gingival grooves in maxillary incisors. A possible predisposing factor to localized periodontal disease. *Br Dent J* 1968;124:14.
6. Simon JHS, Glick DH, Frank AL: Predictable endodontic and periodontic failures as a result of radicular anomalies. *Oral Surg Oral Med Oral Pathol* 1971;31:823.
7. Simon P, Jacobs D: The so-called combined periodontal-pulpal problem. *Dent Clin North Am* 1969;13:45.
8. Tagger M, Massler M: Periapical tissue reactions after pulp exposure in rat molars. *Oral Surg Oral Med Oral Pathol* 1975;39:304.
9. Hiatt WH, Amen CR: Periodontal pocket elimination by combined therapy. *Dent Clin North Am* March 1964, p 133.
10. Hiatt WH: Regeneration of the periodontium after endodontic therapy and flap operation. *Oral Surg Oral Med Oral Pathol* 1959;12:1471.
11. Saunders RL de CH: Microradiographic studies of human adult and fetal dental pulp vessels, in Corslett VE, Engstione A, Pattel HH Jr (eds): *X-ray Microscopy and Microradiography.* New York, Academic Press, 1957, pp 561–571.
12. Cahn LR: The pathology of pulps found in pyorrhetic teeth. *Dent Items Interest* 1927;49:598.
13. Andreasen JO: Treatment of fractured and avulsed teeth. *J Dent Child* 1971;38:29.
14. Clark HB, Tam JC, Mitchell DF: Transplantation of developing teeth. *J Dent Res* 1955;34:322.
15. Counsell LA: Intentional reimplantation of teeth. Reports of two cases. *Oral Surg Oral Med Oral Pathol* 1964;18:681.
16. Cserepfalvi M: Clinical report of homotransplantation. *J Am Dent Assoc* 1963;67:35.
17. Cserepfalvi M, Price PJ: Transplantation of a preserved human tooth to a monkey. Preliminary report of a case. *J Dent Res* 1968;47:641.
18. Rubach WC, Mitchell DF: Periodontal disease, accessory canals and pulp pathosis. *J Periodontol* 1965;36:34.
19. Stahl SS: Pathogenesis of inflammatory lesions in pulp and periodontal tissues. *Periodontics* 1966;4:190.
20. Seltzer S, Sinai I, August D: Periodontal effect of root perforations before and during endodontic procedures. *J Dent Res* 1970;49:332.
21. Seltzer S, Bender IB, Zionitz M: The interrelationship of pulp and periodontal disease. *Oral Surg Oral Med Oral Pathol* 1963;16:1474.
22. Lanjeland K, Rodrigues H, Dowden W: Periodontal disease, bacteria, and pulpal histopathology. *Oral Surg Oral Med Oral Pathol* 1974;37:257.
23. Lowman JV, Burke RS, Pelleu GB: Patent accessory canals: Incidence in molar furcation region. *Oral Surg Oral Med Oral Pathol* 1973;36:580.
24. Koenigs JF, Brilliant JD, Foreman DW Jr: Preliminary scanning electron microscope investigations of accessory foramina in furcation areas of human molar teeth. *Oral Surg Oral Med Oral Pathol* 1974;38:773.
25. Kramer IRH: The vascular architecture of the human dental pulp. *Arch Oral Biol* 1960;2:177.
26. Castelli WA, Dempster WT: The periodontal vasculature and its responses to experimental pressures. *J Am Dent Assoc* 1965;70:890.
27. Carranza FA, Cabrini RL, Itoiz ME, Dotto CA: A study of periodontal vascularization in different laboratory animals. *J Periodont Res* 1966;1:120.
28. Cutright DE, Bhaskar SN: A new method of demonstrating microvasculature. Oral Surgery-Oral Pathology Conference No. 21, Walter Reed Army Medical Center. *Oral Surg Oral Med Oral Pathol* 1967;24:442.
29. Stahl SS, Slavkin HC, Yameda L: Speculations about gingival repair. *J Periodontol* 1972;43:395.
30. Morris ML: The subcutaneous implantation of periodontally diseased roots. *J Periodontol* 1972;43:737.
31. Morris ML: A study of the inductive properties of the organic matrix of dentin and cementum. *J Periodontol* 1972;43:10.
32. Register, AA, Scopp IW, Kassouny DY: Human bone induction by allogeneic dentin matrix. *J Periodontol* 1972;43:459–467.
33. Grossman LI: *Endodontic Practice*, 9th ed. Philadelphia, Lea & Febiger, 1978, p 337.
34. Schilder H: Cleaning and shaping the root canal. *Dent Clin North Am* 1974;18:269.
35. Schilder H: Filling root canals in three dimensions. *Dent Clin North Am* Nov. 1967, p 723.
36. Luebke RG, Glick DH, Ingle JI: Indications and contraindications for endodontic surgery. *Oral Surg Oral Med Oral Pathol* 1964;18:97.
37. Andreasen JO, Rud J: Modes of healing histologically after endodontic surgery in 70 cases. *Int J Oral Surg Oral Med Oral Pathol* 1972;1:148.
38. Baumann L, Rossman SR: Clinical roentgenologic and histopathologic findings in teeth with apical radiolucent areas. *Oral Surg Oral Med Oral Pathol* 1956;9:1330.
39. Bhaskar SN: Periapical lesions—Types, incidence, and clinical features. Oral Surgery-Oral Pathology Conference No. 17, Walter Reed Army Medical Center. *Oral Surg Oral Med Oral Pathol* 1966;21:657.
40. Andreasen JO: *Traumatic Injuries of the Teeth.* St Louis, CV Mosby Co, 1972, p 203.
41. Lenstrup K, Skieller V: Follow-up study of teeth replanted after accidental loss. *Acta Odontol Scand* 1959;17:503.
42. Andreasen JO, Hjorting-Hansen E: Replantation of teeth. I. Radiographic and clinical study of 110 human teeth replanted after accidental loss. *Acta Odontol Scand* 1966;24:263.
43. Herbert WF: A case of complete dislocation of a tooth. *Br Dent J* 1958;105:137.
44. Lindahl B, Martensson K: Replantation of a tooth. A case report. *Odontol Rev* 1960;11:325.
45. Bodecker CF, Lefkowitz W: Replantation of teeth. *Dent Items Interest* 1935;57:675.
46. Burley MA, Crabb HSM: Replantation of teeth. *Br Dent J* 1960;108:190.
47. Myers HI, Flanagan VD: A comparison of results obtained from transplantation and replantation experiments using Syrian hamster teeth. *Dent Abstracts* 1959;4:6.
48. Sherman P: Intentional replantation of teeth in dogs and monkeys. *J Dent Res* 1968;47:1066.
49. Hammer H: Replantation and implantation of teeth. *Int Dent J* 1955;5:439.
50. Henning FR: Reimplantation of luxated teeth. *Aust Dent J* 1965;10:306.
51. Bennett DT: Traumatized anterior teeth. *Br Dent J* 1963;15:346.
52. Kaqueler JC, Massler M: Healing following tooth replantation. *J Dent Child* 1969;36:303.
53. Löe H, Waerhaug J: Experimental replantation of teeth in dogs and monkeys. *Arch Oral Biol* 1961;3:176.
54. Cooke C, Rowbotham TC: Treatment of injuries to anterior teeth. *Br Dent J* 1951;91:146.
55. Ravn JJ, Helbo M: Replantation af akidentelt eksartikulerede taender. En klinisk efterundersolegels af 28 taender. *Tandlaege Badet* 1966;70:805.
56. Prichard JF: Management of the periodontal abscess. *Oral Surg Oral Med Oral Pathol* 1953;6:474.

57. McFall WT Jr: Periodontal abscess. *J NC Dent Soc* 1964;47:34.

Suggested readings

Andreasen JO: *Traumatic Injuries of the Teeth.* St Louis, CV Mosby Co, 1972.

Arens DE, Adams WR, DeCastro RA: *Endodontic Surgery.* Hagerstown, Md, Harper and Row, 1981.

Cohen S, Burns RC: *Pathways of the Pulp.* St Louis, CV Mosby Co, 1976.

Gerstein H: *Techniques in Clinical Endodontics.* Philadelphia, WB Saunders Co, 1983.

Grossman LI: *Endodontic Practice,* 9th ed. Philadelphia, Lea & Febiger, 1978.

Schilder H: Filling root canals in three dimensions. *Dent Clin North Am* Nov. 1967.

Schilder H: Cleaning and shaping the root canal. *Dent Clin North Am* 1974;18(2):269.

Weine FS: *Endodontic Therapy,* 2nd ed. St Louis, CV Mosby Co, 1976.

Chapter 10

Management of Irradiated and Chemotherapy Patients

Eugene W. Dahl / Thomas G. Wilson, Jr

Radiotherapy is a common treatment for patients with cancer of the head and neck region.[1] Radiation therapy may be the preferred treatment for some tumors, whereas other tumors will require radiation combined with surgery or chemotherapy. The intent in any therapy is to cure the patient, but in some instances radiation provides only useful palliation. The dental practitioner faced with maintaining the oral health of patients who are undergoing radiation therapy or who have completed treatment with cancerocidal radiation doses to the head and neck region may be unfamiliar with the regimens needed to maintain these patients. It is the intent of this chapter to provide a realistic and effective treatment approach for these patients.

The generalist should integrate treatment efforts with a maxillofacial prosthodontist or dental oncologist whose clinical judgment is based on sufficient previous experience with irradiated patients.

Principles of radiotherapy

The general dentist who elects to care for irradiated patients must have a fundamental understanding of radiation physics and radiobiology to develop a logical treatment approach. Radiation therapy is defined as the therapeutic use of ionizing radiation.[2] The radiation used in radiotherapy can be classified as either electromagnetic or particulate. Electromagnetic rays commonly used for therapeutic applications are x-rays and gamma rays. Both consist of photons and are identical in nature, but they differ in the manner in which they are produced. X-rays are produced from the linear acceleration of electrons that are bombarded into a metal target. Gamma rays are produced by the radioactive decay of isotopes, usually cobalt 60.

The most commonly used particulate radiation source is the electron beam, which has mass and carries a negative charge. The particles are absorbed within the tissue by colliding with the orbital electrons of the tissue atoms. The electron beam is produced by a linear accelerator. The beam may be used alone or in conjunction with protons to treat certain types of head and neck cancer.

When external beam therapy (electrons, cobalt 60, high-energy protons) is used, it is delivered in a series of treatments as fractions. Fractionation allows regular reoxygenation of the tumor cells, so that they will be as radiosensitive as possible. This procedure also allows more cells to be in the radiosensitive phase of their cell cycle, and normal cells seem to recover better from sublethal damage than do tumor cells between fractions.

Dental therapy for the radiation patient

The goal of the dental management team is to prevent or reduce the severity of the complications associated with radiation therapy (Fig 10-1). Potential complications include[3]:

1. Mucositis
2. Xerostomia
3. Alteration of taste acuity
4. Fungal infections
5. Radiation-induced caries
6. Osteoradionecrosis
7. Trismus and edema

Dental examination

A pretreatment oral and dental examination should be obtained along with data pertaining to the histopathologic diagnosis of the lesion, tumor site, clinical staging, neck node involvement, urgency of treatment,

---

COMPLICATIONS OF RADIOTHERAPY

Diagnosis	Treatment Options

Mucositis
1. Oral lavage salt (1 tsp.) and soda (1 tsp.) dissolved in 1 quart H_2O, swish and spit. (Use with caution in hypertensives.)
2. Viscous Xylocaine Plain, dilute 1:2 with water.
3. 0.5% Dyclone.
4. Kaolin-Pectin mixture.
5. Sucral Fate.
6. Benylin 50/50
7. Codeine-containing compounds.

Xerostomia
1. Frequent sips of water.
2. Sugarless candy or gum.
3. Pilocarpine hydrochloride 5 mg four times daily.
4. Salivary substitutes.

Trismus
1. Forced opening exercises.
2. Bite openers.
   a. Tongue blades.
   b. Threaded screw.
   c. Dynamic bite openers.

Candidiasis
Oral cavity
1. Chlorotrimazole 500 mg vaginal tablets. Dissolve in mouth four times daily for 7 days.

Angular cheilitis
1. Mycolog ointment.

Radiation caries
1. 1% NaF (sensitive oral cavity).
2. 0.4% SnF_2.
   a. Brush-on method (Hodgkins).
   b. Custom fluoride carriers.
3. Conventional endodontic therapy.
4. Crown amputation for nontreatable teeth within the radiation field.
5. Acute periapical infection. Drain area through tooth. Prescribe broad-spectrum antibiotics, e.g., ampicillin.

Osteoradionecrosis
1. Gentle debridement.
2. Mucosal guards.
3. Neomycin sulfate ointment
4. Oral irrigation.
5. Hyperbaric oxygen therapy.
6. Surgical resection.

Fig 10-1

volume of proposed radiation fields, mode of therapy, prognosis, and the dose to be delivered to the tumor site.[4] After these data are collected and the radiotherapist and dental oncologist have been consulted, a treatment plan can be formed that will allow input from the practitioners ultimately responsible for managing the patient.

The generalist is able to manage most of the oral- and dental-related complications of therapy, but knowledge of tumor biology is beyond the scope of the average practitioner. Cancer is a potentially life-threatening disease; if the patient's recovery is to be maximized, optimal management must be provided for the patient through a team approach.

Periodontal examination

The periodontal status of the remaining dentition is the single most important part of the preradiation evaluation.[5] At this stage the periodontist must decide which teeth in the radiation field will be retained. Because these decisions can have a great impact on future morbidity, they should not be made without adequate information. A complete periodontal examination similar to that described in chapter 2 should be performed. A consultation with the radiation oncologist should come next, where details of the amount of radiation and areas to be radiated can be ascertained. Removing a tooth or providing periodontal or endodontic therapy can often delay the start of radiation therapy; failure to remove or treat these teeth before radiation therapy begins can lead to a great number of negative consequences if these teeth later require extraction. The recent conservative approach toward retention of as many teeth as possible has merit, but if a tooth with a questionable prognosis resulting from a restorative periodontal, pulpal, or occlusal problem is located in the radiation field, preradiation extraction is still the treatment of choice. The dental awareness of the patient and his or her existing periodontal status will dictate how aggressive you should be with extracting teeth prior to therapy.

When teeth are extracted, you should get primary closure if possible, prescribe antibiotics, and allow at least 10 to 14 days of healing time prior to the commencement of radiotherapy if the extraction site is within the proposed treatment area.[6] The dentist must give the final approval for commencement of radiotherapy, and his or her clinical judgment is the key to determining when healing has progressed adequately. The minimum healing requirement is a layer of granulation tissue covering the base of the extraction site.

Therapy during radiation

Ulceration and desquamation of the oral mucous membranes in the course of therapy may lead to severe radiation mucositis.[7] The mucositis begins to appear 2 to 3 weeks after the start of therapy and is most severe at the completion of treatment.[8] Alcoholics and heavy tobacco users exhibit the most severe reactions because of the already compromised condition of the oral mucosae. The acute phase will interfere with dietary requirements because of the discomfort associated with swallowing, and normal oral hygiene regimens may become too painful to accomplish.[9] The patient should be instructed to prepare a dilute solution of baking soda (1 teaspoon) and table salt (1 teaspoon) dissolved in a quart of water and rinse the oral cavity as needed to alleviate the discomfort, and the need for good oral hygiene should be stressed.

Secretion of saliva declines when the major salivary glands are within the fields of treatment.[10] Although the glands themselves are radioresistant, changes occur in salivary volume, viscosity, buffering capacity, pH, and salivary components because of the effect on the fine vasculature that supplies the gland. The onset of xerostomia is rapid; it may be persistent and irreversible, depending on the radiation fields and the dosage given. Treatment of xerostomia is essentially palliative and supportive in nature. The patient may be instructed to take frequent sips of water, or to use sugarless mints and gum. Various saliva substitutes also are available and may be used as often as desired. Clinical experience, however, has shown such products to be ineffective in most cases.

The taste acuity of most patients is altered during radiation therapy.[11] Taste is affected because the taste buds undergo atrophy and degeneration. In most cases taste will gradually return to near normal levels after therapy is concluded, but some patients will never regain normal taste sensation and may complain of a metallic sensation. The degree of xerostomia is linked to the patient's ability to experience normal taste. Before therapy begins the patient should be counseled on the possible taste acuity alterations.

Edema of the tongue, buccal mucosa, submental or submandibular area, and cheeks is often clinically apparent shortly after radiation therapy ends. Fibrosis of the connective tissue inhibits adequate drainage of cellular fluids, and surgical resection of lymphatics exacerbates the problem.[12] The patient should be told that the swelling will decrease in severity but will be a persistent problem.

Limited jaw opening results from fibrosis of the connective tissue and the temporomandibular joint.[13,14] The degree of trismus varies and depends on the radiation dose and fields used to treat the tumor. Limited opening can affect the patient's ability to maintain adequate oral hygiene, and his or her nutritional status may deteriorate. Regimens of physical therapy consisting of forced opening exercises to break the adhesions, or mechanical devices to assist opening, are suggested. A recommended therapy is maximal opening 20 times in succession, four times a day. You should encourage and support the patient because regaining the lost opening dimension may take many months.

Osteoradionecrosis is the most devastating complication of radiotherapy and may necessitate a partial or complete bony resection of the affected area.[15] Bone is almost twice as dense as soft tissue and therefore absorbs a greater amount of radiation. Bone virtually becomes a nonvital tissue because of the obliteration of its arteriolar vessels. The repair capacity of the bone is seriously compromised, making it susceptible to infection and trauma. The mandible absorbs more radiation because of its greater density than does the maxilla, and the less generous blood supply to the mandible makes it more susceptible to necrosis.

Osteoradionecrosis can be prevented in most instances by eliminating precipitating factors such as extractions in radiation fields, minor trauma from an ill-fitting prosthesis, periodontal surgery, and surgical endodontic procedures. The conservative treatment of small necrotic areas consists of gentle debridement, irrigation with normal saline solutions, and the use of neomycin sulfate packs. Consultation with a practitioner experienced in managing such lesions is encouraged, because the course of treatment is extended and the general practitioner may not clinically recognize a lesion that is responding favorably or an area of necrosis that is progressing. Hyperbaric oxygen is a therapeutic regimen for osteoradionecrosis that offers hope for lesions that do not respond to conservative measures, but the therapy is expensive and its availability is limited.[16]

Maintenance therapy

Maintenance of the remaining dentition during and following radiation requires that the patient be placed on an adequate oral hygiene routine that includes daily application of topical fluoride preparations.[17,18] Clinical observations indicate that patients treated with radiation to the upper neck fields (submandibular triangle) have the greatest permanent degree of xerostomia. As reported by Keene et al,[19] there is a 100-fold increase in the concentration of the caries-associated Streptococcus mutans bacteria in the postirradiated, xerostomic mouth. It is mandatory that patients be placed on a topical fluoride, either 1% NaF or 0.4% SnF_2 gels.[20–22] Both gels provide adequate fluoride protection, but the stannous fluoride has the additional benefit of plaque inhibition.[23,24] The fluoride gel is applied by a custom-fabricated tray or a "brush on method" (Figs 10-2 and 10-3).

Candida albicans populations may increase up to 100-fold following radiation therapy.[25] These fungal infections appear as erythema and create a burning sensation of the oral mucosae. Angular cheilitis is also a common sequela of therapy and should be treated with antifungal ointments. The acute fungal infection can be treated with chlorotrimazole vaginal tablets until the infection is eliminated.

Routine dental procedures such as oral prophylaxis, routine operative care, fixed prosthodontics, nonsurgical endodontic treatment, and removable prosthodontics may be performed within the irradiated area.[7,26] Periodontal root planing, if needed, should be accompanied by antibiotics. A removable prosthesis should be meticulously fabricated to avoid overextension and microtrauma from occlusal interferences.[27,28] Soft denture liners should be avoided because of the likelihood of deterioration that could precipitate areas of irritation and possible bone exposure.[7] Placement of artificial teeth should be evaluated on an individual basis because of the varied healing potential of each patient. Continual periodic followups are absolutely necessary to evaluate the masticatory mucosa beneath the prosthesis.[10]

In general these patients should be seen every 3 months, have bite-wing radiographs taken every 6 to 12 months, and have a full series of radiographs taken every 2 years.

FABRICATION OF A CUSTOM FLUORIDE CARRIER

Armamentarium

1. Diagnostic cast
2. Vacuum forming machine
3. Polypropylene Staguard mouthguard material 0.150 inch
4. Bunsen burner
5. Band-Parker laboratory knife with No. 25 blade
6. Den Silk
7. Scissors
8. Plaster bowl with cold water
9. No. 7 wax spatula
10. Acrylic trimming bur
11. Hanau alcohol torch

When custom fluoride carriers are to be fabricated for a patient, irreversible hydrocolloid impressions are obtained and poured in dental stone. The casts are retrieved and trimmed in the shape of a horseshoe.

The carriers are made by placing a sheet of mouthguard material in the frame of the vacuum forming machine. Turn on the heating element of the machine and swing it into position over the plastic sheet.

As the polypropylene material is heated to the proper temperature, it will first droop or sag in the frame, and then it will lose its cloudy appearance and become completely clear. The cast should be in position at the center of the perforated stage of the vacuum forming machine. Turn on the vacuum. Grasping the handles on the frame that holds the mouthguard material, forcibly lower the heated material over the cast. Turn off the heating element and swing it off to the side. After 60 seconds turn off the vacuum, dip the Den Silk into the cool water, and adapt the mouthguard material to the cast, using the Den Silk as a separating medium. Allow ample cooling time so the carrier will not distort on removal from the cast.

The sheet should be released from the holding frame with the cast. The Bard-Parker knife blade is heated on the Bunsen burner, and a cut is made 5 mm beyond the tooth-gingival junction. The cut should be beveled into the tissue so the cut edge will not cause irritation or be uncomfortable. The excess material is trimmed with the scissors and an acrylic bur. The edges of the carrier are smoothed with a heated No. 7 wax spatula and flame polished with the Hanau torch.

Fig 10-2

INSTRUCTION SHEET TO BE GIVEN TO THE PATIENT

Radiation Therapy and Your Mouth

Radiation therapy given to the head and neck areas results in <u>permanent changes</u> in your saliva. These changes will cause your teeth to become <u>very sensitive</u> and to <u>decay rapidly</u> unless properly protected by the continued <u>indefinite daily use of fluoride</u>. In addition, frequent rinsing, ideally with a dilute salt and baking soda solution, is necessary to prevent soreness of the oral tissues.

Radiation therapy also has an effect on the portion of the bone that receives radiation. This effect on the bone <u>permanently</u> reduces its ability to heal and resist infection. Therefore, it is strongly recommended that you do not have any elective surgery including gum surgery or extraction of teeth from bone treated with radiation.

Recommended Daily Oral Care:
1. Thorough cleaning of mouth after each meal.
   A. Thoroughly brush with a non-irritating dentifrice of your choice.
   B. Floss teeth carefully.

2. Fluoride application.
   A. Apply fluoride in prescribed manner either using a <u>second</u> toothbrush, or (in special cases) applying a thin coating of the fluoride gel to the inner surfaces of your fluoride carriers, placing these on the teeth and wearing for 5 or preferably 10 minutes.

   B. If you have been instructed to use the specially made fluoride carriers, following the 5- to 10-minute wearing period they are removed, rinsed in cool water to remove residue fluoride gel, and stored in a cool place until the next wearing.

   C. After removing the fluoride carriers or after brushing on your fluoride, <u>do not</u> rinse, eat, or drink for 30 minutes.

Additional Supplies:
1. Additional fluoride can be obtained during your return visits to our office, or the doctor can write a prescription for a similar product available from your local druggist.

2. When required, new flexible fluoride carriers can be obtained by returning the models of your teeth to this office.

Dental Care:
1. You must keep your mouth clean.

2. You must use your fluoride daily for the rest of your life.

3. You must be examined and treated by your dentist on a regular schedule <u>at least</u> every 4 months.

4. You must have your teeth cleaned by a hygienist or dentist at least every 4 months.

5. Dental x-rays, anesthesia, having your teeth filled or crowned, or root canal treatment, will do you no harm.

6. You must not have teeth extracted or gum surgery within the areas of your mouth treated with radiation for fear of serious complications.

Fig 10-3

- Dental and periodontal evaluations are essential before the start of radiation therapy.
- A treatment team consisting of the radiation oncologist, dental oncologist, and general dental practitioner and occasionally a periodontist will ensure proper patient management.
- Perform surgical procedures within the radiation field before the start of therapy.
- Oral hygiene and daily application of fluoride are necessary to preserve the dentition.
- Avoid oral trauma that may expose bone and lead to osteoradionecrosis.
- Frequent maintenance visits are essential.
- When complications arise that are beyond the skills of the general dentist, seek the appropriate specialist.

Chemotherapy

Control of malignancies by chemotherapeutic agents has emerged in recent years as the primary treatment or as an adjunct to surgery and radiation. The increased use of chemotherapy is based on the development of effective anticancer agents that may provide a cure or disease-free interval. The actions of these drugs produce toxic effects on the body both directly at the cellular level and indirectly by myeloimmunosuppression of the hematopoietic and lymphoid tissues.

Chemotherapy was used as a treatment for cancer as early as 1865 when Lessauer used potassium arsenite to treat leukemia. Numerous chemotherapeutic agents are now in use, and new ones are constantly being developed. The chemotherapeutic agents are classified in Table 10-1.

Protocols are combinations of chemotherapeutic agents that have been developed to treat a specific type of tumor. Examples of common protocols are given in Table 10-2.

Oral cavity toxicity

The oral cavity is one of the most accessible areas of the body for clinical examination, and it mirrors the effects of chemotherapy on the rest of the gastrointestinal tract and in many ways on the bone marrow.[29] The cells that line the cavity proliferate at a rapid rate like those of the bone marrow and gastrointestinal mucosa. Toxicity to major organ systems may also show effects in the oral cavity. The toxic effects on the central nervous system from the plant alkaloids may result in facial paresthesia; bone marrow toxicity may result in thrombocytopenia leading to potential bleeding problems or in granulocytopenia leading to potential infectious problems.

Table 10-1 Chemotherapeutic agents and modes of action

Agent type	Mode of action
Alkylating agents	Alkylation of DNA
Antibiotics	Disrupt DNA and RNA synthesis
Antimetabolites	Substitution and competition
Plant alkaloids	Mitotic arrest
Miscellaneous	
Hormones	Disrupt all synthesis
Platinum complexes	Inhibit cell growth
Enzymes	Inhibit cell growth

Table 10-2 Protocols of chemotherapeutic agents

Protocol	Agents
FAC	Fluorouracil, adriamycin, cytoxan
VAMP	Vincristin, actinomycin D, methotrexate, prednisone
MOPP	Mustargen, oncovin, prednisone, procarbazine
POMP	Prednisone, oncovin, methotrexate, mercaptopurine
CHOP	Cytoxan, adriamycin, oncovin, prednisone
CHOP-BLEO	CHOP + bleomycin

Toxicity and complications related to the oral cavity are generally classed together under the term stomatitis. Oral complications related to chemotherapy can be classified into three areas: *(1)* mucositis, *(2)* hemorrhage, and *(3)* infections. Mucositis is an inflammation of the oral mucosal lining. Its severity can range from mild erythema and irritation to severe, painful forms such as ulcerative desquamative gingivostomatitis. Hemorrhaging or bleeding disorders may result from drug-induced thrombocytopenia or from a secondary factor such as a loose tooth, a sharp tooth, toothbrush abrasion, or an ill-fitting prosthesis. Granulocytopenia greatly increases susceptibility to viral, fungal, and bacterial infections.

The multimodal therapy of radiation and chemotherapy is rapidly gaining popular acceptance. If a patient has been treated with both modalities, the net result of the therapy must be considered from a clinical standpoint. The combined therapy may result not only in the selected toxicity from each type of therapy but in an exaggerated response, which from the clinician's viewpoint complicates the patient's overall management. This makes the pretreatment oral evaluation mandatory to eliminate potential problems. Examples of drugs that can cause alterations of tissue response to the radiation/chemotherapy combination are actinomycin D, which accentuates the normal tissue response to ionizing radiation, and metronidazole, which increases the radiation damage to hypoxic cells.[30]

It is sometimes necessary to consider surgical procedures in patients receiving chemotherapy. The dentist must always consider the hematologic status of the patient when a surgical procedure such as a biopsy or extraction is indicated. A coagulation profile and a complete blood count with differential will give most of the routine information a dentist will need. This information, together with knowledge of the chemotherapeutic agents being used[31] and the time in course, will help in making proper decisions as to when manipulative procedures such as surgery or even a dental cleaning can be performed.

When biopsies are needed, consider the location of the site to be operated. Try to select a site where adequate hemorrhage control procedures (such as direct pressure) can be effected.

Combination chemotherapy is rapidly becoming the most common modality used in anticancer treatment. The side effects are usually additive. Proper timing for manipulative procedures in the oral cavity is extremely important. Laboratory tests showing the current hematologic status is a critical factor to observe. The danger of infection even with antibiotic coverage must be considered and a clinical judgment must be made regarding the benefit of the dental procedure versus the risk to the patient.

Chemotherapy patients with periodontal disease

In general these patients present only acute problems during their chemotherapy. The systemic medications that are toxic to the rapidly dividing cancer cells also affect the oral cavity. If the periodontium is healthy, then chemotherapy usually has no noticeable negative effects on the periodontium. If problems arise, they should be treated in conjunction with the oncologist. Frequent prophylaxes are helpful during and for about a year after medication to help the periodontium remain stable.

––––––– *At a glance* –––––––

Chemotherapy

- A dental team approach is suggested for patients receiving chemotherapy.
- Systemic manifestations of chemotherapy such as paresthesia and thrombocytopoiesis leading to potential bleeding problems can show up in the head and neck.
- Local reactions to chemotherapy include mucositis, hemorrhage, and infections.
- If the periodontium is healthy, the effect on these tissues is minimal.
- These patients should be seen at least four times a year for maintenance.

References

1. Brady LW, Davis LW. Radiation therapy in the management of head and neck tumors, in Hamner JE, III (ed): *The Management of Head and Neck Cancer.* New York, Springer-Verlag, 1984, pp 207–218.
2. Moss WT, Brand WN, Batlifora H: *Radiation Oncology,* 4th ed. St Louis, CV Mosby Co, 1983.
3. Ritchie JR, Brown JR, Guerra LR, Mason G: Dental care for the irradiated cancer patient. *Quintessence Int* 1985;12:837–842.
4. Beumer J, Brady F: Dental management of the irradiated patient. *Int J Oral Surg* 1978;7:208.
5. Silverman S, Chierci G: Radiation therapy of oral carcinoma—1. Effects on oral tissues and management of the periodontium. *J Periodontol* 1965;36:478.
6. Beumer J, Curtis TA, Firtell DN: *Maxillofacial Rehabilitation: Prosthodontic and Surgical Considerations.* St Louis, CV Mosby Co, 1979, p 60.
7. Daly TE, Drane JB: *Management of Dental Problems in Irradiated Patients: Refresher Course.* Houston, University of Texas at Houston, M.D. Anderson Hospital and Tumor Institute and Dental Branch, 1972, p 33.
8. Dreizen S, Daly TE, Drane JB, Brown LR: Oral complication of cancer radiotherapy. *Postgrad Med* 1977;61(2):85–92.
9. Chencharick JD, Mossman KI: Nutritional consequences of the radiotherapy of head and neck cancer. *Cancer* 1983;51:811.
10. Dreizen S, Brown LR, Handler S, Levey BM: Radiation induced xerostomia in cancer patients—Effect on salivary and serum electrolytes. *Cancer* 1976;38:273.
11. Conger AD, Wells MA: Radiation and aging effect on taste structure and function. *Radiat Res* 1969;37:31.
12. Engeset A: Irradiation of lymph nodes and vessels: Experiments in rats with reference to cancer therapy. *Acta Radiol* 1964;5(Suppl):229.
13. Brown KE: Dynamic opening devices for mandibular trismus. *J Prosthet Dent* 1968;20:438.
14. Rahn AO, Boucher LJ: *Maxillofacial Prosthetics: Principles and Concepts.* Philadelphia, WB Saunders Co, 1970, pp 39–44.
15. Marx RE: Osteoradionecrosis: A new concept in its pathophysiology. *J Oral Maxillofac Surg* 1983;41:283–288.
16. Marx RE: A new concept in the treatment of osteoradionecrosis. *J Oral Maxillofac Surg* 1983;41:351–357.
17. Daly TE, Drane JB: Preventive oral care for the irradiated cancer patient. *Dent Surv* 1970;46:36–38.
18. Daly TE, Drane JB, MacComb WS: Management of problems of the teeth and jaws in patients undergoing irradiation. *Am J Surg* 1972;124:539.
19. Keene HJ, Daly T, Brown LR, Dreizen S, Drane JB, Horton IM, Handler SF, Perkins DH: Dental caries and *Streptococcus mutans* prevalence in cancer patients with irradiation-induced xerostomia: 1-13 years after radiotherapy. *Caries Res* 1981;15:416.
20. Shannon IL, Cook JM, Henson WT: Reduction of enamel solubility by stannous fluoride. *J Houston Dist Dent Soc* 1968;40:7–10.
21. Shannon JS: Water-free solutions of stannous fluoride and their incorporations into a gel for topical application. *Caries Res* 1969;3:339–347.
22. Alexander WE, McDonald RE, Stookey GK: Effect of stannous fluoride on recurrent caries: Results after 24 months. *J Dent Res* 1973;52:1147.
23. Rollo G: Effect of fluoride on initiation of plaque formation. *Caries Res* 1977;11(Suppl 1):243.
24. Mazza JE, Newman MG, Sims TN: Clinical and antimicrobial effect of stannous fluoride on periodontitis. *J Clin Periodontol* 1981;8:203–212.
25. Chen TY, Webster JH: Oral monilia study on patients with head and neck cancer during radiotherapy. *Cancer* 1974;34:246.
26. Hoar RE: *Investigational Analysis to Develop Oral Preventive and Supportive Care of the Pediatric Oncology Patient.* Thesis. University of Texas Health Science Center at Houston, Dental Branch, 1980.
27. Rahn AO, Matalon V, Drane JB: Prosthetic evaluation of patients who have received irradiation to the head and neck regions. *J Prosthet Dent* 1958;19:174.
28. Curtis T, Griffith MR, Firtell DN: Complete denture prosthodontics for the radiation patient. *J Prosthet Dent* 1976;36:66.
29. Lockhart PB, Sonis ST: Relationship of oral complications to peripheral blood leukocytes and platelet counts in patients receiving cancer chemotherapy. *Oral Surg Oral Med Oral Pathol* 1979;48:21–28.
30. Dreizen S: Stomatotoxic manifestations of cancer chemotherapy. *J Prosthet Dent* 1978;40:650.
31. Dreizen S, McCredie K, Keating M: Chemotherapy-induced oral mucositis in adult leukemia. *Postgrad Med* 1981;69:103–108, 111–112.

Chapter 11

Diagnosis and Maintenance for Dental Implants

Thomas G. Wilson, Jr / Frank L. Higginbottom

There has been a tremendous amount of new interest in dental implants within the last few years. This has been stimulated by the work of Dr P.-I. Brånemark, a Swedish physician. Brånemark's studies show a high percentage of successes of over 10 years in edentulous mandibles.[1] The genesis of this success seems to be his discovery of osseointegration. He originally described the process as the intimate contact between bone and implant seen at the light microscopic level. This is to be differentiated from implant systems surrounded by thick connective tissues, which are termed fibro-osseous integration systems.[2] The closer coaptation of bony tissue to implant seen in osseointegrated systems seems to provide increased stability and longevity. Diagnosis and maintenance are different for these two groups because of the differences in attachment. As a group, fibro-osseous systems have a more guarded prognosis and therefore need more aggressive maintenance.

Fibro-osseous integrated implants

At present, because of the high failure rate, you should assume that tissue breakdown is occurring from the time of placement and treat the implant accordingly.[3]

Diagnosis of peri-implantitis around fibro-osseous implants

1. *Radiographs.* It is appropriate to use periapical radiographs for diagnosing problems around fibro-osseous integrated implants. These should be supplemented with panographic radiographs where needed (Figs 11-1a and b). If evidence occurs that structures such as the nasal floor, maxillary sinuses, or contiguous nerves are in danger, you should con-

sider removing the device. In addition, protracted pain, mobility, or unmanageable infection warrant removal of the implant.

2. *Probing.* Use of a periodontal probe in the early phases after placement of fibro-osseous integrated implants could be of some benefit; however, as the proliferation of the epithelium progresses, it becomes less and less effective because of the design of most of these devices.

3. *Gingival bleeding, color, and tone.* Look for the same situations that are seen around a healthy tooth; therefore, no bleeding upon probing is the norm. The color of the peri-implant tissues should be analogous to that seen around a healthy tooth. The tissue surrounding the implant should be tight and preferably made up of keratinized gingiva, not alveolar mucosa. Suppuration should not be present (Fig 11-2).

4. *Patient comfort.* The patient should be comfortable. This should include function, esthetics, and access for oral hygiene efforts on the patient's part.

5. *Mobility.* In a number of successful fibro-osseous integrated implants, mobility is present. The 1978 Consensus recommends that the mobility be less than 1 mm buccolingually, mesiodistally, or vertically.[4]

6. *Microbiological monitoring.* Little or no research has been done using monitoring of the bacteria around this class of implants; however, the possibility is that this would be helpful in some failing situations. It is not recommended as a routine procedure (see chapter 2).

7. *Occlusion.* Fibro-osseous integrated implants should have good centric relation–centric occlusion balance, no balancing interferences or fremitus, and light contact on the prosthesis. Contrary to statements by some authors, these implants do not generally accept lateral forces well.

8. *Plaque and calculus.* These parameters should be noted at each maintenance visit and the patient counseled where improvement is needed.

9. *Prosthesis.* Check the prosthesis on top of the implant for fit, cleansibility, and intact interface.

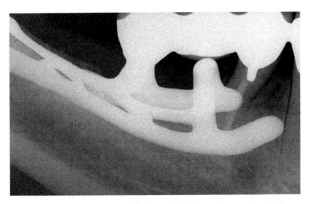

Fig 11-1a Where possible, a right-angle periapical radiograph should be used.

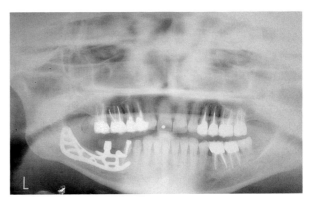

Fig 11-1b Panographic radiographs or a series of periapical radiographs can be used when an overview of the implant is needed.

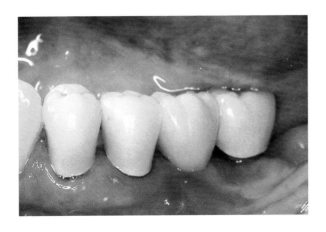

Fig 11-2 The tissues around this unilateral subperiosteal implant (the terminal abutment) remain clinically healthy several years after placement. This is a result of effective cleaning on the part of the patient and access for plaque removal provided by the restorative dentistry.

Maintenance treatment

Treatment at maintenance visits around these implants consists of the following possibilities:

1. *Curettage.* It is possible to do soft-tissue curettage around these implants. It is not advised that the implant itself be touched during these procedures. At present little research has been done in this area, but using a curette with the blade toward the soft tissues will help to reduce inflammation.

2. *Peri-implant tissues.* The amount and type of the peri-implant tissues may need to be modified to enhance patient comfort and facilitate home care. This often necessitates a free gingival graft. Grafting should be performed only after improved oral hygiene has failed to achieve a positive resolution.

3. *Occlusal adjustment.* Light contacts in centric occlusion with no lateral (if possible) contacts are suggested for this class of implants. These parameters should be routinely checked.

4. *Chemotherapeutic treatment.* The amount of microbial plaque can be dramatically reduced in these patients by using a chlorhexidine mouthrinse twice a day. This approach should usually be applied only for the short term. Systemic antibiotics can also be helpful in acute situations.

5. *Recall interval.* The interval should be varied depending on the health of the peri-implant tissues, but in general once every 3 months is suggested for these patients.

Osseointegrated implants

Osseointegrated implants have an intimate association with the bone when viewed under a light microscope. The Brånemark implants have a greater longevity than do their fibro-osseous counterparts.[5,6] This longevity could be related both to the bony interface with the implant and, in those made from titanium, to the hemidesmosomal attachment seen between implant and soft tissue.[7] This is an epithelial attachment similar to that seen around teeth.

The few studies done on the microbiology of the ecosystem around osseointegrated implants[8,9] suggest that periodontal-like breakdown is possible around these teeth, which should be treated accordingly.

Diagnosis of peri-implantitis around osseointegrated implants

1. *Radiographs.* Periapical radiographs are helpful in diagnosing problems around these implants. If you need to see the entire implant it may be necessary to remove the overlying prosthesis or to have a specially designed holder. Right-angle radiographs are needed because the thin line that shows up around failing implants can be easily obscured by small changes in angulation. Brånemark implants can be expected to lose about 0.5 to 1 mm of bone the first postoperative year and then 0.06 to 0.08 mm per year afterwards.[10]

2. *Sound.* A titanium osseointegrated implant when struck with a metal instrument produces a ringing sound. This can be used as one of the diagnostic criteria for health. To accomplish this, the overlying prosthesis must be removed, which may not be possible at each maintenance visit (Fig 11-3).

3. *Probe.* There is a question about whether these implants should be probed or not, because there doesn't seem to be a direct connective tissue interface and probing may strip away the epithelial attachment. However, it seems reasonable at this time to probe. This would be especially helpful if a consistent, known probing force was used so that you could tell how much soft tissue compression was occurring. Great care should be used to avoid scratching the implants.

4. *Gingival bleeding, color, and tone.* No bleeding should be seen upon probing (Fig 11-4). This parameter is particularly important because patients with poor oral hygiene tend to have more rapid breakdown around implants than patients who clean well.[10] Gingival color should be the same as around a healthy tooth. The tissue tone should be tight even though there are occasions when osseointegrated implants do well without having keratinized gingiva around them. It has been observed that they do better with a surrounding band of keratinized gingiva.[11]

5. *Plaque and calculus.* The presence or absence of plaque and calculus on these implants should be noted at each maintenance visit. These deposits should be removed at each maintenance visit.

6. *Occlusal factors.* Osseointegrated implants can handle more loading than fibro-osseous implants. However, you should still avoid excessive occlusal loads because excessive force (in the form of bruxing) may accelerate breakdown,[10] even though some would argue that the quantity of bone actually increases around the implant in the typical bruxer.

7. *Prosthesis check.* The prosthesis should be checked to make sure there is no movement and that the screws that retain the prosthesis are tight and intact, because fracture may occur.[11] Small changes in the prosthetic device can be translated into very detrimental effects on the implants themselves.

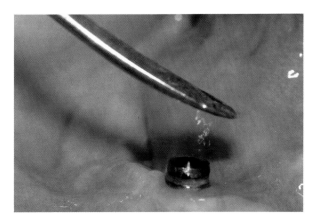

Fig 11-3 A "healthy" osseointegrated implant will produce a ringing sound when struck with a metal instrument, whereas a duller tone is produced by an implant that is not integrated. This diagnostic test should be performed after the overlying prosthesis has been removed.

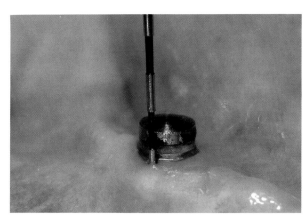

Fig 11-4 Probing should produce no bleeding when the peri-implant tissues are healthy. If available a plastic probe can be used around titanium implants.

8. *Microbiologic monitoring.* A recent study by Mombelli and co-workers[9] studied healthy and failing titanium implants in the same mouth. They found microbes similar to those seen in healthy sulci around teeth in the successful implants. Around failing implants they saw bacteria much like those found around teeth with periodontitis. This type of monitoring may be useful in the recalcitrant case but is not suggested for routine use.

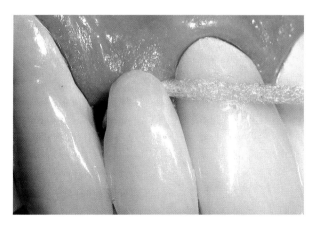

Fig 11-5 Super Floss® (Oral-B) or gauze can be used to clean around implants as well as the tissue surface of the prosthesis.

Treatment and prevention of peri-implantitis—prophylaxis of osseointegrated implants

Supra- and subgingival deposits should be removed at each maintenance visit. Plaque can be easily removed using Super Floss® (Oral-B) or gauze[12] (Fig 11-5). Calculus on these surfaces is not as tenacious as on natural teeth and can be readily taken off. Use of plastic instruments is suggested for this purpose (Fig 11-6). Avoid ultrasonic scalers, interdental brushes with exposed metal, and titanium scalers.[13] A chlorhexidine mouthrinse (Peridex®) helps to clean the large areas of the prosthesis found approximating the soft tissues and cleans the implants themselves. This mouthrinse, along with metronidazole, may help to reduce gingival hyperplasia seen around these implants[14]; however, sometimes a gingival graft is necessary to eliminate this condition (Figs 11-7a to c).

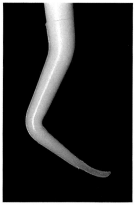

Fig 11-6 This plastic instrument (Nephron Corp) is shaped like a 4R/4L and allows easy access for removing supragingival and subgingival deposits on implants.

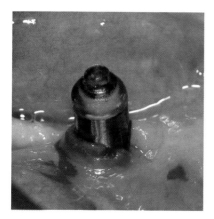

Fig 11-7a This proliferative tissue did not respond to improved oral hygiene, chemotherapy, or gingivoplasty.

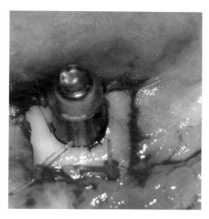

Fig 11-7b A free gingival graft was placed with the abutment cylinder in place.

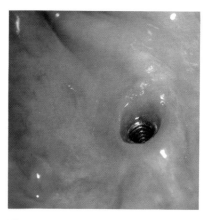

Fig 11-7c After healing (with the abutment cylinder removed), the tissue is healthy and no longer bothers the patient.

At a glance

Osseointegrated implants

- ■ Potential problems can be diagnosed in the following ways:
  - Right-angle parallel periapical radiographs provide accurate information on the implant bone interface
  - A well-osseointegrated implant will emit a sharp ring when tapped with a metal instrument (remove any overlying prosthesis prior to the test)
  - Probe (using a constant force, if possible)
  - Monitor gingival bleeding (or suppuration), color, and tone
- ■ Prophylaxis:
  - Remove plaque with gauze or Super Floss®
  - Remove calculus with plastic instruments
  - In patients who do not effectively clean their implants, use chlorhexidine (Peridex)
  - Where necessary, remove and replace hyperplastic tissue with keratinized tissue

---

Implant failure

Some implants fail early in treatment, but many continue to serve for years. Early failure is usually accompanied by increased mobility, positional change of the implant, and occasionally pain. Early in therapy, if the failing implant cannot be stabilized or the patient relieved of pain, the implant should be removed.

Fibro-osseous systems

Criteria for long-term failure of fibro-osseous implant systems were adopted at the National Institute of Health/Harvard Consensus Development Conference in 1978.[4] They are as follows:

1. Movement considered significant
2. Unmanageable infection
3. Bony fracture
4. Medical or psychological problems
5. Implant fracture that cannot be managed
6. Implant endangers adjacent teeth
7. Severe cosmetic problems
8. Paresthesia that cannot be tolerated by the patient
9. Significant bone loss
10. Pain

Because these implants are treated like a periodontally compromised tooth, various forms of periodontal therapy, including gingival grafting, flap operations, and bone grafting (not hydroxyapatite), may be needed. Oral hygiene seems to be of utmost importance in retaining these implants.[3]

Osseointegrated systems

Long-term information is available only on the Brånemark system at present.

These implants fail in one of two ways, very rapidly or very slowly. The rapid failures (most within the first year) are usually because of failure to osseointegrate or prematurely placing strong mechanical forces on the fixtures. Other failures due to material breakdown have been reported. The rapidly failing implant is usually doomed; however, removal of excess loads, if discovered early, may halt breakdown. Slowly progressing bone loss can be treated by more conventional methods to control the inflammatory process. These include reinforcement of oral hygiene, soft-tissue curettage, and flap operations. This slow bone loss appears radiographically like that seen around a tooth.

References

1. Brånemark P-I, Breine U, Adell R, Hansson BO, Lindström J, Olsson A: Osseointegrated implants in the treatment of the edentulous jaw. Experience from a 10-year period. *Scand J Plast Reconstr Surg* 1977;16:1.
2. Weiss CM: A comparative analysis of fibro-osteal and osteal integration and other variables that affect long-term maintenance around dental implants. *J Oral Implantol* 1987;13:467.
3. Smithloff M, Fritz ME: The use of blade implants in a selected population of partially edentulous adults. A ten-year report. *J Periodontol* 1982;53:413.
4. Schnitman PA, Shulman LB, eds: *Dental Implants: Benefit and Risk.* US Dept of Health and Human Services publication No. 81-1531, December 1980.
5. Smithloff M, Fritz ME: The use of blade implants in a selected population of partially edentulous adults. A 15-year report. *J Periodontol* 1987;58:589.
6. Adell R, Lekholm U, Rockler B, Brånemark P-I: A 15-year study of osseointegrated implants in the treatment of the edentulous jaw. *Int J Oral Surg* 1981;10:387.
7. Gould TR, Westburg L, Burnette DM: Ultrastructural study of the attachment of human gingiva to titanium in vivo. *J Prosthet Dent* 1984;52:418.
8. Lekholm U, Ericsson I, Adell R, Slots J: The condition of the soft tissues at tooth and fixture abutments supporting fixed bridges. A microbiological and histological study. *J Clin Periodontol* 1986;13:558.
9. Mombelli A, Van Oosten MAC, Schurch E, Lang NP: The microbiota associated with successful or failing osseointegrated titanium implants. *Oral Microbiol Immunol* 1987;2:145.
10. Lindquist LW, Rockler B, Carlsson GE: Bone resorption around fixtures in edentulous patients treated with mandibular fixed tissue-integrated prostheses. *J Prosthet Dent* 1988;59:59.
11. Albrektsson T: A multicenter report on osseointegrated oral implants. *J Prosthet Dent* 1988;60:75.
12. Balshi TJ: Hygiene maintenance procedures for patients treated with the tissue integrated prosthesis (osseintegration). *Quintessence Int* 1986;17:95.
13. Thomson-Neal D: *A Pilot Study to Evaluate the Effects of Various Prophylactic Treatments on Titanium, Sapphire and Hydroxylapatite Coated Implants via SEM,* master's thesis, Louisiana State University School of Dentistry, 1988.
14. Newman MG, Flemmig TF: Periodontal considerations of implants and implant-associated microbiota, in NIH Consensus Development Conference: Dental Implants, 1988, p 57.

Chapter 12

Maintenance for the TMJ Patient

Charles Holt

The dental profession is constantly gaining knowledge about temporomandibular joint (TMJ) disorders. These problems overlap in a number of areas with the periodontal patient. These areas include the patient who bruxes, those who receive treatment splints, and orthognathic surgery patients. In addition, long dental appointments need to be modified for these patients.

The relation of trauma from the occlusion has been discussed in chapter 7. What follows is an overview of TMJ disorders that provides guidelines for the dental maintenance of the TMJ patient.

Advances in the diagnosis and treatment of TMJ disorders have resulted in a need for clarification of posttreatment maintenance. In the recent past, most TMJ problems were treated with "shotgun"-type therapy that was basically designed to reduce pain and discomfort with little attention given to long-term maintenance. Improved understanding of stress, myofascial disease, internal derangements, bruxism, and occlusion has provided the dentist with increased knowledge with which to provide improved maintenance care.

Maintenance and active treatment should be based on an accurate diagnosis of the patient's problem. Maintenance for stress-induced diurnal bruxism is certainly treated differently than degenerative joint disease. It must also be understood in treating head and neck pain that acute pain is a symptom of disease, whereas chronic pain is the disease itself.[1]

Classification of TMJ problems is difficult because of the wide range of signs, symptoms, and disease processes that may be present. The term *myofascial pain-dysfunction syndrome* (MPD) that was first used by Laskin[2] is familiar to the dentist, but "in the dental literature, the term has largely lost its meaning when we see it frequently used to designate all types of temporomandibular disorders, even structural joint disease."[3]

For the purpose of this chapter, TMJ disorders will be divided into two categories: *(1)* pain-dysfunction syndromes (ie, etiology related to factors other than joint pathology; Table 12-1) and *(2)* internal derangements of the TMJ (ie, etiology directly related to joint pathology; Table 12-2). Pain-dysfunction syndromes and microtrauma to the joint from structural and functional disharmonies may lead to internal derangements by excessive passive interarticular pressure.[4] Many patients exhibit a combination of these two categories and this must be considered in treatment and maintenance, especially in nonpainful internal derangements. The symptoms of internal derangements without the complaint of pain should not be taken lightly when dealing with maintenance of the TMJ patient, because anterior disk displacements set the stage for a long series of events that culminate in degenerative arthritis.[5]

Table 12-1 Factors contributing to pain-dysfunction syndromes

Stress
Bruxism
Occlusal disharmonies
Structural problems (ie, poor posture, scoliosis, etc)
Tongue habits
Chewing habits
Breathing obstructions
Allergies
Endocrine disorders
Infections
Sleep apnea and other sleep disturbances
Collagen diseases
Myofascial trigger points
Fibromyositis
Myositis

Table 12-2 Internal derangements

Disk displacements
Damaged articular disk
Damage to the joint capsule
Damage to ligamental attachments of the disk-condyle
   mechanism (always present in disk displacements)
Damage to the retrodiskal tissue
Adhesions
Condylar subluxation
Capsular fibrosis
Fibrous ankylosis
Osseous ankylosis
Synovitis
Capsulitis
Osteochondritis (ideopathic condylar osteonecrosis)
Synovial chondromatosis
Gout
Arthritis
   Degenerative osteoarthritis
   Rheumatoid arthritis
   Traumatic arthritis
   Infectious arthritis
   Psoriatic arthritis
Developmental abnormalities
Steroid necrosis
Tumors

Splints

Orthotic devices of various types are extensively used in treating and maintaining TMJ patients. Splints that place the mandible in centric relation or centric occlusion position and forward repositioners are the most common. The uses, advantages, and disadvantages are shown in Table 12-3.

General considerations

The occlusal splint, in addition to providing stability for the TMJ patient, is helpful in the periodontal patient to prevent tooth movement and distribute the forces of bruxism. For this reason, the occlusal splint should cover all teeth in the arch on which it is placed.

Maxillary or mandibular splints may be used. The mandibular appliance has superior esthetics and phonetics and is preferred if eating in an appliance is required. In cases of deep overbite, improved anterior guidance and less stress to periodontally involved teeth are usually obtained with a maxillary appliance. If a mandibular forward repositioner is used for day wear, a maxillary forward repositioner with long anterior ramp should be used at night.

Maintenance

Obviously, many of the factors involved in pain-dysfunction syndromes and internal derangements will require assistance from other health care practitioners. It is beyond the scope of a discussion on maintenance of the TMJ patient to elaborate on the differential diagnosis and treatment of all the aforementioned conditions, but assuming that the initial problem has been resolved, certain guidelines for maintenance may be given. The main factors to be considered in the maintenance of the TMJ patient are stress, bruxism, occlusal disharmonies, myofascial disease, disk displacements, degenerative joint disease, and proper postsurgical care.

Stress

The influence of stress in the TMJ patient is well documented in the dental and medical literature. A caring doctor is essential in the maintenance of the TMJ patient, along with appropriate referrals to a psychologist or psychiatrist. In acute problems, careful explanation by the dentist is usually sufficient in reducing the stress involved. In cases of chronic pain or difficult stress situations, it is appropriate to refer the patient for biofeedback training or counseling. The main factor is that the patient must be made aware of the effect of stress in TMJ disorders. Centric occlusion splints to disengage the occlusion and reduce stress to the joints should be used in high-stress patients. The patient should wear the appliance at night and during identified high-stress activities.

Bruxism

Bruxism is a central nervous system-induced phenomenon. Rugh[6] has shown that bruxism is not induced by occlusal disharmony, as once believed. Various portable electromyographic instruments are now available to establish whether the patient is a diurnal and/or nocturnal bruxist. Diurnal bruxism patients should be evaluated for stress management by appropriate medical personnel. Nocturnal bruxism patients should use a centric occlusion splint during sleep periods. The appliance should be adjusted at 6- or 12-month intervals to maintain proper balance and evaluate wear. When bruxism is severe, muscle relaxants, tranquilizers, and tricyclic antidepressants are sometimes indicated. Proper medical consultation should be provided if long-term use is proposed.

Table 12-3 Comparison of three splinting devices used in managing TMJ patients

Splint	Uses	Advantages	Disadvantages
Centric relation	Myofasical pain dysfunction (MPD) Relieve myospasm before reconstructive dentistry Determine the effect of functioning in centric relation condylar position Bruxism	Can make anterior jig portion quickly for use as diagnostic aid when using maxillary appliance Reversible treatment May use canine protection or group functioning principles May vary changes in vertical dimension	May precipitate dislocation or subluxation of disk if internal derangement exists May increase TMJ pain and swelling in cases of severe inflammation of the retrodiskal tissue May cause posterior condylar displacement if splint is not constructed properly Esthetics is a problem in anterior open bite cases
Centric occlusion	Myofascial pain dysfunction (MPD) Dislocation of disk Subluxation of disk when treating position brings mandible into severe Class III position Degenerative joint disease Relieve myospasm in cases of internal derangement Bruxism Postsurgical cases	Reversible treatment Definitive aid in determining condylar position Prevents posterior condylar displacement May vary changes in vertical dimension Increases joint space to allow proper positioning of disk Aids in determining functional centric position May use varying degrees of canine and/or group function Relieves pressure on retrodiskal tissue Allows for remodeling condyle Extremely useful in differential diagnosis	May present misleading information in case of subluxation of disk (ie, patients with mid to late subluxation may have reduction of pain but the disk is not captured with the splint) Esthetics is a problem in anterior open bite cases
Forward repositioner	Subluxation of disk Following manipulation of dislocated disk	Provides stable position for captured disk Easy to adjust as disk repositions to a more normal position	Esthetics Phonetics Difficult to use in patients with severe tongue thrust if maxillary appliance used Maxillary forward repositioner cannot be adjusted for functional movements.

Occlusal disharmonies

All patients, but especially TMJ patients, should be provided with stable occlusion. In maintenance of the TMJ patient, it is assumed that occlusal dysfunction has been corrected and a stable occlusal position has been established. Proper anterior guidance, posterior bite support, canine guidance, and no balancing interferences are basic to the maintenance of the TMJ patient. A centric occlusion splint that incorporates these factors should be worn at night. The preexisting occlusal problems and restored occlusion should be considered when additional restorative needs are necessary for a patient in maintenance. In some instances dental implants can be used to restore lost function. In these patients, quadrant or unilateral restorative dentistry should be considered if extensive procedures are contemplated. If changes in vertical dimension are considered, a fully adjustable articulator and hinge axis determination should be utilized.

Myofascial disease

An understanding of myofascial disease is one of the most important considerations in maintenance of the TMJ patient. The interrelationship between myofascial disease and TMJ dysfunction has been well established.[7] The problem encountered in maintenance of the TMJ patient is not always a lack of joint stabilization or improper restoration of adequate occlusion, but the existence of unresolved myofascial disease.

Thermography is one of the more recent advances in the diagnosis of myofascial disease, and it may prove to be the most helpful aid in maintenance of the TMJ patient.[8] Thermograms, which are pictures of the distribution of heat being emitted from the body, provide a physiologic evaluation of autonomic dysfunction of sensory nerve distribution. They give diagnostic information regarding myofascial disease, musculoligamentous injury, trigger points, peripheral nerve entrapments, and nerve fiber irritation. Treatment may then be initiated on a physiologic basis. It is possible to monitor therapeutic response during and following treatment. If pain and dysfunction return during maintenance, additional thermograms are helpful when compared with pretreatment thermograms.

Portable transcutaneous electrical nerve stimulation (TENS) units for home use can aid greatly in management and maintenance of the TMJ patient. Most practitioners think of TENS use as a pain control device, but used properly it is a physiologically specific device for resolving myofascial and neurogenic disease processes. Techniques are available for its use in headaches, myofascial disease, atypical facial pain, trigeminal neuralgia, bruxism, internal derangements, and postoperative pain and edema.[9]

Many modalities are available in the treatment of myofascial disease. Those who treat TMJ patients should be well versed in allopathic, osteopathic, and chiropractic principles.

Disk displacement

The most common internal derangement encountered by the dentist is disk displacement. Careful review of the anatomic structures of the disk-condyle mechanism makes it apparent that disk displacements cannot occur without damage to the lateral collateral ligament of the articular disk to the mandibular condyle. Farrar and McCarty[10] indicate that untreated disk displacements invariably lead to degenerative changes in the joint. Therefore, maintenance for patients with disk displacements is extremely important in clinical practice.

Several synonyms for disk displacements exist in the literature. Reciprocal clicking, dislocation with reduction, and subluxation of the articular disk represent one category. Closed lock, dislocation without reduction, and dislocation of the articular disk are synonyms for complete displacement of the articular

disk. The most complete classification for these disorders is described by Bell.[4]

For maintenance purposes, these patients can be divided into four categories.

Disk captured or repositioned

These patients have responded to treatment to the point that the disk is stable and proper occlusion has been established. An orthotic appliance for night use, which prevents any possibility of distalizing the mandible, should be provided. It is also beneficial to have the patient wear the appliance during high-stress times and physical activities. The occlusion should be checked at each maintenance visit and the principles involved in the previous discussion regarding occlusal disharmonies should be applied.

Unstable displacements

Patients who have been treated and are pain free but in whom the disk is not stable will experience continued subluxation. Minimum treatment to provide occlusal stability should be provided and orthotic appliance therapy continued during high-stress times, physical activity, and sleep periods. Radiographs of the TMJs should be taken every 1 to 2 years. Following initial treatment and then as indicated by symptoms, close monitoring of symptoms and patient education must be provided.

Nonreducible dislocations of the disk

This category includes patients diagnosed as having dislocation without reduction that has been refractory to reduction and is not painful. Vertical dimension should not be changed, and occlusal stability should be provided with minimum treatment. As in the other categories, an orthotic appliance in centric occlusion position with prevention of distalization of the mandible should be worn during high-stress times, physical activities, and sleep.

Disk displacements that do not respond to treatment

This includes patients in whom pain continues and surgery is necessary. Postsurgical maintenance will be discussed later in this chapter.

Degenerative joint disease

The vast majority of patients with degenerative joint disease respond well to conservative care without joint surgery. Once the patient has stabilized, which normally follows 4 to 6 months of orthotic appliance wear and resolution of myofascial disease, maintenance must be continued for life. Centric occlusion splints should be utilized as in the previous categories (ie, during high-stress times, physical activities, and sleep). Thick splints are not necessary because disocclusion of cuspal interdigitation is the main purpose of the appliance. Lower orthotic appliances are more esthetically pleasing and make speaking easier, thereby encouraging frequent wear. If proper long centric and canine disocclusion cannot be provided with the mandibular appliance because of occlusion, a maxillary appliance should be used. Any attempt at changing the vertical dimension, if restorative treatment is needed, should be avoided if at all possible. If a patient with degenerative joint disease is comfortable, adaptive changes have occurred in the joints and the occlusal position should not be violated. If it does become necessary to change the vertical dimension, hinge-axis and fully adjustable articulators should be used. Dentures should be fabricated with lingualized occlusion. Radiographs of the joints should be taken at 1- to 5-year intervals.

Postsurgical care

Recent advances in surgical techniques and knowledge of internal derangements have led to an increase in surgical procedures for TMJ dysfunction. Disk tie-back, menisectomy, fossa implants, total joint replacement, arthroscopic procedures, and various other surgical techniques are being performed successfully. Postsurgical maintenance is an important determinant of treatment success in addition to routine postsurgical care such as a liquid diet for 2 to 3 weeks. Provide instruction regarding oral hygiene following joint surgery. Decreased opening may prevent proper oral hygiene for a short time. Chlorhexidine mouth rinses can be helpful during this period.

The following factors are essential to proper postsurgical maintenance.

Resolution of myofascial disease

Evaluation and treatment of myofascial problems should be addressed before surgery, if at all possible. Orthotic appliances, physical therapy, orthopedic evaluation, neurologic evaluation, and stress evaluation should be used as indicated. After surgery the patient must be monitored and treated as necessary to resolve any myofascial problems that arise.

Occlusion

The decision whether to correct occlusal problems before or after joint surgery is difficult. In most cases successful occlusal treatment cannot be done until the joint position has been stabilized. Some techniques, such as total joint replacement, should be preceded by correction of the occlusion if possible. Concurrent orthognathic procedures and joint surgery are indicated in some cases. Consultation and understanding among the surgeon, restorative dentist, orthodontist, and periodontist are essential.

Postsurgical splints

Thin, mandibular centric occlusion splints are preferred for most joint surgery cases. The splint should be placed immediately in arthroscopic surgery patients and whenever gross malocclusion is present, but most open joint surgery patients are best treated by placement of the orthotic appliance 3 to 4 weeks after surgery. If the orthotic appliance is placed at surgery, it should be worn 24 hours a day, even while eating, for the first 2 to 3 weeks. Wear while eating may then be discontinued, and splint therapy should continue for 3 to 4 months. Two to 4 months after surgery, mounted models should be prepared to evaluate the occlusion. After occlusal stability is obtained, the patient should wear an orthotic appliance at night indefinitely.

Joint mobilization

Physical therapy and exercises should be initiated as soon as healing allows. The importance of increasing range of motion in opening, lateral, and protrusive movements should be stressed to the patient, and range-of-motion measurements should be charted at each postoperative appointment.

Long term

Joint radiographs in closed and open positions should be taken at 6 months and then every 1 to 2 years. After 6 months the night orthotic appliance and occlusion should be checked on a routine basis.

Our current level of knowledge in dentistry does not provide us with absolutes in the treatment and maintenance of the TMJ patient. In light of the advances of recent years, the future is exciting in regard to our ability to manage successfully the patient suffering from TMJ dysfunction and craniofacial pain.

─────── *At a glance* ───────

■ Those involved in the maintenance of the periodontal patient should be made aware of the essentials of maintenance of the TMJ patient.

■ Factors in maintenance include:
Stress
Bruxism
Occlusal disharmonies
Myofascial disease
Disk displacements
Degenerative joint disease
Post-TMJ surgery considerations

References

1. Sternbach RA: Chronic pain as a disease entity. *Triangle* 1981;20:27.
2. Laskin DM: Etiology of the pain-dysfunction syndrome. *J Am Dent Assoc* 1969;79:147.
3. Bell WE: *Orofacial Pains: Classification, Diagnosis, Management,* 3rd ed. Chicago, Year Book Medical Publishers, 1985, p 162.
4. Bell WE: *Clinical Management of Temporomandibular Disorders.* Chicago, Year Book Medical Publishers, 1982, pp 140–159.
5. Farrar WB, McCarty WL Jr: *A Clinical Outline of Temporomandibular Joint Diagnosis and Treatment,* 7th ed. Montgomery, Ala, Normandie Publications, 1982, p 16.
6. Rugh JD, Barghi N, Drago CJ: Experimental occlusal discrepancies and nocturnal bruxism. *J Prosthet Dent* 1984; 51:548.
7. Travell JG, Simons DG: *Myofascial Pain and Dysfunction: The Trigger Point Manual.* Baltimore, Williams & Wilkins Co, 1982, pp 168–173.
8. Finney JW, Holt CR, Pearce KB: Thermographic diagnosis of temporomandibular joint disease and associated neuromuscular disorders. Postgraduate Medicine: Custom Communications, Academy of Neuro Muscular Thermography. Clinical Proceedings, Dallas, Texas 1985—Special Report, March 1986, pp 93–95.
9. Holt CR: *TENS in the Management of Craniofacial Pain.* Protocol Booklet. St Paul, Minn, Health Care Specialties Division/3M, 1986.
10. Farrar WB, McCarty WL Jr: Inferior joint space arthrography and characteristics of condylar paths in internal derangements of the TMJ. *J Prosthet Dent* 1979;41:548.

Chapter 13

Selected Topics

I. Dental Hypersensitivity

Janice Barone / Thomas G. Wilson, Jr

Dentinal or cervical hypersensitivity is an ongoing concern for dental therapists and patients. It is a problem frequently encountered and can be a troublesome clinical complaint. Hypersensitivity not only can be painful but can interfere with good oral hygiene practices, leading to caries and periodontal diseases. Many symptoms and characteristics are associated with tooth root hypersensitivity. A variety of stimuli can elicit a painful response, and several theories have been advanced to explain dentinal sensitivity and how it occurs. Areas of research have included mechanisms of pain transmission through dentin and how naturally occurring or other environmental desensitizing mechanisms inhibit or reduce pain. This chapter covers a number of the studies that have been conducted to evaluate treatment agents or compounds and their effect on hypersensitivity, and presents specific recommendations for dealing with the problem of hypersensitivity.

Common causes and symptoms

Root surface hypersensitivity is frequently seen with gingival recession. Recession can occur as a result of incorrect toothbrushing or a lack of attached gingiva, after periodontal therapy, or as a sequela to periodontitis.[1-3]

When the soft tissue and cementum are lost, the dentin is exposed, and pain may be elicited by a variety of stimuli. Thermal, tactile, chemical, and osmotic stimulation of exposed root surfaces can produce painful dental sensations of variable severity and frequency. In most patients the pain is instantaneous when the offending stimulus is applied, is short-lived, and usually disappears immediately when the stimulus is removed. Hypersensitivity may be present on most teeth, or it can develop in one region or tooth and be absent elsewhere despite seemingly similar conditions. Although many individuals have exposed dentin, not all experience hypersensitivity symptoms. There is no definite explanation for this apparent anomaly, although certain factors such as age of the individual, rate of exposure of the dentinal surface, and effect of natural or other environmental desensitizing mechanisms may be responsible.[4] Research has shown that areas of cervical dentin display patent tubules.[5] In individuals who experience no sensitivity with exposed dentin, occlusion of these tubules may have blocked transmission of stimuli to the pulp.[6,7]

――――― *At a glance* ―――――

Causes and symptoms

- Not all areas of exposed root surface are hypersensitive.
- Currently it is assumed that dental root sensitivity is preceded by removed cementum and exposed dentinal tubules.

Theories of sensitivity

Intensive research has been done on how certain stimuli influence nerve fibers. Several theories have been proposed to explain the mechanism of pain transmission across dentin. Three main theories have emerged, although each remains somewhat controversial.

Direct stimulation of sensory nerve endings

This theory suggests that dentinal sensitivity is due to direct stimulation of sensory nerve endings in the dentin.[8] Electron microscopy has revealed nerve fibers in dentin, but it is still not clear what percentage of dentinal tubules contain nerves. A number of studies[9-14] indicate that nerves occur only in the most pulpal part of the dentin and not near the periphery. It remains unclear how a stimulus applied to the dentin could influence nerve fibers that apparently do not penetrate all the dentinal tubules or even the bulk of the dentin.[15] Nerves in the dentinal tubules are pain receptors, but because they exist only in the circumpulpal part of the dentin, they alone cannot account for dentinal sensitivity.

Dentinal receptor mechanism

A mechanism may exist whereby stimuli are transferred through the dentin to the tissue areas where nerves have been demonstrated and/or to the pulp. This theory suggests that odontoblasts and their processes act as dentinal receptor mechanisms. The odontoblast may therefore have a special sensory function, and the functional complex with the nerve ending in or near the odontoblastic layer may act as an excitatory synapse. The odontoblast and its process have been perceived as a transducer mechanism.[4] However, it is believed that odontoblastic processes do not occupy the full length of the dentinal tubules. Thus dentinal sensitivity cannot be fully explained on the basis of the odontoblast-receptor theory.

Hydrodynamic mechanism

A more widely accepted theory is that a hydrodynamic mechanism transmits stimuli to the pulp. Rapid fluid flow within the tubules could mechanically stimulate nerve receptors in the pulp.[16] Brännström[11,17-21] theorized that pain is produced by the rapid displacement of the tubular contents at the pulpodentinal border due to a stimulus causing a change in the slow outward fluid flow that seems to occur normally. Brännström and Astrom[19] have claimed that all stimuli known to cause dentinal pain, with the exception of electric stimuli, will cause movement of the fluids within the dentinal tubules, and that if this movement is rapid, it will mechanically stimulate nerve endings in the dentin-pulp border zone.

───── *At a glance* ─────

Theories of sensitivity

■ Pain may be perceived following application of a noxious stimulus for one (or a combination) of the following reasons:
- There may be nerve endings that are directly affected
- Odontoblasts may transfer the stimulus to the pulpal tissue
- Rapid fluid flow within the tubule may transfer the message

Requirements and properties of treatment agents

Whatever mechanisms cause dentin hypersensitivity, mechanical blocking of the tubules by precipitation of compounds or by surface coating is an essential requirement of a desensitizing agent. In 1935 Grossman[22] suggested an ideal desensitizer is: (1) nonirri-

tating to the pulp, (2) relatively painless when applied, (3) easily applied, (4) rapid in action, (5) effective for a long time, (6) produces no discoloration, and (7) consistently effective. Despite extensive research, no universally accepted or definitely predictable desensitizing agent or treatment has been found that satisfies all of these criteria. Numerous agents and treatments have been used and studied for their effectiveness. Many of the agents used to treat dentinal sensitivity have an obtunding action and are used because of that property. Some agents supposedly stimulate the formation of secondary dentin, whereas other agents such as adhesive or bonding materials have been used simply to cover the sensitive areas. An agent may be effective in one individual but not in another and for one stimulus but not for another. A positive effect in some form may be found in every agent tested. Nevertheless, many placebo responses have been obtained and must be considered in evaluating results from treatment agents.

Variables that affect treatment agent assessment

Several factors may affect the evaluation of a treatment agent because of the symptomatic nature and variability of the condition. Studies estimating improvement in hypersensitivity have been handicapped by an inability to observe patient response objectively[23]; most investigations depend on the patient's interpretation. A number of devices have been developed[24-26] to quantitate patient responses to different stimuli. However, most of these instruments allowed accurate measurement of the applied stimulus, but the evoked response was still subjective in nature. Other variables that also may alter the degree of hypersensitivity and treatment assessment include age, emotional temperament, and general health status of the patient.[4] No single method of evaluation is reliable when used alone; correlation between the patient's history of the condition and his or her response to the test stimuli is also necessary when assessing treatment.

At a glance

Requirements for treatment agents

- They must make the dentinal tubules impermeable to the various stimuli that elicit a hypersensitive response.
- They must do no harm.

Treatment agents

Sodium fluoride

Much attention has been given to fluorides as desensitizing agents. Fluoride was first proposed as a desensitizing agent by Lukomsky in 1941.[27] Working with various preparations of sodium fluorides, Hoyt and Bibby in 1943[28] concluded that a 33% sodium fluoride paste (incorporating equal parts of kaolin and glycerin) was extremely effective in reducing hypersensitivity. In a recent study, Tarbet et al[29] found that a 33% sodium paste produced a significant reduction in hypersensitivity at 3- and 7-day intervals following application, but this desensitizing effect was no longer significant at day 10. Gedalia et al[30] placed a 2% sodium fluoride solution on exposed cervical dentin after pretreatment with 10% strontium chloride. They noted a significant decrease in sensitivity after treatment with sodium fluoride with or without pre-

treatment with 10% strontium chloride solution. Sodium fluoride alone was still significantly effective. There have been favorable results with concentration levels ranging from 0.7% to 2% solutions of sodium fluoride.[31-33] Sodium fluoride in gel form has been widely recommended; however, there are insufficient controlled studies documenting its use in topical application. Use of sodium fluoride in a dentifrice specifically to treat dentin sensitivity is a relatively new approach. In 1984 Collins and Perkins[34] revealed that the efficacy of sodium fluoride in a special dentifrice to treat dentin sensitivity remains questionable.

Sodium fluoride with or without iontophoresis

The effectiveness of sodium fluoride on tooth hypersensitivity with and without iontophoresis also has been evaluated. Iontophoresis is the process of influencing ionic motion by electric current. The use of an electric current could enhance ion uptake by dentinal tissues and aid in achieving desensitization. An electrical potential may increase fluoride penetration and retention of the ion within tooth structure.[35] Zardok et al[36] observed whether iontophoresis causes a greater increase in dentin's fluoride uptake than topical fluoride alone; fluoride concentrations in the surface and subsurface layers of the iontophoretically treated teeth were significantly higher than in those treated only topically. Murthy et al[37] compared 33% sodium fluoride paste with iontophoresis using 1% sodium fluoride; iontophoresis with 1% sodium fluoride provided more relief after one application and was preferable to treatment with the paste. Minkov et al[38] compared 2% sodium fluoride with and without iontophoresis and found no appreciable difference between the two forms of treatment; however, in this study a positive electrode was applied to each tooth. Gangarosa and Park[39] advocate using a negative charge because a positive charge at the tooth surface would hinder penetration of the fluoride into the tooth. By applying 2% sodium fluoride to exposed root surfaces and a positive electrode to each tooth, they obtained 80% moderate reduction of sensitivity and 20% good reduction. When they applied iontophoresis with a negative electrode, their results showed 100% good reduction. Gangarosa and Park also found that the use of a positive electrode is a cardinal error in fluoride iontophoresis. In a recent study using mechanical and thermal devices to evaluate patient responses quantitatively, Lutins et al[35] also evaluated the effectiveness of iontophoresis with and without electric current and sodium fluoride on tooth hypersensitivity. Teeth received a 2% neutral sodium fluoride solution applied with an electrode iontophoresor. Test teeth received the solution with current, and control teeth (in the same individual) did not receive current with the solution. Fluoride was applied at days 0 and 7; this is a short time span for evaluation, but this is the period recommended for use of the iontophoresor. It had been previously suggested that application of fluoride at these intervals provides maximum fluoride uptake.[39] Because many hypersensitive teeth show reduced sensitivity over time, the researchers used this short evaluation period for more meaningful evaluation of this technique. The study participants were tested at days 0 and 7. Statistically, the test teeth showed more improvement than the control teeth. Only slight improvement was noted in response to temperature change, indicating that patient comfort will be only partially enhanced with this technique.

Another iontophoretic technique that has been evaluated involves the use of an iontophoretic toothbrush. Manning[40] described a brush with an aluminum handle powered by batteries that is designed for use with fluoride dentifrices. The rationale is that if a desensitizing agent (in this case the fluoride ion) can be attracted to a hypersensitive root through the creation of a positive charge at the tooth, desensitization may be enhanced.[41] The iontophoretic toothbrush in combination with a fluoride dentifrice can be effective in reducing hypersensitivity.[42–44]

On the whole, iontophoresis is an effective and safe method for treating hypersensitive root surfaces. Iontophoresis has demonstrated no detrimental effect on pulpal tissue, odontoblasts, and/or nerves.[45] The effects of fluoride by iontophoresis have been attributed to more effective penetration of the dentinal tubules by the fluoride and to possible stimulation of secondary dentin formation.[37] Available studies show that teeth subjected to a current of 1 mA per minute remain vital.[45,46] This amount of current is adequate to promote ion transfer of fluoride to the tooth. The electrolyte of choice is 1% to 2% sodium fluoride with the preferable application of a negative electrode.

Stannous fluoride

Stannous fluoride has been more recently advocated as an effective agent in treating cervical hypersensitivity. Miller et al[47] demonstrated that a water-free 0.4% stannous fluoride gel was effective in reducing pain associated with dentinal hypersensitivity. However, an adequate pain response grading system, which is necessary to quantify the effectiveness of a treatment agent, was not used in this investigation.

Another study[48] assessed the use of a gel containing 0.4% stannous fluoride as a desensitizing agent using the "methods of limits" with a standardized and repeatable cold thermal and electrical stimulus. After initial sensitivity ratings were recorded, the study participants were given an unmarked sample of a gel containing 0.4% stannous fluoride or a placebo. The placebo was an identical gel minus the 0.4% stannous fluoride. Participants were asked to apply the gel to the sensitive area with a clean, dry toothbrush or cotton-tipped applicator twice daily. Each was also instructed not to rinse for 30 minutes following the application. Reduction in sensitivity was evaluated by comparing the mean sensitivity scores at the initiation of the study with the mean scores at various test intervals after initial ratings. The testing intervals were done at 2, 4, and 8 weeks. Participants whose gel contained the 0.4% stannous fluoride noted significantly less sensitivity than those whose gel did not contain 0.4% stannous fluoride at the 4- and 8-week measuring periods for both electrical and thermal stimuli. A fully active 0.4% stannous fluoride gel was determined to be an effective agent in controlling pain associated with hypersensitive dentin. However, prolonged (up to 4 weeks) and consistent use was necessary in order to achieve this effect.[48]

Other research[49] indicated that the use of a stable aqueous stannous fluoride solution containing 0.717% fluoride and 0.303% tin was an effective agent in treating dentinal hypersensitivity. In contrast, Penney and Karlsson[50] demonstrated that tin diffuses less readily than fluoride into the dentin. The molecular size of fluoride is similar to that of the hydroxyl group it is believed to replace. Because tin is a larger atom, the ionic exchange for tin and its chemical role in reducing hypersensitivity appears negligible.

Favorable results have been seen in areas of research evaluating stannous fluoride in precise concentrations as an effective treatment agent.

Calcium hydroxide

Calcium hydroxide also has been studied for its antalgic effect in hypersensitive cervical areas. Green et al[51] treated patients complaining of hypersensitivity after periodontal surgery with calcium hydroxide and potassium nitrate. They evaluated these agents using controlled applications of quantitative stimuli. Results for mechanical and hot stimulation revealed that calcium hydroxide was the more successful agent in relieving hypersensitivity immediately upon application. However, at the end of the testing period the calcium hydroxide and potassium nitrate results appeared to be similar. Over a 3-month period all results were statistically significant relative to the control group. In cold stimulation calcium hydroxide was again more successful than potassium nitrate in its immediate effect and continued to be the best agent throughout the testing period. Calcium hydroxide may be a recommended treatment for patients who are sensitive only to cold. Patients in this study reported relief up until the 2-week to 1-month interval; this appears to support the concept that calcium hydroxide produces only a superficial blockage of the dentinal tubules and that, with time, this blockage is worn away. Studies have shown that reapplications were often necessary because of the transient action of calcium hydroxide.[20,51,52] Green et al have suggested that calcium hydroxide be used as a desensitizing agent initially following periodontal treatment to reduce pain so that proper oral hygiene can be reestablished.[51]

An office procedure in clinical practice may consist of mixing calcium hydroxide (0.4 g) with sterile water in a dappen dish, making a paste. A fresh mixture is prepared for each patient. Isolate and dry the teeth with cotton rolls and apply paste to the entire exposed root surface. Because of the highly alkaline nature of the calcium hydroxide paste (pH 12), the gingival mucosa must be isolated to avoid gingival ulceration. Remove the paste in 5 minutes and have the patient rinse with sterile water.

Potassium nitrate

Potassium nitrate has recently received more scrutiny in clinical studies to evaluate its therapeutic effect on hypersensitive root surfaces. Tarbet et al[26] studied the effectiveness of 5% potassium nitrate delivered in a low-abrasive toothpaste as a daily home treatment of dentinal hypersensitivity. In the 4-week, double-blind, parallel, comparative study of 27 adults, hypersensitivity levels in affected teeth were evaluated by two quantifying methods. Electrical stimulus and cold air stimulus were used to acquire objective data. Subjective data, derived from responses of the study participants to changes perceived in their general tolerance to normal daily stimuli of their hypersensitive teeth, were also analyzed. Objective data showed that after 2 weeks, use of the potassium nitrate paste had a significantly greater desensitizing effect than the vehicle (control) paste. The therapeutic response to potassium nitrate increased continuously for the length of the study period. Subjective data at 2 weeks also showed that the potassium nitrate toothpaste was significantly superior to the control toothpaste. Correlations between the objective and subjective data strongly support the validity of the methods Tarbet et al used and the accuracy of the resulting data. Prior to this study no desensitizing agent suitable for daily home use had passed the test of objective evaluation, nor had any produced objective results that could be correlated with broadly perceived subjective effectiveness. Other published data have shown that a strong placebo effect is present in strictly subjective evaluations.

Hodosh et al[52,53] also advocate regular use of a toothpaste containing 5% potassium nitrate for desensitizing teeth. In patients with extremely sensitive teeth, application of a 5% potassium nitrate gel via a plastic sleeve or tray was a synergistic treatment to the 5% potassium nitrate toothpaste. This office and/or home treatment regimen was effective and easy to use. The approach was especially effective as a preprophylaxis procedure, rendering the teeth notably less sensitive during scaling and other tactile procedures.

In another study by Tarbet et al,[54] four commercially available toothpastes were evaluated for their effectiveness on dentinal hypersensitivity. In this double-blind parallel study, the toothpastes containing the following active ingredients were examined: 5% potassium nitrate, 10% strontium chloride, 2% dibasic sodium citrate in a pleuronic gel, and 1.4% formaldehyde (this last toothpaste at the time of the study contained 1.4% formaldehyde, but it has since been reformulated into a strontium chloride dentifrice). Both quantitative and subjective data were acquired, and sensitivity levels were measured weekly for 4 weeks. In response to electrical stimulation, all four treatment groups showed less sensitivity at all four evaluation periods. For cold air evaluations, the potassium nitrate and dibasic sodium citrate groups showed less sensitivity at all weekly evaluations when compared with baseline data. The strontium chloride and formaldehyde groups were each less sensitive at weeks 2, 3, and 4. Subjective response scores reflect the same pattern as the objective scores for the potassium nitrate group (ie, significance at all evaluations). The strontium chloride group had significant differences from baseline at weeks 2, 3, and 4; the formaldehyde group at weeks 3 and 4; and the dibasic sodium citrate group achieved less sensitivity only at the 4-week evaluation. In comparing the four toothpastes and their ability to desensitize hypersensitive root surfaces, all the objective and subjective response scores from the potassium nitrate group showed significantly greater reductions in sensitivity than the scores obtained from the other toothpastes. In conclusion, the data showed potassium nitrate to be the superior desensitizing toothpaste.

A 5% potassium nitrate dentifrice has been shown to be an effective and quick-acting agent for the daily home treatment of dentinal hypersensitivity. However, recent clinical evaluations of two potassium nitrate dentifrices failed to show superiority of potassium nitrate over the placebo dentifrice during a 12-week period. Stimuli used consisted of a dental explorer and cold air blast, and a discomfort scale scoring system was employed.[55,56] Further studies are needed to determine the mechanism of action of potassium nitrate, because it is not known exactly how this compound acts to produce a desensitizing effect in dentinal hypersensitivity, though an oxidizing effect has been proposed.[52]

Resins and adhesives

Several investigators have studied the effect of resins and adhesives on exposed hypersensitive root surfaces[23,57] as potential means of sealing the dentinal tubules. Results from these studies have shown immediate and long-lasting blockage of sensitivity on most surfaces between 1 month and 1 year. However, where the adhesive sheared off, sensitivity (baseline level) returned. The importance of root surface conditioning prior to resin impregnation and the clinical technique of applying the resin is emphasized by Brännström et al.[57] Resins and adhesive materials appear to be most appropriate in cases where specific areas of persistent hypersensitivity are present, rather than for more generalized root surface hypersensitivity.

Newman[58] suggested sealant impregnation for treating hypersensitive teeth. The Newad sealant system was used in this technique. However, it was noted that portions of the procedure may be painful (the preparation of the root surface by pumicing and acid etching). This pain factor, combined with the possible need to reapply the sealant every 6 months, does not make this method of desensitization a prime choice. Wycoff[59] concludes that the glass ionomer cements are the kindest to the pulp, and no etching is required. Properties include excellent adhesion, good mechanical strength, placement without mechanical tooth preparation, and hydrophilia. In addition, glass ionomer is esthetic and seems to be nonirritating to the pulp. Doering and Jensen[60] have investigated the placement of a light-cured dentin bonding agent. Of 12 participants with hypersensitivity, 74% reported no pain 3 months after placement of this agent.

Although the resin-adhesive systems, especially the new light-cured dentin bonding agents, appear immediately to be effective, further research is needed to evaluate the effect on the pulp.

Other treatment agents

The literature cites many other compounds that have been studied for their usefulness in treating root hypersensitivity. Sodium silicofluoride, acidulated sodium fluoride phosphate, sodium citrate and pluronic gel (F127), sodium monofluorophosphate, potassium oxalate, and strontium chloride are some of the many treatment agents that have been used. Each has shown some degree of efficacy in reducing hypersensitivity.

Another factor that is generally believed to aid in reducing sensitivity is effective plaque removal. Keeping the teeth free of plaque is an important element in all other efforts as well.

Conclusion

The compounds that have been tried are highly diverse, yet all are supposedly effective for treating dental sensitivity. The mechanisms of action of the various desensitizing agents are not completely understood. For example, the use of fluoride or strontium may result in a deposition of insoluble salts in the exposed tubules.[28] In iontophoresis, the application of a current may result in the formation of reparative dentin[61] or may produce paresthesia by altering the sensory mechanism of pain conduction.[39] Calcium hydroxide may cause a beneficial increase in dentinal microhardness.[62] A lack of understanding of the exact mode of action of most of the so-called "active" desensitizing agents, together with insufficient data on the mechanism of pain transmission through the dentin, makes it difficult to select the most suitable treatment. The relative lack of comparative studies between treatment agents compounds this difficulty.

Other factors to be considered are the ease of use or application of the agent, the ability of the agent to reach all sensitive surfaces, such as furcation areas, and patient cooperation and acceptance of the agent.

To date there is no generally accepted group of agents for office use that is consistently effective in treating dentinal hypersensitivity. However, various fluoride compounds, such as sodium fluoride and/or stannous fluoride, seem to be most widely used. At-home agents used exclusively or as adjuncts to professional therapy appear to be very effective and easily used and accepted by patients. A desensitizing toothpaste and/or a fluoride gel or solution are the agents most commonly recommended.

———— At a glance ————

Treatment agents

- Various agents have been used in treating dental sensitivity, but none has proven ideal.
- Studies are hampered by the fact that while the delivery agent can be standardized, patient response is subjective and highly variable.
- A number of agents have some success as desensitizers. Among them are sodium fluoride (with and without iontophoresis), calcium hydroxide, potassium nitrate, resins and adhesives, and stannous fluoride.

The role of occlusion

Teeth that are subjected to trauma become more sensitive (especially to cold stimuli). Relief or reduction of sensitivity often occurs gradually after trauma has been reduced or removed from the teeth. For this reason patients with dental sensitivity presenting for periodontal therapy are often treated with occlusal adjustment, habit devices, or splinting before procedures that will expose more root surface. In some cases it may be weeks (or months) before the patient is ready to proceed with therapy.

Clinical applications

No one treatment agent or method will provide total desensitization for all stimuli in all individuals; a combination of agents or treatments may be necessary.

We should approach the problem with this fact in mind. Following are the steps and the order in which they are taken in our practice.

1. Improve patient oral hygiene where possible.
2. Check for and eliminate any occlusal prematurities with occlusal adjustment or a habit appliance.
3. Check for and eliminate defective restorations or caries.
4. Place the patient on a dentifrice containing potassium nitrate.
5. If sensitivity still exists 30 days later, place the patient on 0.4% stannous fluoride gel twice a day (used in place of their regular dentifrice).
6. If sensitivity still exists 30 days later, use topical application of a 0.717% stannous fluoride gel.
7. If sensitivity continues and pain and problems are unbearable to the patient, suggest endodontic therapy for the tooth.

II. Maintenance for the Diabetic Patient*

Thomas G. Wilson, Jr

Relationship between diabetes and periodontal diseases

Any factor that can tip the scales in favor of the pathogenetic bacteria is to the host's detriment. A continuing debate exists about what role diabetes plays in modifying host resistance. The discussion that follows is a review of the current knowledge.

Most people who have teeth also have some form of periodontal disease. Diabetics are no exception. One study screened 25,672 patients who presented for therapy at a large clinic.[63] Of this group 126 were diabetic and 64 (51%) of these had some form of periodontitis.

Diabetics seem to have more periodontal diseases than patients without diabetes, and the poorer the control, the worse the periodontal disease.[64] Age and length of time the patient has had the disease seem to affect severity of the periodontal problem. Glavind and co-workers[65] studied 102 males between the ages of 20 and 40. Half were diabetic and half were not. They found the severity of gingival involvement was the same for both groups. This was independent of duration of diabetes or insulin dosage. Up to age 30 both groups had similar levels of bone loss. The group age 30 to 40 had more bone loss (with a positive relation to duration of diabetes) than controls.

Eighteen female diabetics age 18 to 35 years studied by Cohen et al[66] were found to have greater pocket formation, more gingival involvement, and more tooth mobility than controls.

After an extensive review of the literature, Saadoun[67] concluded the following:

1. In uncontrolled diabetics, periodontal diseases are more severe than those found in controls.
2. On the whole, controlled diabetics seem to have about the same incidence of periodontal diseases as the general population.
3. Once diabetics have a periodontal disease, they fare worse than their nondiabetic counterparts.

What causes the negative change seen in diabetics?

There are probably numerous factors that make periodontal problems worse in the diabetic. Three factors seem to be closely associated with these negative changes.

1. *Microangiopathy.* The same changes seen in the retina, kidney, and muscle vessels are found in the gingival tissues,[68–70] and patients who have retinopathy exhibit more severe periodontal lesions than those who don't.[65]
2. *Altered polymorphonuclear chemotaxis.* This problem is found in diabetics,[71] and, as previously discussed, patients with this problem tend to have more aggressive periodontal disease.
3. *Bacterial plaque formation.* Supragingival plaque causes gingivitis and sets up an environment for the formation of the subgingival growth of the bacteria responsible for periodontitis. It has been demonstrated in one study that insulin-dependent diabetic children have higher plaque scores than nondiabetic controls.[72]

How to deal with the diabetic patient who has or may have periodontal disease

Diabetics should have an examination that includes the periodontium. When a patient is found to have a periodontal problem, it should be treated more aggressively and monitored more closely than it would be in a nondiabetic patient. In addition, they should understand that they must comply to suggested oral hygiene and maintenance schedules in an above-average manner in order to reduce the chances for recurrence.

After therapy, these patients should initially be placed on a maintenance interval similar to that of other periodontal patients. This interval will be modified as needed (see chapter 6).

*Portions of this section were originally published by and are reproduced with the permission of *The Diabetes Educator*, 1989;15:343–345.

─────── *At a glance* ───────

- Diabetics suffer from periodontal diseases at about the same rate as the general population.
- Once a diabetic has periodontitis, he or she loses attachment more rapidly than a nondiabetic counterpart.
- The negative change may be caused by
  - Microangiopathy
  - Altered polymorphonuclear chemotaxis
  - Increased bacterial plaque formation
- As a rule, diabetics with periodontal diseases should be treated aggressively and placed on frequent maintenance.

III. Prophylactic Coverage for Prevention of Bacterial Endocarditis and Periprosthetic Infections

Thomas G. Wilson, Jr

Prevention of bacterial endocarditis

With more sophisticated methods of detection currently in use, the number of heart murmurs discovered grows yearly. When this is added to the increased number of patients having cardiac prostheses and those surviving longer with previously fatal cardiovascular problems, the number of patients needing prophylactic antibiotics before dental procedures has grown. Recommendations from the American Heart Association for these patients are shown in Fig 13-1.[73,74]

Recently it has been suggested by some that the intramuscular or intravenous medications suggested for higher-risk patients can be replaced with oral medications. In these cases, consultation with the patient's physician is recommended before altering suggested regimens.

Prevention of periprosthetic infections

More and more patients are receiving prosthetic joints. Cases have been reported where these devices have become infected with organisms that could have come from the oral cavity.[75] Consequently, antibiotic coverage for these patients before dental procedures has been suggested.[76] At present there is no consensus about the proper antibiotic or dosage or indeed whether this is appropriate. The patient's physician should be consulted. If antibiotics are to be used, the following regime has been suggested:

Cephalexin (Keflex) — 2 g orally 1 hr before procedure, then 1 g orally 6 hrs later
For patients allergic to cephalexin, clindamycin (Cleocin) — 600 mg orally 1 hr before procedure, then 600 mg orally 6 hrs later

**AMERICAN HEART ASSOCIATION
SCIENTIFIC STATEMENT SUMMARY**

In December 1984, the American Heart Association issued a special report entitled "Prevention of Bacterial Endocarditis." The Council on Dental Therapeutics of the American Dental Association also approved the statement as it related to dentistry.

The purpose of this report was to recommend regimens of prophylactic antibiotics for patients at risk for developing bacterial endocarditis while undergoing dental treatment, surgical procedures or instrumentation involving mucosal surfaces or contaminated tissue. Table 1 lists common cardiac conditions for which prophylaxis is or is not recommended. Certain patients, such as those with prosthetic heart valves and surgically constructed systemic-pulmonary shunts or conduits, are at higher risk of endocarditis than others.

Table 1

Cardiac Conditions A

Endocarditis Prophylaxis Recommended:
    Prosthetic cardiac valves (including biosynthetic valves)
    Most congenital cardiac malformations
    Surgically constructed systemic-pulmonary shunts
    Rheumatic and other acquired valvular dysfunction
    Idiopathic hypertrophic subaortic stenosis (IHSS)
    Previous history of bacterial endocarditis
    Mitral valve prolapse with insufficiency B

Endocarditis Prophylaxis Not Recommended:
    Isolated secundum atrial septal defect
    Secundum atrial septal defect repaired without a patch six or more months earlier
    Patent ductus arteriosus ligated and divided six or more months earlier
    Postoperative coronary artery bypass graft (CABG) surgery

---

AThis table lists common conditions but is not meant to be all inclusive.

BDefinitive data to provide guidance in management of patients with mitral valve prolapse are particularly limited. It is clear that in general such patients are at low risk of development of endocarditis, but the risk-to-benefit ratio of prophylaxis in mitral valve prolapse is uncertain.

The procedures for which endocarditis prophylaxis is indicated are listed in Table 2. Antibiotic regimens given to patients as continuous rheumatic fever prophylaxis are inadequate for the prevention of bacterial endocarditis.

Table 2

Dental and Upper Respiratory Tract Surgical
Procedures for Which Endocarditis Prophylaxis Is Indicated

All dental procedures likely to induce gingival bleeding (not simple adjustment of orthodontic appliances or shedding of deciduous teeth)
Tonsillectomy and/or adenoidectomy
Surgical procedures or biopsy involving respiratory mucosa
Bronchoscopy, especially with a rigid bronchoscope
Incision and drainage of infected tissue

A
    The risk with flexible bronchoscopy is low, but the necessity for prophylaxis is not yet defined.

Fig 13-1

A summary of recommended antiobiotic regimens for dental/respiratory tract procedures is given in Table 3 . . . .

It should be noted that in patients with compromised renal function, it may be necessary to modify or omit the second dose of antibiotics. Intramuscular injections may be contraindicated in patients receiving anticoagulants. Children's doses should not exceed adult doses.

Table 3
For Dental Procedures and Surgery of the Upper Respiratory Tract

1. For most patients: **Oral Penicillin***	**Adults:** 2.0 g of penicillin V one hour prior to procedure and then 1.0 g six hours after initial dose. **Children less than 60 pounds:** 1.0 g of penicillin V one hour prior to procedure and then 500 mg six hours after initial dose.
2. For those <u>allergic to penicillin</u> (may also be selected for those receiving oral penicillin as continuous rheumatic fever prophylaxis): **Erythromycin****	**Adults:** 1.0 g orally one hour prior to procedure and then 500 mg six hours after initial dose. **Children:** 20 mg/kg orally one hour prior to procedure and then 10 mg/kg six hours after initial dose.
3. For those patients at <u>higher risk</u> of infective endocarditis (especially those with prosthetic heart valves) who are not allergic to penicillin: **Ampicillin** plus **Gentamicin**	**Adults:** Ampicillin 1.0-2.0 g plus gentamicin 1.5 mg/kg IM or IV both given 30 minutes before procedure, then penicillin V 1.0 g (500 mg for children under 60 lbs) orally six hours after initial dose. (Alternatively, the perenteral regimen may be repeated eight hours after initial dose.) **Children:** Timing of doses is same as for adults. Dosages are ampicillin 50 mg/kg and gentamicin 2.0 mg/kg.
4. For <u>higher risk</u> patients (especially those with prosthetic heart valves) who are <u>allergic to penicillin</u> **Vancomycin**	**Adults:** Vancomycin 1 g IV slowly over 60 minutes, begun 60 minutes before procedure; no repeat dose is necessary. **Children:** Vancomycin 20 mg/kg IV slowly over 60 minutes, begun 60 minutes before procedure; no repeat dose is necessary.

* For patients unable to take oral penicillin, 2 million units of aqueous penicillin G (50,000 units/kg for children) IV or IM 30-60 minutes prior to the procedure and 1 million units (25,000 units/kg for children) six hours after initial dose may be substituted.

**For patients unable to tolerate oral erythromycin, changing to a different erythromycin preparation may be beneficial. For those who can tolerate neither penicillin nor erythromycin, an oral cephalosporin (1.0 g one hour prior to the procedure plus 500 mg six hours after initial dose) may be useful, but data are lacking to allow specific recommendation of this regimen. Tetracyclines <u>cannot</u> be recommended for this purpose.

WARNING

The Committee recognizes that it is not possible to make recommendations for all possible clinical situations. Practitioners must exercise their clinical judgment in determining the duration and choice of antibiotic when special circumstances apply. Furthermore, since endocarditis may occur despite antibiotic prophylaxis, physicians and dentists should maintain a high index of suspicion regarding any unusual clinical events following dental or surgical procedures.

Fig 13-1 Continued.

References

1. Woofter C: The prevalence and etiology of gingival recession. *Periodont Abstr* 1969;17:45–50.
2. Carranza FA (ed): *Glickman's Clinical Periodontology*. Philadelphia, WB Saunders Co, 1979, pp 103–104.
3. Schluger S, Yuodelis RD, Page RC: *Periodontal Disease: Basic Phenomena, Clinical Management, and Occlusal and Restorative Interrelationships*. Philadelphia, Lea & Febiger, 1977, p 213.
4. Addy M, Dowell P: Dentine hypersensitivity—A review. Clinical and in vitro evaluation of treatment agents. *J Clin Periodontol* 1983;10:351.
5. Ishikawa S: A clinico-histological study on the hypersensitivity of dentine. *J Jpn Stomatol Soc* 1969;36:278.
6. Johnson NW, Taylor BR, Berman DS: Ultrastructure of tubular sclerosis in human carious deciduous dentin. *J Dent Res* 1971;50:685 (Abstr No. 97).
7. Brännström M, Garberoglio R: Occlusion of dentinal tubules under superficial attrited dentine. *Swedish Dent J* 1980; 4:87.
8. Fernhead RW: Innervation of dental tissues, in Miles AEW (ed): *Structural and Chemical Organization of Teeth,* Vol. 1. New York, Academic Press, 1967, pp 247–281.
9. Anderson DJ: The pulp as a sensory organ, in Finn SB (ed): *Biology of the Dental Pulp Organ. A Symposium*. Birmingham, University of Alabama Press, 1968, pp 273–280.
10. Anderson DJ, Naylor MN: Chemical excitants of pain in human dentine and dental pulp. *Arch Oral Biol* 1962;7:413.
11. Brännström M: The elicitation of pain in human dentine and pulp by chemical stimuli. *Arch Oral Biol* 1962;7:59.
12. Dellow PG, Roberts ML: Bradykinin application to dentine: A study of a sensory receptor mechanism. *Aust Dent J* 1966; 11:384.
13. Scott D Jr, Tempel TR: A study in the excitation of pulp nerve fibres, in Anderson DJ (ed): *Sensory Mechanisms in Dentine*. New York, MacMillan Co, 1963, pp 27–46.
14. Scott D Jr, Tempel TR: Neurophysiological response of single receptor units in the tooth of the cat. *J Dent Res* 1965; 44:20.
15. Seltzer S: Hypothetic mechanisms for dentine sensitivity. *Oral Surg Oral Med Oral Pathol* 1971;31:388.
16. Brännström M: A hydrodynamic mechanism in the transmission of pain producing stimuli through the dentine, in Anderson DJ (ed): *Sensory Mechanisms in Dentine*. New York, MacMillan Co, 1963, pp 73–79.
17. Brännström M: Sensitivity of dentine. *Oral Surg Oral Med Oral Pathol* 1966;21:517.
18. Brännström M, Johnson G: The sensory mechanism in human dentine as revealed by evaporation and mechanical removal of dentine. *J Dent Res* 1978;57:49.
19. Brännström M, Aström A: Study on the mechanism of pain elicited from the dentin. *J Dent Res* 1964;43:619.
20. Brännström M, Aström A: The hydrodynamics of the dentine, its possible relationship to dentinal pain. *Int Dent J* 1972; 22:219.
21. Brännström M, Linden LA, Aström A: The hydrodynamics of the dental tubule and pulp fluid. A discussion of its significance in relation to dentinal sensitivity. *Caries Res* 1967; 1:310.
22. Grossman LI: The treatment of hypersensitive dentin. *J Am Dent Assoc* 1935;22:592.
23. Dayton RE, De Marco TJ, Swedlow D: Treatment of hypersensitive root surfaces with dental adhesive materials. *J Periodontol* 1974;45:873.
24. Naylor MN: A thermo-electric tooth stimulator. *Br Dent J* 1961; 110:228.
25. Smith BA, Ash MM: Evaluation of a desensitizing dentifrice. *J Am Dent Assoc* 1964;68:639.
26. Tarbet WJ, Silverman G, Stolman JM, Fratarcangelo PA: Clinical evaluation of a new treatment for dentinal hypersensitivity. *J Periodontol* 1980;51:535.
27. Lukomsky EH: Fluorine therapy for exposed dentine and alveolar atrophy. *J Dent Res* 1941;20:649.
28. Hoyt WH, Bibby BG: Sodium fluoride for desensitizing dentine. *J Am Dent Assoc* 1943;30:1372.
29. Tarbet WJ, Silverman G, Stolman JM, Fratarcangelo PA: An evaluation of two methods for the quantitation of dentinal hypersensitivity. *J Am Dent Assoc* 1979;98:914.
30. Gedalia I, Brayer L, Kalter N, Richter M, Stabholz A: The effect of fluoride and strontium application on dentine: In vivo and in vitro studies. *J Periodontol* 1978;49:269.
31. Massler M: Desensitization of cervical cementum and dentin by sodium silicofluoride. *J Dent Res* 1955;34:761 (Abstr No. T36).
32. Stout WC: Sodium silico-fluoride as a desensitizing agent. *J Periodontol* 1955;26:208.
33. Ehrlich J, Hochman N, Gedalia J, Tal M: Residual fluoride concentrations and scanning electron microscopic examination of root surfaces of human teeth after topical application of fluoride in vivo. *J Dent Res* 1975;54:897.
34. Collins JF, Perkins L: Clinical evaluation of the effectiveness of three dentifrices in relieving dentin sensitivity. *J Periodontol* 1984;55:720.
35. Lutins ND, Greco GW, McFall WT Jr: Effectiveness of sodium fluoride on tooth hypersensitivity with and without iontophoresis. *J Periodontol* 1984;55:285.
36. Zadok J, Gedalia I, Weinman J, Daphni L: Fluoride uptake by root dentin after immersion in 2% NaF solution with iontophoresis. *J Dent Res* 1976;55:310.
37. Murthy KS, Talim ST, Singh I: A comparative evaluation of topical application and iontophoresis of sodium fluoride for desensitization of hypersensitive dentine. *Oral Surg Oral Med Oral Pathol* 1973;36:448.
38. Minkov B, Marmari I, Gedalia I, Garfunkel A: The effectiveness of sodium fluoride treatment with and without iontophoresis on the reduction of hypersensitive dentin. *J Periodontol* 1975;46:246.
39. Gangarosa LP, Park NH: Practical considerations in iontophoresis of fluoride for desensitizing dentin. *J Prosthet Dent* 1978;39:173.
40. Manning MM: New approach to desensitization of cervical dentin. *Dent Surv* 1961;37:731.
41. Johnson RH, Zulqar-Nain BJ, Koval JJ: The effectiveness of an electro-ionizing toothbrush in the control of dentinal hypersensitivity. *J Periodontol* 1982;53:353.
42. Jensen AL: Hypersensitivity controlled by iontophoresis: Double blind clinical investigation. *J Am Dent Assoc* 1964; 68:216.
43. Collins EM: Desensitization of hypersensitive teeth. *Dent Digest* 1962;68:360.
44. Schaeffer ML, Bixler D, Yu PL: The effectiveness of iontophoresis in reducing cervical hypersensitivity. *J Periodontol* 1971;42:695.
45. Walton RE, Leonard LA, Sharawy M: Effects on pulp and dentin of iontophoresis of sodium fluoride on exposed roots in dogs. *Oral Surg Oral Med Oral Pathol* 1979;48:545.
46. Scott HM: Reduction of sensitivity by electrophoresis. *J Dent Child* 1962;29:225.
47. Miller JT, Shannon IL, Kilgore WG, Bookman JE: Use of a water-free stannous fluoride-containing gel in the control of dental hypersensitivity. *J Periodontol* 1969;40:490.
48. Blong MA, Volding B, Thrash WJ, Jones DL: Effects of a gel containing 0.4 percent stannous fluoride on dentinal hypersensitivity. *Dent Hygiene* 1985;59:489.
49. Thrash WJ, Dorman HL, Smith FD: A method to measure pain associated with hypersensitive dentin. *J Periodontol* 1983; 54:160.
50. Penney DA, Karlsson UL: Fast desensitization of tooth roots by topically applied stannous fluoride and strontium chloride in dogs. *Arch Oral Biol* 1976;21:339.
51. Green BL, Green ML, McFall WT Jr: Calcium hydroxide and potassium nitrate as desensitizing agents for hypersensitive root surfaces. *J Periodontol* 1977;48:667.
52. Hodosh M: A superior desensitizer—Potassium nitrate. *J Am*

Dent Assoc 1974;88:831.

53. Hodosh M, Hodosh S, Hodosh A, Shklar G: Potassium nitrate gel-sleeve: An effective procedure for dentinal hypersensitivity. *Quintessence Int* 1982;13:1251.

54. Tarbet WJ, Silverman G, Fratarcangelo PA, Kanapka JA: Home treatment for dentinal hypersensitivity: A comparative study. *J Am Dent Assoc* 1982;105:227.

55. Manouchehr-Pour M, Bhat M, Bissada N: Clinical evaluation of two potassium nitrate toothpastes for the treatment of dental hypersensitivity. *Periodont Case Reports* 1984; 6:25.

56. Manouchehr-Pour M, Bhat M, Bissada N: Clinical evaluation of potassium nitrate toothpastes for treatment of dentinal hypersensitivity. *J Dent Res* 1984;63:248 (Abstr No. 696).

57. Brännström M, Johnson G, Nordenvall KJ: Transmission and control of dentinal pain: Resin impregnation for the desensitization of dentin. *J Am Dent Assoc* 1979;99:612.

58. Newman GV: Sealant impregnation for treatment of hypersensitive dentin. *J Clin Orthod* 1982;16:457.

59. Wycoff SJ: Current treatment for dentinal hypersensitivity. In-office treatment. *Compend Cont Educ Dent* 1982; (Suppl 3):S113.

60. Doering J, Jensen ME: A new photocuring dentin bonding material: Six month clinical results. *J Dent Res* 1985;64:276 (Abstr No. 916).

61. Lefkowitz W, Burdick HC, Moore DL: Desensitization of dentin by bioelectric induction of secondary dentin. *J Prosthet Dent* 1963;13:940.

62. Mjor IA, Finn SB, Quigley MB: Effect of calcium hydroxide and amalgam on non-carious, vital dentine. *Arch Oral Biol* 1961;3:283.

63. Motegi K, Nakano Y, Ueno T: Clinical studies on diabetes mellitus and diseases of the oral region. *Bull Tokyo Med Dent Univ* 1975;22:243.

64. Galea H, Aganovic I, Aganovic M: The dental caries and periodontal disease experience of patients with early onset insulin dependent diabetes. *Int Dent J* 1986;36:219.

65. Glavind L, Lund B, Löe H: The relationship between periodontal state and diabetes duration, insulin dosage and retinal changes. *J Periodontol* 1968;39:341.

66. Cohen DW, Friedman LA, Shapiro J, Kyle GC, Franklin S: Diabetes mellitus and periodontal disease: Two year longitudinal observations. *J Periodontol* 1970;41:709.

67. Saadoun AP: Diabetes and periodontal disease: A review and update. *Periodontol Abstr* 1980;28:116.

68. Stahl S, Witkin G, Scopp I: Degenerative vascular changes observed in selected gingival specimens. *Oral Surg Oral Med Oral Pathol* 1962;15:1495.

69. McMullen J, Legg M, Gottsegen R, Camerini-Davalos R: Microangiopathy within the gingival tissues of diabetic subjects with special reference to the prediabetic state. *Periodontics* 1967;5:61.

70. Keene J Jr: A histochemical evaluation for small vessel calcification in human nondiabetic and diabetic gingival biopsy specimens. *J Dent Res* 1969;48:968.

71. Goteiner D, Vogel R, Deasy M, Goteiner C: Periodontal and caries experience in children with insulin dependent diabetes mellitus. *J Am Dent Assoc* 1986;113:277.

72. Mowat AG, Baum J: Chemotaxis of polymorphonuclear leukocytes from patients with diabetes mellitus. *New Engl J Med* 1971;284:621.

73. Shulman ST, Amren DP, Bisno AL, Dajani AS, Durack DT, Gerber MA, Kaplan EL, Millard HD, Sanders WE, Schwartz RH, Watanakunakorn C: Prevention of bacterial endocarditis. A statement for health professionals by the committee on rheumatic fever and infective endocarditis of the council on cardiovascular disease in the young. *Circulation* 1984; 70:1123A.

74. American Heart Association: Prevention of bacterial endocarditis: A committee report of the American Heart Association. *J Am Dent Assoc* 1985;110:98.

75. Grogan TJ, Dorey F, Rollins J, Amstutz HC: Deep sepsis following total knee arthroplasty. Ten-year experience at the University of California at Los Angeles Medical Center. *J Bone Joint Surg* 1986;68:226.

76. Cioffi GA, Terezhalmy GT, Taybos GM: Total joint replacement: A consideration for antimicrobial prophylaxis. *Oral Surg Oral Med Oral Pathol* 1988;66:124.

Chapter 14

Improving Patient Compliance

Thomas G. Wilson, Jr

Throughout this book it has been shown that patients' health is improved when they comply to maintenance therapy. Failure to comply often leads to failure of therapy. Are these problems unique to dentistry? And more important, how can we encourage our patients to improve their compliance?

What is compliance?

The traditional term has meant "the extent to which a person's behavior coincides with medical or health advice."[1] The word compliance has come to represent a situation in which the patient is a passive responder to the practitioner's rules. In truth, to be successful you must establish communication that will lead to a bond of trust between you and the patient. This union has been termed adherence[2] or therapeutic alliance.[3] The term compliance is used throughout this text because of the overwhelming preference for the term in the literature.

Compliance in medicine

The medical literature is filled with studies on compliance. A recent search showed over 7,000 articles published within the last few years. Most studies found noncompliance to be the rule and not the exception. In general, patients comply best to changes that require only short-term behavioral modification. They also do well when they perceive their disease to be acute or feel it a threat. The less threatening the problem and the longer the required behavioral changes must continue, the less likely a patient is to comply. Even in the short term, compliance is not perfect for the average patient.[4] The decline of compliance over time was graphically demonstrated by Hedstrand and Abery[5] when they studied taking prescribed medication for hypertension in middle-age men. They found that compliance slid from 94% in the first year to 65% in year 2 to 34% in year 3. In another study, diabetics also tended to comply poorly to recommended medications and diets even when they understood that noncompliance could detrimentally affect their health.[6]

Patients with other potentially life-threatening problems such as smoking[7] and previous myocardial infarcts[8] tend not to comply to suggested life-style modifications and therefore worsen their prognosis.

At a glance

Compliance in medicine

- Compliance is better with acute problems.
- The greater the perceived threat, the greater the compliance.

Compliance in dentistry

Most of us feel that our therapy works well, and we would like to believe that most patients do what we ask. Patients don't make long-term behavioral changes to problems they consider relatively non-threatening, and because we deal for the most part with chronic problems that are not usually threatening in an immediate sense, our chances of success in significantly changing our patients' behavior are slim.[9]

In dentistry, studies on the subject of compliance have been primarily in two areas: oral hygiene and what keeps the patient in (or away from) the dental office.[10] We know that the most common dental diseases are caused by plaque, and that when plaque is removed and the damage repaired, these diseases tend not to recur as long as patients comply to suggested oral hygiene or maintenance.[11,12] The critical question is, Do patients do what we suggest? When we look at oral hygiene, the answer seems to be an overwhelming "no." Patients use a toothbrush most often, with aids used to clean interproximally falling far behind.[13–15] Where dental visits are concerned, the record is not much better. Patients give a number of reasons for noncompliance: fear, self-destructive behavior, economic concerns, lack of rapport with the dentist.[16–19]

At a glance

Compliance in dentistry

- Most patients don't comply to suggested oral hygiene.
- Most dental offices experience a very high patient turnover.

Compliance in periodontics

The studies done in periodontics are limited.[20–22] While the results may not be typical, those studies give us some idea of patient compliance to maintenance. One study dealt with all the patients seen on recall during the first 8 years of my practice.[20] Of the approximately 1,000 patients reviewed, only about 16% complied with their suggested recall intervals, whereas 35% never returned for any follow-up care.

Of these patients, we were able to follow 162 for 5 years and found that none of the individuals who were in complete compliance lost any teeth, whereas erratic compliers lost 60 teeth.[21] Our other research showed that patients who comply best with suggested maintenance schedules have less gingivitis as measured by bleeding upon probing.[21] At least in these periodontal patients, those who comply tend to do better than those who do not.

At a glance

Compliance in periodontics

- Patients who comply to suggested maintenance do better than those who don't.
- The better one complies, the better the periodontium fares.
- In one study only 16% of the patients in a periodontal office complied to maintenance intervals as suggested.

Improving patient compliance

We would all like to improve patient compliance, but how do we achieve this goal? Success in compliance is relative. To expect perfect compliance from all patients is unrealistic, but to strive for improvement can only benefit everyone involved. The guidelines that follow are generalities and do not work for every patient, or even for the same patient over time. They should be modified for each individual and each practitioner. You should be forewarned that increasing patient compliance may necessitate behavioral changes on your part as well as the patient's.

Guidelines

1. *Establish goals.* These could include no bleeding upon probing, no new carious lesions, etc. It is then important to reinforce positive performance. To tell how the patient is progressing, accurate records must be kept (see chapter 2), and the results (positive or negative) should be communicated to the patient. It may prove helpful to show patients charts on their performance or even provide them with a copy.

2. *Modify barriers that reduce patient compliance.* This may involve modifying office schedules, office hours, changing office personnel, or changing the attitude of the dental professional. The better and more timely the service, the more likely people are to return. This is especially true of "middle and upper class" individuals. If these patients consistently have to sit in the waiting room, their compliance is likely to dwindle. A short questionnaire given to the patient can provide feedback. Many patients avoid dental work because of fear. Questions on the health history designed to bring these fears to light may help the therapist and the patients to deal with their problem (see chapter 2). Providing "pain-free" services can also increase compliance; this may involve use of outpatient hospital facilities or in-office sedation.

3. *Provide personalized service.* The more you can do to make patients feel at ease in your office, the more likely they are to do what you suggest. It is best to have the patient see the same person every time, hence staff turnover should be minimized. In our office the use of personality testing for all of our staff (including the periodontist) has resulted in a more compatible group of individuals, which has reduced intraoffice stress and turnover. Other ways to make the patient feel more accepted are to write notes about things of special interest (or dislike) in the patient's chart and to take photographs of each patient and affix them to the front of the chart so they will be recognized when appearing for their appointment. The list is limited only by your imagination.

4. *Remind patients of their scheduled appointments.* Studies show that either the mail or a telephone call will do, but we prefer the telephone because it is more personal, and because it ensures that contact with the patient has been made. Most patients schedule their next appointment while still in the office. They are given a card (we keep a copy) containing their appointment time and a note reminding them that we appreciate a call if they cannot keep their appointment. They are then reminded beforehand by telephone. Even with all these systems, we have found it difficult to keep much above 80% compliance on an average day of maintenance visits. To improve, we may need to use more sophisticated tracking devices (such as the computer) to identify the patients who habitually break appointments.

5. *Write down any instructions for the patient.* Retention of information is greater when the patient can read directions at his or her leisure and does not need to retain verbal instruction.

6. *Simplify.* The simpler the request, the more likely the patient is to comply. This can run the spectrum from providing medication that the patient takes once daily (instead of four times) to giving him or her an interproximal brush in place of dental floss.

7. *Modify the patient's general and specific health beliefs.* A prediction of the patient's compliance can be obtained by questioning or testing. Patients should be asked about their attitude toward dental health, whether they think their problem is serious, whether they think the practitioner's suggestion will work, and whether they think the suggested regime will be difficult to follow. The professional should then deal with each patient's misconceptions. In some cases a verbal or written contract dealing with compliance is helpful.

8. *Monitor compliance.* Monitoring compliance in dentistry can be easier than in other health professions because of the demonstrable and observable changes that occur. The patient who follows recommended oral hygiene procedures will have fewer caries and periodontal problems. The patient who wears elastics as suggested will have more orthodontic movement, and so on. These are clinical end points that can be monitored, and that allow feedback to be given to the patient. Examples would include monitoring probing depths and bleeding seen after probing. When these parameters improve, the patient should be informed and positively reinforced. Compliance with scheduled appointments presents a special challenge in record keeping; the number of patients changing or missing appointments can be substantial in a busy practice. If you are to be successful in monitoring compliance, make every attempt to keep accurate records.

- ■ Establish goals and give positive feedback.
- ■ Modify barriers to compliance.
- ■ Provide personalized service.
- ■ Remind patients of appointments.
- ■ Write down instructions.
- ■ Simplify.
- ■ Change the patient's health beliefs.
- ■ Monitor compliance.

Compliance is an intricate subject. Greater understanding, and therefore better ways of dealing with the problem, are continually being found. The more we know about the subject, the greater our success.

References

1. Haynes RB: Introduction, in Sackett DL, Haynes RB (eds): *Compliance With Therapeutic Regimes.* Baltimore, Johns Hopkins University Press, 1979, p 1.
2. Turk DC, Salovey P, Litt MD: Adherence: A cognitive behavioral perspective, in Gerber KE, Nehenkis M (eds): *Compliance—The Dilemma of the Chronically Ill.* New York, Springer Publ Co, 1986, p 44.
3. Barofsky I: Compliance, adherence and the therapeutic alliance: Steps in the development of self care. *Soc Sci Med* 1978;12:369.
4. Malins AF: Do they do as they are instructed? A review of outpatient anaesthesia. *Anaesthesia* 1978;33:832.
5. Hedstrand H, Abery H: Treatment of hypertension in middle-age men. A feasibility study in a community. *Acta Med Scand* 1976;199:281.
6. Rosenstock IM: Understanding and enhancing patient compliance to diabetic regimes. *Diabetes Care* 1985;8:610.
7. Pederson LL: Compliance with physician advice to quit smoking: A review of the literature. *Prev Med* 1982;11:71.
8. Oldridge NB: Compliance and exercise in primary and secondary prevention of coronary heart disease: A review. *Prev Med* 1982;11:56.
9. Ice R: Long-term compliance. *Phys Ther* 1985;65:1832.
10. Wilson TG: Compliance: A review of the literature with possible applications to periodontics. *J Periodontol* 1987;58:706.
11. Axelsson P, Lindhe J: Effects of controlled oral hygiene procedures on caries and periodontal disease in adults. *J Clin Periodontol* 1978;5:133.
12. Suomi JD, Greene JC, Vermillion JR, Doyle J, Chang JJ, Leatherwood EC: The effect of controlled oral hygiene procedures on the progression of periodontal disease in adults: Results after third and final year. *J Periodontol* 1971;42:152.
13. Johansson L-Å, Öster B, Hamp S-E: Evaluation of cause-related periodontal therapy and compliance with maintenance care recommendations. *J Clin Periodontol* 1984;11:689.
14. Boyer EM, Nikias MK: Self-reported compliance with a preventive dental regimen. *Clin Prev Dent* 1983;5:3.
15. Strack BB, McCullough MA, Conine TA: Compliance with oral hygiene instructions and hygienist's empathy. *Dent Hyg* 1980;54:181.
16. Friedson E, Feldman JJ: The public looks at dental care. *J Am Dent Assoc* 1958;57:325.
17. Farberow NL: Noncompliance as indirect self-destructive behavior, in Gerber KE, Nehenkis M (eds): *Compliance—The Dilemma of the Chronically Ill.* New York, Springer Publ Co, 1986, pp 24–43.
18. Ball RM: National health insurance: Comments on selected issues. *Science* 1978;200:864.
19. Davis P: Compliance structures and the delivery of health care: The case of dentistry. *Soc Sci Med* 1976;10:329.
20. Wilson TG, Glover ME, Schoen J, Baus C, Jacobs T: Compliance with maintenance therapy in a private periodontal practice. *J Periodontol* 1984;55:468.
21. Wilson TG, Glover ME, Malik AK, Schoen JA, Dorsett D: Tooth loss in maintenance patients in a private periodontal practice. *J Periodontol* 1987;58:231.
22. Wilson TG, Glover ME, Barraque B, Schoen J, Dorsett D: Bleeding upon probing in maintenance patients in a private periodontal practice. Unpublished data.

Index